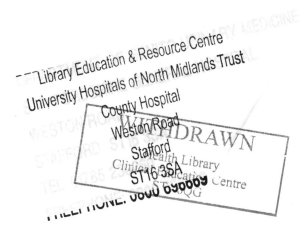

The
New Dictionary
of
Medical Ethics

The
New Dictionary
of
Medical Ethics

edited by
Kenneth M Boyd

Senior Lecturer in Medical Ethics
Edinburgh University Medical School
and Research Director, Institute of Medical Ethics

Roger Higgs

Professor and Head of Department
Department of General Practice and Primary Care
King's College School of Medicine, London

Anthony J Pinching

Louis Freedman Professor of Immunology
St Bartholomew's and The Royal London School
of Medicine and Dentistry
Queen Mary and Westfield College, University of London

BMJ
Publishing
Group

© BMJ Publishing Group 1997

First published in 1997
by the BMJ Publishing Group, BMA House, Tavistock Square,
London WC1H 9JR

British Library Cataloguing in Publication Data

A catalogue record for this book is available from the British Library
ISBN 0–7279–1001–9

Typeset, printed and bound by
Latimer Trend & Company Ltd, Plymouth

This dictionary is dedicated to
Edward Shotter
Dean of Rochester
and pioneer in medical ethics

Preface

On reviewing the landmark *Dictionary of Medical Ethics* edited by AS Duncan, GR Dunstan, and RB Welbourn, first published in 1977, we were struck by the distance which medicine and medical ethics have moved in the intervening years. New techniques and new approaches to health care have altered the focus of moral analysis and broadened its scope. Since that time, ethics has become a standard part of daily clinical work, discussion, and teaching in hospitals and the community. While we acknowledge the enormous influence of the previous volume, it is clear that a different approach is now needed. New areas have to be covered, new ways of looking at things explored. Our predecessors agreed that the editors of a new dictionary should have a free hand to fashion it as we thought fit. We thank Gordon Dunstan, Richard Welbourn, Barbara Duncan, and the publishers, Darton, Longman and Todd, for this. Although this new dictionary differs in many ways from the earlier work, it has been prepared in the same spirit of interdisciplinary cooperation and concern for the practicalities of medical ethics.

Our approach has been to make this more than simply a dictionary of definitions. On most major topics we have included some pointers to related ethical issues, inevitably treating these illustratively rather than comprehensively. For many important subjects, we have invited contributors who are highly experienced in their fields to write short essays, encouraging them to give a personal flavour to their pieces. Apart from giving a healthy diversity in style and approach, this serves to emphasise that in many areas there is no simple right or wrong ethical view on a subject – rather that the ethical issues are resolved by people making judgments in a particular medical and social context using appropriate frameworks.

We have tried to use cross reference as much as possible, to reflect the way in which topics are connected, or to display differences. This has enabled us to offer further coverage of some subjects and, where different authors are involved, to demonstrate a variety of points of view. The book is largely grounded in experience in the United Kingdom, but the issues are universal. It is aimed at everyone, from the healthcare professions or from the public at large, who is interested in clarifying moral issues in medical and nursing care and who would like some help in structuring his or her thinking, or who has found some concept either in medicine or ethics unclear or confusing in the process of doing this. A form of signposting as well as a reference book, we hope the dictionary will prove interesting and a helpful introduction to the extraordinary range of ethical issues that interweave with the day to day specifics of clinical practice.

The interested reader is encouraged to go beyond these brief glimpses, and we have indicated some useful texts as well as the specific references given in entries. We have tried to use titles for main entries that are most likely to be sought for a particular topic, but appreciate that usage varies and changes. The listing has focused on subjects where there is a particular ethical component to be highlighted. Inevitably, however, there will be some omissions, which we would be glad to rectify in future editions.

We have elected to use a new system for coping with the use of singular personal pronouns to avoid sexism and the inappropriate use of "their" or cumbersome devices such as (s)he or he/she, which only draw attention to themselves and away from the subject matter. We have chosen to use "she" in entries from A to L and "he" from M to Z. We hope that readers find this acceptable and equitable.

Authors are identified by their initials at the end of each entry and a full list of authors follows this preface. Where the editors made substantive additions, they are shown as joint contributors. We are enormously grateful to our many authors, who have worked so hard to meet our instructions and to compress their accounts into such necessarily brief pieces. The book relies heavily on their contributions and we hope that they are pleased with the overall result.

We are deeply indebted to Mary Banks of the BMJ Publishing Group for her unstinting support and practical help throughout the preparation of this book. She has catalysed some extremely productive and enjoyable editorial meetings, where we all learnt a great deal, but also managed to produce the book in its present form. Ann Lloyd has done all the technical editing and we are greatly indebted to her for applying all her skill and experience in refining the final product.

RH would particularly like to thank Lesley Higgins, Jayne Martin, and their colleagues for their skill, and Costas Kyriakos for his encouragement at all times. AJP would like to give very special thanks to Zöe Wright for reading all his draft entries and making extremely valuable suggestions to enhance their clarity and compass, as well as removing some of the more obvious hobby-horses. He is also most grateful to Esther Fernandes for skilful and elegant secretarial assistance. KMB would like to thank his Institute of Medical Ethics colleagues, especially Raanan Gillon and Hazel McHaffie, for their continuing support and encouragement, and he is especially grateful to Pat for allowing her holiday listening to be punctuated by recitals of dictionary entries.

KENNETH M BOYD
ROGER HIGGS
ANTHONY J PINCHING

How to use the dictionary

Readers will find an index of entries beginning on page 279 to help them locate quickly the word they seek.

Cross references within entries are in italics. These will not always be the exact word sought but will lead the reader to the relevant entry. For example, the word *family*, in the entry on abortion—ethical aspects is italicised to lead to the entry *Families*.

Contributors' initials are at the bottom right of each entry; their full names can be found in the list of contributors on page xi.

In the interests of economy and simplicity all the third person singular pronouns in entries from A to M are feminine, ie, she, her, hers and all those from L to Z are masculine, ie, he, him, his (see the editors' note in the Preface).

There is a short bibliography on page 277.

Contributors

Contributors are listed alphabetically under their abbreviations, as they appear in the dictionary.

AA	Amanda Amos
DA	David Armstrong
HA	Helen Alexander
JAl	John Alderson
JAn	Jane Anderson
PA	Peter Abrahams
SA	Sheila Adam
WA	Waqar Ahmad
AB	A Busuttil
ACB	Anne C Bayley
CB	Colin Blakemore
DB	Douglas Black
HB	Howard Brody
JBo	John Bowker
JBr	Joanna Breach
KMB	Kenneth M Boyd
MB	Martin Butwell
NBe	Neil Betteridge
NBr	Nicky Britten
PBo	Paul Booton
PBr	Peter Braude
PJFB	Peter JF Baskett
RMB	RM Burstall
RSB	Raj S Bhopal
SB	Susan Bewley
VNB	Virginia N Bolton
AC	Alleyna Claxton
AVC	Alastair V Campbell
BC	Brendan Callaghan
CTC	Colin T Currie
DC	Daniel Callahan
GC	Graham Clayden
JC	Jeremy Coid
KC	Kenneth Calman
MC	Margaret Cushen
RCr	Roger Crisp
RCo	Roslyn Corney
VC	Vanessa Crawford
CD	Christopher Dare
JRD	Jeremy R Dale
RD	Raymond Davern
RSD	Robin S Downie

SD	Sophie Day
SPBD	Stuart PB Donnan
CAE	Charles A Erin
FEE	FE Edwards
GE	Grimley Evans
ME	Martyn Evans
TE	Tyrrell Evans
AMF	Anna M Flynn
DF	David Freestone
GF	Greta Forster
KWMF	KWM Fulford
PF	Peter Fenwick
AG	Andrew Grubb
CG	Caroline Gooding
GG	Grant Gillett
PG	Paul Goulden
RG	Raanan Gillon
WJG	WJ Gallagher
AH	Andrew Harris
AMH	Anita Mitchell-Heggs
BHe	Barbara Hedge
BHo	Bernard Hoose
JSH	J Stuart Horner
KH	Kenneth Howse
PH	Patrick Hoyte
RH	Roger Higgs
RHa	R Hangartner
RHf	Raymond Hoffenberg
RHl	Ruth Holt
SH	Søren Holm
TH	Tony Hope
BJ	Bryan Jennett
EMJ	E Mary Judge
MHJ	Martin H Johnson
MJ	Margot Jefferys
PK	Peter Kelleher
ALl	Ann Lloyd

ALo	Adrian Lower		**PP**	Patrick Pietroni
DL	David Lamb		**RLP**	RL Palmer
DRL	Desmond R Laurence		**RTP**	Richard T Penson
GL	George Lewith		**WP**	William Plant
HL	Harold Lambert			
LL	Lucio Luzzatto		**BQ**	Bashir Qureshi
ML	Malcolm Lader			
SL	Stephen Lock		**ASR**	Arnold S Relman
VL	Vic Larcher		**FR**	Fiona Randall
			IR	Ian Ross
AM	Aubrey Manning		**JAR**	JA Raeburn
AMy	Alan Maynard		**RR**	Rosalind Ramsay
FM	Fiona Moss		**WR**	William Reid
HM	Hazel McHaffie			
JAM	JA McEwan		**ASa**	Adam Sampson
JKM	JK Mason		**AMS**	Alexander McCall-Smith
JMa	Jonathan Mann		**ASo**	Ann Sommerville
JMo	Jonathan Montgomery		**CSc**	Crispian Scully
MJM	MJ Michell		**CSk**	Celia Skinner
MM	Mary Midgley		**DS**	David Shapiro
PHM	PH Millard		**EFS**	Edward F Shotter
PM	Peter Maguire		**GS**	Gamal Serour
RM	Roy Meadow		**JAS**	Jane A Smith
RJM	Robert J Maxwell		**JCS**	JC Stoddart
SM	Sandy Macara		**LJS**	Lesley J Southgate
SAMM	Sheila AM McLean		**LS**	Lorraine Sherr
TSM	T Stewart McGregor		**MS**	Marilyn Strathern
VM	Veronica Moss		**PS**	Peter Speck
			RAS	Robert A Sells
JN	Julia Neuberger		**RSi**	Ruth Siefert
PN	Patrick Nairne		**RSm**	Richard Smith
RN	Richard Nicholson		**SJS**	Sue J Studdy
VHN	Vivienne H Nathanson			
			AT	Anthony Thorley
JDO'H	JD O'Halloran		**JLT**	Janet Treasure
DO	David Oxenham		**KRT**	Klaus-Rüdiger Trott
AJP	Anthony J Pinching		**DW**	David Weatherall
BP	Brian Potter		**EW**	E Whelan
DMP	David Malcolm Potts		**JW**	J Williamson
GCP	Gillian C Penney		**PDW**	Peter D White
MP	Mike Porter		**PW**	Pat Wilkie
			ZW	Zoë Wright

A

As, rule of Previous generations of medical students were given instruction in medical ethics based on the prohibition of *abortion, addiction, adultery, advertising,* and *association* with *unqualified practitioners*. It will be possible from this to gauge the influence and progress of modern medical ethics. "Si monumentum requieris, circumspice": or at least, read on.

RH

Abortion The termination of a pregnancy either spontaneously or by intervention before the *fetus* reaches *viability* (currently regarded as 24 weeks of gestation in the UK). The term "miscarriage" is now preferred in relation to spontaneous pregnancy loss and the term "abortion" reserved for induced termination.

Abortion may be induced legally (by medical or surgical means) or illegally. There is great variation among nations in relation to the grounds for legal abortion but currently over 40 per cent of the world's population live in countries where abortion on request is legally permissible. The UK abortion law may be regarded as in the "middle ground" of liberality. It does not allow for abortion on request but permits abortion on socio-economic grounds providing two registered medical practitioners certify in good faith that continuation of the pregnancy would constitute a risk to the physical or mental health of the woman, or of her existing children, greater than if the pregnancy were terminated.

Advances in techniques for legal abortion now mean that maternal mortality associated with legal, first trimester abortion is around one tenth of that associated with term pregnancy. Such advances include techniques for preparing, or priming, the cervix prior to surgical abortion and the development of non-surgical drug regimens for terminating both very early and second trimester pregnancies.

Unsafe abortion continues to be a major contributor to maternal mortality and morbidity in countries where abortion is illegal. The issue of abortion continues to excite considerable controversy with powerful and vocal lobbies on both sides. There is evidence that research and development of new techniques of contraception and abortion are hindered by this political controversy.

GCP

Abortion – ethical aspects The morality of purposeful destruction of a human *fetus* has been of major concern since at least the time of Hippocrates. In our decades, with political and religious alignments added to personal scruple, disagreement has intensified almost to the point where ethical arguments are submerged and vital compromise becomes impossible.

Abortion might be sought because of threat to the life of the mother, her state of mind, the effect on the *family*, the initiation of the pregnancy (such as *rape*), the fetus's exposure to noxious drugs or infection, prenatal potential or actual defects, or simply because the new baby was not desired or could not be afforded. Whether such reasons render abortion justifiable, however, is widely contested, from those who would consider it never to be so, or only if the life of the mother were at stake, to those who would respond positively to a request from a woman for a termination whatever her reasons; and many positions in between.

A series of themes is detectable in the justification of these positions. One is the concept of humanity.

1

Human life is in some senses overwhelmingly special. If it is God's creation, it is called sacred, and respected as such and to such an extent as not to allow interference from man. Unbelievers also consider that human life has unique moral value: destruction of actual human life is almost always a crime. But where does life begin? The point of birth is convenient: but there is little to choose between the newborn and the nearly born. *Viability*, the ability to pursue a separate existence, is blurred by the need for nurture of newborns, relates to the individual fetus, and changes with changes in the technological environment. It may be a helpful concept when the baby is severely damaged (as in anencephaly), and in practice it forms a point of no return for an individual decision maker who finds herself pregnant.

At the other extreme, the moment of conception where male and female gametes join to produce the embryo has obvious logic but depends on the concept of what the fetus will become, of potential. Can potential be assumed, or must it be proved in some way? The actual embryo at this time is hard to distinguish from surrounding tissue and is often lost without moral concern at menstruation. A later moment, when the central nervous system begins to develop, or can be seen to have developed, could be chosen: from such a moment on the fetus may feel pain, and most would agree experimental procedures should cease. Thus the question has changed to "When does life begin to matter morally?" This approach considers what sort of entities fetuses are (ontological status). Is the fetus an individual organism, a human being (biologically or psychologically) or a person? Even if full *personhood* or humanity is not attributed to fetuses, their status can still be best described in terms of *potential*. However, we do not usually treat a "potential entity" exactly as if it were the real thing, nor necessarily feel that every potential entity should fulfil that potential (the "acorns and oaks" argument).

Thus the ontological status of the fetus is intertwined with its moral status. The environmental debate has begun to challenge the concept of human beings in general being an unalloyed good, while the prevalent desire of parents to limit family size ("every child a wanted child") represents similar thinking in micro. But *morality* has a duty to ensure that the rights of those who are vulnerable or who have difficulty in getting their rights recognised should be particularly protected. Whatever the status of the fetus, the future generation is of inestimable value: yet its bringing to pass is in the hands of only half the population, women. *Feminism* would suggest that women's views are not sufficiently canvassed or respected. The next generation may be foisted on them as a parasite, without proper choice, thought or support (even if this "stranger" eventually becomes accepted and deeply loved): a woman, in this view, should "have the right to choose". But what of the rights of the fetus, unable to articulate them and therefore even more requiring of protection? Who should be the protector – medicine, law, or some other force in society? Some maintain against this that any intrusion into the decision of the mother acts against women. In practice, it has been shown that women usually take great thought and pains to identify and minimise the harms, balancing different or competing harms in a nuanced way when considering whether to keep or terminate a new pregnancy. Such down-to-earth examples of compromise might put ethicists, politicians, campaigners, and religious leaders to shame, and convert the general question to the particular:

"How much should this possible new life matter, in this situation and at this stage?"

See also: Conscientious objection; ensoulment; reproduction.

References
Dworkin R. *Life's dominion*. London: Harper Collins, 1993.
Gilligan C. *In a different voice*. Cambridge, Mass: Harvard University Press, 1993.

RH

Absolutism suggests that a rule, *duty* or *concept* always applies as an ethical imperative, and admits of no compromise or exception. *Deontology* or duty-based thinking (to tell the truth for instance) is sometimes presented thus. However, because by their nature, ethical questions suggest doubt, debate or conflict, an absolutist approach seldom seems helpful, particularly in the complexities of health care and in modern multicultural life where few accept a single rule or duty which underpins all other decisions. But if we can rule out absolutism in debate, it is hard to do so absolutely in logic.

See also: Complexity.

RH

Abuse is used to suggest that a person, service, substance or object is being used wrongly. It has the overtone of disapproval and negative judgment from the speaker's perspective: "misuse" is the term to describe a wrong use in a more objective or factual sense. Thus abuse already contains the content of disapproval, and views of this may change, eg, the judgmental "self-abuse" has changed to the more neutral "masturbation". Recently the mistreatment of people by others in a position of trust has become a major social and ethical issue (*child abuse*, elderly abuse) and can be extended to those in less powerful positions being mistreated by

superiors. Which substances are legitimately "used" and which "abused" may also be subject to shifts in societal views and values.

See also: Drug misuse.

RH

Accident implies something that happens by chance, but in the medical field usually involves a physical injury rather than the process of a disease, or something otherwise seen as an illness. Superficially it may imply that the sufferer bears no *responsibility*, but observation may question this (inattention, carelessness, *alcoholism* and so on) and government funding agencies may see the possibility of alternative sources of accident care funding (*insurance*, personal responsibility). *Compensation* for injury is a linked issue, and usually requires that someone else should be at fault. "No fault compensation", as pioneered in New Zealand, has led to the broadening of the use of the word.

RH

Accountability Taking responsibility for one's actions in a way that is demonstrable to others and with the prospect of being held to account in terms of public redress, financial penalty, professional censure, or legal action. In clinical *decision-making*, accountability means making clinical and ethical judgments in a way that can withstand external scrutiny according to defined or implicit moral or professional codes. In health service terms, it is the demonstrable responsibility to utilise, or oversee, the use of public or private funds in the cost-effective delivery of appropriate treatment and care. This accountability is ultimately owed to public and patients in the effective stewardship of *resources*. It is exerted more literally between the various layers of management: providers, purchasers, and government departments and agencies.

3

The concept of moral accountability may spread the use wider to involve a more general *responsibility*. Some writers use the word to describe the ability to give an account of oneself in the sense of describing or reporting one's personal history and goals.

See also: Purchasing; transparency.

AJP/RH

Active/passive distinction The difference between (actively) doing something and (passively) allowing it to happen is sometimes given as a reason not only (a) why (as in the more formal *acts and omissions doctrine*) it is always wrong for doctors to kill patients but in some circumstances may be right to allow them to die, but also (b) why it is morally less acceptable to withdraw than to withhold life-sustaining *treatment*. This psychologically appealing distinction has a moral basis – normally we are held responsible for the foreseeable consequences of our own actions, but not for failing to prevent many things that happen in the world or are done by others. But morally (and sometimes legally), we can be held responsible for allowing those things to happen or be done by others which we were in a position, or had a special responsibility, to try to prevent. Thus the active/passive distinction, considered in isolation from the particular responsibilities and circumstances of the *moral agent*, is often an insufficient ethical criterion. In practice too (again as with acts and omissions), the distinction may be problematic – it can be argued, eg, that a decision to withhold treatment is just as active as one to withdraw it later.

KMB

Acts and omissions doctrine The distinction between acts and omissions is often made in discussions about "end of life" issues. It is widely held that, although clinicians may sometimes justifiably allow patients to die (by withdrawing or withholding treatment from them), they should never indulge in anything that amounts to active and intentional killing.

Rachels argued that the distinction between the two is not always morally significant.[1] What we foresee, what we intend, and our motives would seem all to be part of the moral picture.

See also: Active/passive distinction; euthanasia; extraordinary and ordinary means; treatment.

BHo

Reference
1 Rachels J. Active and passive euthanasia. N Eng J Med 1975, **292**: 78–80.

Acupuncture is an ancient Chinese medical art that involves both the diagnostic system of traditional Chinese medicine and the therapeutic needling of specific acupuncture points. Modern acupuncture includes electrical point measurement as well as point therapy with lasers, electrical stimulation and magnets. Body acupuncture is the commonest form of acupuncture, although other systems such as ear acupuncture are widely available. Acupuncture is utilised as a method of treatment for a whole variety of conditions, but is commonly available in a number of National Health Service (NHS) settings (pain clinics and physiotherapy departments) for the management of *pain*. In the UK many non-medically qualified acupuncturists now work closely with their conventional colleagues in both hospital and general practice settings. As far as the General Medical Council is concerned, if a medical practitioner refers a patient to an acupuncturist then she must do so with a clear diagnosis and must bear responsibility for the acupuncture treatment provided, in spite of the fact that qualified non-medical acupuncturists carry appropriate professional indemnity.

See also: Complementary medicine.

GL

Addiction Physical and/or psychological dependence on a licit or illicit substance or an activity, such as gambling. Aetiological mechanisms combine biological, psychological, environmental, and iatrogenic factors. Addiction is linked with risk taking in criminal, sexual, and injecting activity, and evokes an emotive response from both the medical profession and the lay population.

Reference
Ghodse AH. *Drugs and addictive behaviour. A guide to treatment* (2nd edn). Oxford: Blackwell Science, 1995.

See also: Drug misuse; order of preferences.

VC

Ad hominem or ad personam (i) For a specific individual (eg, an applicant for a particular post); (ii) a common logical fallacy – making a person's (supposed) qualities or character the crucial step in an argument about truth or morality. "Subjects will not be harmed by Dr A's research project, because Dr A is kind to his patients."

KMB

Adolescence The period between childhood and adulthood when there are great physical and psychological changes, with potential conflicts with parents and/or society, and turmoil in emerging sexuality. The answer to the question: "What sort of person am I?" is in doubt. The key ethical issue concerns whether a person at this time of life is in full control of decisions which concern her, or whether parents still have overriding authority. As in decisions about childhood, there is a balance to be struck between protection or welfare and respecting a person's informed wishes. British law is particularly confused, suggesting age limits for full decision-making competence in different circumstances which make little sense in ethics. The starting point sensibly seems to be – does this person understand enough about this decision to be able to make a reasonably informed choice? If so, the choice made should not be negated just because an adult does not agree with it.

See also: Child, status of; competence; identity; responsibility.

RH

Adoption and fostering Adoption is the permanent legal assumption of parental rights and responsibilities by a person or persons who are not the birth (biological) parents. Legally, adoption puts an adopted child in the same position as a child born in lawful wedlock in terms of the right to inheritance (except of a peerage). There is an underlying tension between whether the main aim of adoption is to find a family for a child or to provide a child for a family.

There may be conflicting issues amongst the four parties involved: the child, the birth parents, the adoptive parents, and the social/legal system representing society's role. Even in the most straightforward situation where the birth parents have no objections to the child being permanently removed from their care, there are problems related to the process of adoption. It is now acknowledged that the child has the right to some knowledge of the birth parents. The benefits to the child include a sense of historical continuity or "roots" but this must be balanced against the disturbing effect that this may have on the adoptive parents and the adopted young person. Careful collaborative planning can offset a number of these problems.[1]

In any dealings with children the first priority is the child's best interest. Adoption appears to be more beneficial to the child than residential or foster home placement.[2] The publication of photographs of children awaiting adoption may increase the chances of finding an adoptive *family* but is the child competent to agree to this or to understand its significance? Issues of *confidentiality* also arise when information is both sought and disclosed about the child (birth family, behavioural or medical history). It may involve *screening* by means of invasive tests which themselves may be considered an unjustifiable burden when the main benefit is information for the adoptive family. The information that may be obtained from screening is increasing in its magnitude. *Consent* for any procedure or disclosure of personal information cannot be given competently by the child and those giving this in proxy may only do this if they believe that the child would have given this *consent* if she had been competent. It could be argued that because an eventual breakdown of the adoptive relationship is a definite possibility (success rate of 53–97%)[3] and that this is very traumatic for a child and significantly reduces the success of future adoption,[4] it justifies any factors that might lead to this being openly disclosed. This would certainly be compatible with an adoption agency's responsibility to be honest and truthful with both sets of clients. The birth parents forfeit their parental rights and *autonomy* when deemed to have failed to meet their responsibilities and where this is detrimental to the child. The court decides. This involves a guardian ad litem being appointed to represent the child and providing evidence for the court.

Some circumstances raise serious ethical questions, namely the adoption of infants from poorer countries where the risk of exploitation of the birth mother's state of deprivation (giving up one child for the sake of her others) renders her consent invalid, and adoption of a child from a surrogate mother. In both these circumstances any exchange of money would appear to increase the risk of exploitation.

In England and Wales, anyone over 25 years of age, a relative of the child over 21 years of age or the mother or father of the child irrespective of age may adopt a child. Agencies try to match the child with the adoptive parents as closely as possible but this may lead to a number of children remaining unplaced as a result of race or disability, when either adoptive parents of their own race cannot be found, or parents willing to manage a child with a physical or mental disability cannot be found. The adoptive parents must be sufficiently informed so that they can judge the effect on their existing children who may feel disadvantaged by even short term fostering.[5] More serious harm to the adoptive parents' children must be avoided, eg the adoption of a sexually abused and abusing young teenager may significantly put younger children in the family at risk.

Lesbian or gay couples who by the nature of their relationship cannot have a child may still want to adopt in order to experience the challenge of parenthood. It can be argued that they would be using the child as an instrument for their own needs but this is equally true for heterosexual parents. However, the deliberate choice of exposing the child to single gender parenting and hence the reduction of that child's experience of role models may not be justified if other adoptive parents who might provide this were available. Adoption of orphans from one culture to another risks cultural confusion and isolation as the child grows up in a society alien to her own. However, the advantage for the child transferring to a country with a very low risk of death cannot be ignored.

References
1 Feast J, Marwood M, Seabrook S, Warbur A, Webb E. *Preparing for reunion – adopted people, adoptive parents and birth parents tell their stories.* London: The Children's Society, 1994.
2 Barth RP, Berry M. Behaviour problems of children adopted when older. *Children Youth Serv Rev* 1989; **ii**: 221–38.
3 Thorburn J. *Success and failure in permanent family placement.* Aldershot: Avebury, 1990.
4 Partridge S, Hanby H, McDonald T. Legacies of loss, visions of gain. An inside look at adoption disruption. In: Westhues A, Cohen JS, eds. *Preventing disruption of special needs adoptions.* Portland: ME University of Southern Maine, 1986.
5 Part D. Fostering as seen by the carers' children. *Adoption Fostering* 1993; **17,1**: 26–31.

See also: Child, status of.

GC

Adultery refers to sexual relations outside marriage, a subject of intense interest in most societies, and both the cause and result of personal *conflict*. Is your duty to follow your promises, your desires, or your need to grow and develop as a person? Medical ethics traditionally keeps out of these turbulent waters by relating in total confidence to that person who is the patient. However, the clinician attending three or more people in such relationships may have conflicting duties if there are children at risk or a *sexually transmitted disease* is present, and so needs to be clear about *boundaries*. Sexual relations between doctor and patient have long been outlawed by the profession because of the *power* and intimacy of a clinical encounter, although this is a hard rule for an isolated country doctor or other professional and appears to be increasingly questioned.

See also: Confidentiality; doctor–patient relationship; faith, bad faith and faithfulness; families.

RH

Advance directives (living wills) A person can anticipate losing the mental capacity to decide or communicate how she wishes to be treated by drawing up a formal advance statement of her *values* and preferences or by naming a person who can be consulted. It will increasingly be unwise to ignore these directives, and they can be helpful to clinicians. But there can be difficulties in interpreting an advance statement which is drawn up either in too general or in too specific terms, and requests for illegal or clinically inappropriate treatment cannot be complied with. However, a competent adult's advance refusal of (a) a specific treatment (eg, *Jehovah's Witnesses*) has legal force, and of (b) life sustaining *treatment* in specific circumstances (eg, *persistent vegetative state*) can have legal force.

Reference
British Medical Association. *Advance statements about medical treatment.* London: BMA, 1995.

KMB

Advertising, if self promotion to obtain patients, traditionally is seen as unethical and may constitute serious professional misconduct. But publicising what services a medical practice offers and at what times, can be helpful to patients. In the UK, *National Health Service* doctors must provide practice leaflets, publicising "general medical services", but those offering only specialised services may not publicise these. In part this reflects the distinction between *primary care*, which patients can access directly (*general practice*, community services, *sexually transmitted disease* clinics) and specialist care, generally provided in *hospital medicine*. The latter have been allowed only to provide information to primary care services and health authorities to enable referral for consultation, but recent guidance suggests that information on specialists may now be provided to the public. The issue is less clear cut for specialists practising *private medicine*. It is essential to avoid suggesting that a particular practitioner is superior to others and to avoid disparagement, which are practices outlawed by the *General Medical Council*. Doctors may not acquiesce in publication of their names in directories which purport to make recommendations as to their quality.

AJP/KMB/BP

Advocacy/activism A professional may have a role in speaking or acting on behalf of an individual patient or a group because of the professional's greater knowledge, power, or influence (for instance, within the *health-care system*), but pursuing the interests of the patient, not the professional. *Nurses* and *general practitioners* or other primary care workers increasingly see personal advocacy as a major component of their individual clinical tasks.

Activism suggests that this work can also be done for a group of people who are at a disadvantage. That this has in the past sometimes been questioned as part of a professional *role* may reflect ambivalence about political involvement, lack of understanding of the health care of groups of people (public health, epidemiology), confusion, or medical *quietism*.

See also: Pressure groups.

RH

Afterlife Belief in life beyond death (in more or less desirable forms) has been widely held throughout history – resurrection, reincarnation, reunion with loved ones, return to the One. Such beliefs cannot normally be proved or disproved and those who hold them nowadays often do not speak of them publicly. But they can have practical implications that those

caring for the dying should tactfully ascertain and respect.

See also: Reincarnation; suffering.

KMB

Agape (pronounced agapay) This, one of the Greek words for love (Latin caritas, English *charity*), denotes a more caring and less self-interested emotion than eros, whose sexual connotation it also lacks. Agapeistic ethics emphasises that individuals are unique, contexts particular and the spirit of love superior to the letter of the law.

See also: Context; love, moderated; situation ethics.

KMB

Age and aging Health care of the elderly assumes increasing importance in developed societies as their populations age and serious illness and hence health care utilisation tends to concentrate increasingly in later life. In addition to degenerative diagnoses traditionally associated with old age such as osteoarthritis, cerebrovascular disease, and dementia, older patients are vulnerable to the full range of acute adult pathologies and are pro rata the heaviest users of acute in-patient services such as internal medicine, general surgery, and trauma orthopaedics.

Healthcare systems have responded variously to these challenges, most successfully where community health and social services are adequate and where strongly developed primary care services and the specialty of geriatric medicine have provided accessible general medical care in circumstances that also allow appropriate access to more expensive organ-based specialties.

Where a mismatch occurs between the health care needs of older people and the provision for such needs, older people may be denied potentially helpful high technology interventions, and where rehabilitation and placement issues are not well addressed, the efficiency of acute hospital facilities may be compromised by "bed-blocking".

Ageism – defined as "discrimination against the old on the grounds of their being old" – has been noted among health care professionals, but there is also evidence to suggest that a better understanding of the special needs of elderly patients results in more positive attitudes to their care.

Ethical issues that arise in relation to the care of the elderly include considerations of costs and benefits of aggressive investigation and *treatment* towards the end of life; questions of impaired *autonomy* by reason of *dementia*; conflicts of interest between impaired dependent patients and their carers; and, at the level of national policy, the proportion of *resources* to be devoted to the care, particularly the *long term care*, of the elderly.

See also: Conflicts of interest.

CTC

AIDS Acquired Immune Deficiency Syndrome is an epidemic immunodeficiency caused by HIV, Human Immunodeficiency Virus. HIV spreads in three ways: by sexual contact (first identified in *homosexuals*, but commonest worldwide among *heterosexuals*); by blood contact (notably among injecting drug-users who share equipment, through unscreened *blood transfusion* and rarely by inoculation injury to health care workers); and by vertical spread from an infected mother to *fetus* or infant. There is a long asymptomatic period between infection and onset of disease, which can be detected by *screening* for HIV antibodies, but 50% of those infected will have progressed to AIDS by ten years. HIV replicates actively even

during clinical latency, leading to an infectious *carrier* state. AIDS is characterised by opportunist infections and tumours that cause an episodic illness, leading to death in about three years from AIDS diagnosis. HIV may cause a form of *dementia*.

AIDS has probably raised more ethical issues than any other single disease, although none is unique to it. Many relate to a perceived tension between the rights of the individual and protection of the public health. The relative responsibilities of those who are infected, or suspect they are, in preventing infection of sexual partners and other contacts, and of uninfected individuals in protecting themselves, underpin the dilemmas. The *confidentiality* of personal health information, heightened by the sensitivity of the behaviours involved, may present problems in balancing duties to the patient as well as to the public health. A clinician, aware of a person's status and behaviour, is in a position to influence behaviour and thus to effect risk reduction, consequently benefiting others. However, the clinician may sense that there is also a duty to warn a third party of risk, if the patient will not. Yet if this is discharged by a breach of the duty of *confidentiality* to the patient, the loss of trust may mean that such information will not be revealed in the future, impeding the clinician's unique role in helping the patient reduce risk to others. Particular problems arise if the same clinician is also involved in care of a contact. *Partner notification* or *contact tracing* are means of following up those who have been exposed to risk that may resolve some difficulties. In antenatal care, there may be tensions between duties to the mother and to the fetus.

Sex education and risk reduction by *condoms* present problems for some religious groups. HIV mainly affects people/communities who are already alienated or *disadvantaged*, eg, homosexuals, drug users, and *prostitutes*; its spread and impact may be exacerbated by *poverty* or *war*. These contexts increase *stigma* and the potential for *blame* and punitive social measures, ostensibly to protect others, but which may be driven by a social agenda. The potential risk of health care workers acquiring HIV occupationally has re-opened debate about what are acceptable risks. The largely theoretical risk to patients from HIV *infected doctors* or dentists has led to guidelines that attempt to balance the rights of staff and their patients.

The care of people with AIDS, especially in industrialised countries, has led to a greater *empowerment* of patients, which has influenced other areas of health care. Choices between therapies are more explicitly a matter for the informed patient and often encompass both conventional and *complementary medicine*. Early access to experimental drugs for patients with advanced disease and modification of *clinical trials* to accommodate their immediate needs have been urged; yet these may promote unproven or even harmful therapies and may impede determination of their efficacy. The debate has been stimulated by strong public *advocacy/activism* by patients and groups representing them. AIDS has prompted more explicit discussion of a patient's right to refuse life-sustaining therapy and the use of *advance directives*. Worry, generally misplaced, about potential effects of HIV encephalopathy and AIDS have raised concerns among employers, the media and the public about employment of those perceived to be at risk of HIV infection. AIDS, increasingly an issue predominantly for the *developing world*, highlights the lack of *equity*, within and between countries in the distribution of *resources*, access to information, prevention, and therapy.

Vaccines have yet to be shown to provide protection, but research into their effectiveness presents ethical problems, because trials need the subjects to be at continuing risk if they are to demonstrate efficacy. Yet this risk can be reduced by health education. Furthermore, the very conduct of a vaccine trial could lead to a false sense of security, if the vaccine proves partly or wholly ineffective. There are also concerns about the use of endangered primate species that may be the only valid model for evaluating challenge by the mucosal route in pre-clinical efficacy studies.

See also: Drug misuse.

AJP

Aims (personal) There is the suggestion that choice in health care may reflect an individual's own long-term aims for herself or a personal value set. These are often unspoken or difficult to articulate, and may need to be searched for by the professional faced with an apparently idiosyncratic or unwise choice. Such choices, if they do not harm others, should normally be respected.

See also: Autonomy.

RH

Akrasia Greek for weakness of will. Can one act, under no external or internal compulsion, against one's own better judgment? If so, some say, such moral weakness is irrational, a sign that *autonomy* is absent. Others deny the possibility, arguing that the relevant judgment must lack depth, or sufficient knowledge and/or experience to understand the implications. Others again observe that few people if any always act totally rationally.

Reference
Gillon R, McKnight CJ. *J Med. Ethics* 1993; **19**: 195–96, 206–10.

KMB

Alcoholism Dependency on alcohol is widespread and so raises particular ethical concerns. There may be pressure on a clinician from others to take *paternalistic* action (which by its very nature may therefore be ineffective), particularly because of the high risk of *suicide* among drinkers. *Tolerance* in society of drink related motoring and other offences is declining, and concerns about public safety may appear to justify breaking *confidentiality* in extreme cases. Doctors, both in training and later, often drink very heavily, so the medical profession does not come to the table with clean hands (or a clear head).

There is considerable disagreement as to whether this should reasonably be considered an *illness*. A genetic predisposition or a shift to the medical model might make "treatment" a more valid option but might at the same time reduce the drinker's own personal *responsibility* to take the only known effective action: not to drink.

See also: Addiction.

RH

Alternative medicine *See* Complementary medicine.

Altruism This describes an attitude or action for the good of someone other than the actor: and this is of interest in health care. In a diluted form it appears as the dictum, "always put the patient's interests first", but though superficially a laudable aim this clearly has limits. The stress on the economic vulnerability of the health service appears to some to put further strain on the individual worker by giving a higher profile to the issue of making or saving money in any particular encounter, and by suggesting that a professional's first loyalty is to the service rather than the patient.

See also: Beneficence; cost containment; donation; egoism; health economics; National Health Service.

RH

Ambiguity Two or more different meanings in one statement or situation is something of which both philosopher and scientist are wary: clarity is an important aim too in health care work. But ambiguity is important in poetry, humour and daily life to give richness and nuance and to suggest rather than confront. Eastern philosophy, able to accept something both being and not being at the same time, has attraction for some. Ethically, however, the important issue may be to be able to understand enough of the ambiguities of a situation or an exchange to enable a rounded assessment to be made; each of the possible meanings or aims may then require analysis. The skill of a good decision-maker may then reside in putting together the different strands of analysis to make the best decision.

See also: Decision-making capacity; religion and philosophy, Eastern; yin yang.

RH

Amniocentesis is a procedure for *prenatal diagnosis* by which a small amount of amniotic fluid is sampled during early pregnancy in order to detect *genetic disorders* in the *fetus*. Cells from amniotic fluid are cultured and the chromosomes analysed to look for disorders such as Down's syndrome. Amniocentesis is performed where there is an increased risk of such abnormalities – eg where the parents are above 35 or if they have had a previously affected child or other family history. With the information, parents and clinicians can discuss whether to continue the pregnancy or whether to induce an *abortion*. The procedure itself carries a small risk of inducing abortion, which

11

will also need to be taken into account. It is best that, before the procedure, parents are prepared for the decisions that will follow.

Genetic counselling may help in assessing risk and in considering possible courses of action, before and after a result. The range of genetic disorders that can now be identified by DNA analysis and a preference for earlier diagnosis has led to increasing use of *chorionic villus sampling* and fetal blood sampling.

See also: Abortion – ethical aspects.

AJP

Anaesthesia (i): general anaesthesia. A pharmacologically induced state of the central nervous system, characterised by a reversible loss of *consciousness* and loss of recall of events occurring during the period of anaesthesia. This state is considered to be part of a continuum of levels of consciousness, ranging from fully conscious, through analgesia, amnesia, loss of responsiveness, loss of motor function, loss of central reflexes, and ending in *death*. There is evidence that some forms of external information, such as auditory stimuli, may be processed and stored by the brain at clinically acceptable levels of anaesthesia.

Regional anaesthesia: pharmacological blocking of sensory nerve fibre transmission to produce analgesia in a particular region of the body.

Anaesthesia (ii): a medical specialty. In the UK, anaesthetics are administered exclusively by medically qualified anaesthetists. Such physicians typically undergo a training period lasting six to ten years, which includes holding training posts and passing postgraduate examinations. The duties of an anaesthetist to a patient include: preoperative medical assessment and preparation; giving appropriate information concerning anaesthesia and gaining *consent*; the

induction, maintenance and reversal of anaesthesia; safeguarding the patient's safety and comfort during anaesthesia and recovery; and providing advice on postoperative care. Many anaesthetists also have commitments to *intensive care* units and *pain* management services; some specialise as well in anaesthesia for particular patient groups, such as obstetric, paediatric and neurosurgical patients.

Anaesthesia is an unusual specialty in so far as it is facilitative rather than diagnostic in nature: it is concerned with the *welfare* of a vulnerable group of patients. When combined with intensive care duties, this often results in anaesthetists being involved in ethical dilemmas, such as those concerning the withdrawing or withholding of *treatment*, the obtaining of consent from incompetent individuals, organ *donation* issues, resource allocation, and the management of ill or incompetent colleagues.

References

Rosen, M, Lunn JN. *Consciousness, awareness and pain in general anaesthesia*. London: Butterworths, 1987.
Scott T, Vickers MD, Draper H. *Ethical issues in anaesthesia*. Oxford: Butterworth-Heinemann, 1994.

EW

Ancillary staff The practice of medicine involves many people other than nurses, doctors, and patients and this term is used to cover some of these. Their contributions to the personal care of patients beyond the immediate limits of their task has often been underestimated: many people, frightened and lonely on a hospital ward or anxious about coming to see a doctor, have given accounts of how the ward cleaner was the only person who would listen, or that they were able to sort out their feelings with a porter or a *receptionist*. Such staff may have different backgrounds, training, and expectations from doctors or nurses but the assumption has been that they work under the same rules and are guided by the same ethical principles as the traditional medical professions. Thus, breach of medical *confidentiality* is usually seen as grounds for instant dismissal for a receptionist, yet the reality is more complex: while groups with socially sensitive conditions such as *AIDS* often declare that the reception system in *general practice* is unacceptably "leaky", receptionists see themselves as "piggy in the middle" between other professionals and patients, and between related patients. The more rigid positions that can be adopted by a doctor, sequestered in a consulting room, are less easy to use when negotiating around a reception desk: extreme skill in communication and tact may be required. This example is one of many that suggest that more research, thinking, and teaching are needed in the ethical issues facing those who work in jobs related to medicine.

See also: Gatekeeping; paramedical professions.

RH

Anger is an emotional reaction to a perceived threat with physiological concomitants akin to those of fear – the body is prepared for "fight or flight". Humans, however, have a much wider range of options than do trapped animals. They may deny the anger and become depressed; they may lose control and resort to *violence*; or they may become bitter and resentful towards others, nursing a grudge. A more positive approach involves, first, **acknowledging** rather than denying the reaction, second, **identifying** the source of threat or frustration, and, third, **communicating** with the person against whom the anger is felt. Anger in health care relationships, if it is even admitted, is usually perceived as disruptive and unhelpful. *Difficult patients* are penalised for their lack of compliance,

and angry staff resort to avoidance or to subtle abuses of their *power* to relieve their feelings. But anger, once brought out into the open, can have a positive effect, improving the quality of the care given or received. Professionals should allow patients to express their anger and should find ways of letting patients know their reactions to them in a non-intimidating way. The gain is a more honest and empowering form of *communication* between patients and their care-givers.

Reference
Campbell AV. *The gospel of anger*. London: SPCK, 1986.

See also: Doctor–patient relationship; emotion.

AVC

Anguish/angst An important concept in *existentialism* denoting a state of distress which may appear dysfunctional but nevertheless offers the opportunity for change or movement. In a similar way, psychological therapists, when a client has a "breakdown", have seen the possibilties for a "break-through". In ethics, a sense of concern may be required to initiate thought.

RH

Animal experiments Living animals are used for various scientific purposes, including: development of medical and veterinary pharmaceuticals; safety testing of non-medicinal products; study of disease and pathology; development of surgical procedures; production of antisera and vaccines; ecological studies, and the advancement of fundamental biological knowledge.

Of the vertebrate species used in experiments, by far the majority (over 80 per cent) are rodents – mainly mice and rats. The remainder are mostly other mammalian species and birds.

Data on the use of invertebrates are unavailable.

It is widely agreed that many kinds of animals (especially mammals and birds) can suffer *pain*, distress, anxiety and other states that humans find unpleasant, sometimes intolerable. Debate centres on the moral significance of animal suffering. While many of the scientific procedures in which animals are used cause only mild *harm*, others can involve more substantial suffering; and in most procedures the animals are killed at the end of the experiments. Those opposed to animal experiments tend to argue that human and animal suffering deserve equal consideration, and that therefore it is unacceptable to harm animals for human ends. Some also argue that animals have a "right" not to be caused such harm.[1] Those supportive of animal experiments contend that the benefits gained can justify the harms caused to the animals – provided that the benefits are sufficiently serious given the harms, and that there is no alternative means of achieving the object of the experiments.

Animal experiments undoubtedly have led to benefits for human and veterinary health and *welfare*; but deciding the importance of the different kinds of potential benefits in order that they might be weighed against animal harm remains contentious.[2]

Researchers, it is widely accepted, have duties to limit the harm caused to animals in experiments; specifically by applying the "3Rs" of reduction, refinement and replacement of animal use. That is, they must use the least number of animals, and cause the least possible harm consistent with the object of the experiments (including appropriate use of *anaesthesia* and analgesia); and, wherever possible, replace the use of animals with non-sentient alternatives. In many countries, such duties are enshrined in legislation regulating the use of animals in experiments.

References
1 Regan T, Singer P, eds. *Animal rights and human obligations* (2nd ed). Englewood Cliffs, NJ: Prentice Hall, 1989.
2 Smith, JA, Boyd KM, eds. *Lives in the balance: the ethics of using animals in biomedical research.* Oxford: Oxford University Press, 1991.

See also: Clinical research and trials; experimentation; research; speciesism; suffering; vivisection.

JAS

Anorexia nervosa *See* Eating disorders.

Antenatal *See* Fetus and embryo; prenatal diagnosis.

Anthropology Biological anthropology and social anthropology study human diversity from the twin vantage points of evolutionary and social differentiation. Whether the particular subject is primate development or community politics, genetic variation or religious practices, both disciplines afford perspectives on contemporary human behaviour. Ethics directly enters social anthropology with its concern for the *moral* bases of social conventions and for the way people translate conventions into personal practice. Social anthropological method endorses the significance of social and cultural *context* for understanding the choices people have and make. Its investment in the study of non-European societies gives it a unique comparative perspective.

MS

Apology Still sometimes found in its original philosophical sense as an explanation or vindication of a point of an argument, this is usually used to indicate a statement acknowledging *fault*. The power of the medical professions (and the advice of some insurers) often leads to medical *mistakes* not being properly acknowledged. There is evidence that this in turn causes the sharpening of *complaints* and *litigation*. The creative aspects of the human interaction in apologising may need to be re-emphasised if health care is to remain healthy and caring. But a third usage, as abuse ("this is an apology of a dictionary"), may lurk uncomfortably below the surface.

See also: Argument, moral.

RH

Appeals An appeal is a call to some person, body or process for authoritative vindication of a position or decision. Appeals can be to a higher court in law, to reason, or to someone's better nature. Often used against what is considered an unjust decision.

See also: Claims; rights.

RSD

Appropriate technology Scientific advance in the field of medicine enables doctors to investigate and treat by high-technology means. This may lead to simple conditions receiving a complex and expensive response (such as a headache being investigated with a CT scan). The balance of cost and benefit, the requirement to minimise harm (to the service and thus to the patients as well), the principle of *parsimony* and an overall aesthetic in health care, combine to suggest that simple, low, or no technology is appropriate in the care of simple, self-limiting conditions that do not endanger life. Such judgments may require good *doctor–patient relationships* with education flowing both ways and a gatekeeper function in *primary care* involving weak *paternalism*.

The tests of new technologies in health care are that they should be effective (and proven to be so), culturally acceptable and affordable, and sustainable in the context for which they are designed. Some would add "politically responsible" to this list, in acknowledgment that giving by rich countries or groups to the poor is sometimes intended to create social *change*, and the motivation must be examined.

See also: Culture; gatekeeping; resources.

RH

A priori/a posteriori from Latin for what comes before/after – either in time or necessarily. Traditionally, a priori arguments work from cause to effect (the fact that the patient has liver disease explains the yellow discoloration of her skin), while a posteriori arguments work from effect to cause (from the patient's yellow skin, dark urine and pale stools, the doctor diagnoses obstructive jaundice). Some (especially Kantian) but not other modern philosophers argue that there can be a priori (including mathematical and logical) knowledge, not derived from experience (a posteriori, as is empirical knowledge) but inherent in the mind, structuring it so as to make experience possible.

KMB

Argument *See* Moral argument.

Arrogance is an accusation often levelled at health care workers who are not sensitive to the balance of *power* in their work, and believe that *competence* earned in the medical sphere enables them to claim it in other fields. Experience suggests that pressure of work reduces good communication and increases the impression of arrogance, which in turn, if things go wrong, leads to increased *litigation*.

See also: Apology; experts and expertise.

RH

Artificial insemination This involves the placing of fresh, unprepared semen into the vagina in the region of the cervix (cervical insemination) or washed and prepared semen high into the uterine cavity (intrauterine insemination) in order to facilitate pregnancy. Its use is advocated in cases of unexplained *infertility* or where a "hostile cervical mucus" is postulated. Artificial insemination using semen from an anonymous donor is used to treat some types of male infertility (*semen donation*).

Ethical dilemmas may arise, eg, when single women request artificial insemination; where semen may be infective; where sperm is commercially advertised; or where a resulting child seeks to identify the donor.

ALo

Artificial organs are used to replace critical functions of a diseased organ, as temporary measures (while awaiting organ recovery or definitive replacement by *transplantation* or (potentially) as a long-term intervention. Research and development costs are enormous. Most devices will inevitably be used in ageing populations in the developed world. This raises questions of *distributive justice*. These devices will usually be tested initially in non-human animal species. *Informed consent* is difficult for experimental and non-proven therapies. The technological *paradigm* may force repeated interventions when such devices fail, often in circumstances of diminished patient *autonomy* and to the point of futility.

WP

Assault If a patient is approached physically ("touched" in English law) without her consent, actual or implied, unless the action can be justified as being necessary to prevent *harm*, an assault may have taken place. This may be part of a routine physical examination, an internal examination, or a blood test, and some would consider being looked at without consent a form of potential assault.

See also: Invasive.

RH

Assisted suicide Putting fatal drugs into a patient's hand may be morally preferable (because more likely to be *voluntary*) but less certain, than *euthanasia* – putting fatal drugs into a patient's arm.

Reference
Battin MP, Lipman AG. *Drug use in assisted suicide and euthanasia.* Binghampton, NY: Haworth Press, 1996.

KMB

Association, rule against The distinction made between orthodox medical practitioners and healers working on other systems has in the past led to confusion and disputes about *responsibility*. As a result, there grew up a rule within orthodox medicine that doctors should not send patients (through referral or consultation) to non-medical healers. This embargo no longer seems appropriate.

See also: Complementary medicine.

RH

Asymmetry/symmetry arguments can be used to test analysis in at least two ways: (a) to compare the different phases of life, such as birth and death, to see if arguments about the status of the fetus or newborn, for instance, can be illuminated by parallel thinking about the status of the terminally ill or recently deceased; or (b) to see if claims made for one side of a relationship are mirrored on the other. For instance, if a doctor has a duty to be truthful to a patient, does the same apply to the patient's statements to the doctor?

RH

Attempted suicide *See* Parasuicide.

Attitudes commonly used to refer to a state of mind with an evaluative element concerning an issue, object, or person. But the literature is replete with different definitions and uses in research, so much so that some reviewers have felt unable to distinguish between attitudes, opinions, values, and even beliefs.

Of the three components – knowledge, feeling, action tendency – usually attributed to attitudes, action tendency (validity as a predictor of behaviour) attracts most controversy, particularly over complex issues. This is perhaps, at least partly, because attitudes are essentially inferred, often from responses to scales or questionnaires, and could simply be artefacts of a research design. A related problem is the tendency to present a single attitude in isolation, outside the context of other relevant attitudes, some of which may conflict. The adoption of wider contextual approach is but one of several requirements for progress in attitudinal research.

JDO'H

Attitudes, knowledge, skills These are considered to be the three components of required professional education and training in health care, forming an interlocking whole in professional excellence. Deficiency in one may be blameworthy in law and in medical ethics. For instance, a highly competent and clever professional may still be considered by most to be acting less than correctly if delivering care accompanied by a patronising, hypercritical or arrogant attitude. One of the problems for professional commentators and educators is that people with deficiencies in professional skill and in current knowledge can be identified without great difficulty but that attitudes are less easily tested in training and less easily noted as right or wrong. It may be that the professional assessor can be rescued here by the lay person: for instance, where it may be difficult to censure a gynaecological colleague who clearly despises women, lay panels may have clearer judgment and no such qualms.

Reference
Education Committee of the General Medical Council. *Tomorrow's doctors: recommendations on undergraduate medical education.* London: Education Committee of the General Medical Council, 1993.

RH

Audit, clinical A formal means of assessing whether actual clinical performance conforms to good clinical practice. By showing whether what clinicians do is what they intend to do, it is a means of maintaining or raising standards and forms an increasing part of medical practice. For a long time, the *autopsy* has served as the ultimate medical audit with feedback through reports or formal clinico-pathological conferences. Medical audit, as now performed, requires that a certain standard or *guideline* has been or can be set, based on current knowledge and opinion, against which performance can be assessed. It usually involves examining *medical records* and necessarily evaluates the adequacy of record-keeping as well as what has been done. The audit cycle or spiral is achieved by ensuring that the results are used to inform or enhance clinical performance and/or to modify guidelines, enabling later re-audit. Conduct of medical audit is increasingly a requirement by professional bodies and health commissioners as a means of ensuring *accountability.* Formally, audit is distinct from *research*, which sets out to test a hypothesis – eg, about what might be a more efficacious way of treating a disorder than current practice, as opposed to determining

17

whether clinical practice is successfully applying what is already known. While the conduct of clinical research requires the prior approval of a *research ethics committee*, it is generally considered that medical audit does not. In reality, the distinction may prove somewhat arbitrary and there may be a necessary overlap, though this may only be evident after the work has been done; this may raise difficult issues if prior approval was not sought and research ethics committees may need to set guidelines about the extent to which audit may need such approval. Medical audit is part of the wider clinical audit, comprising audits of *nursing* and organisational aspects of health care, such as clinic waiting times, for which external targets may be set, as in the UK *Patient's Charter*.

See also: Quality assurance.

AJP

Authenticity Understanding and acceptance of real emotion keeps a professional in touch with her own value set. Such genuineness or authenticity appears to be detected by *patients* and highly prized. "My doctor cried with me when mother died". However, the requirement of a professional to "play a part", eg to care for a patient she doesn't like, may lead to an individual being unsure of what she actually feels or believes in, and so make ethical judgments more difficult. Some existentialists describe as authentic the style of life of someone who understands the meaninglessness of the world but chooses to act consistently.

See also: Existentialism.

RH

Authoritarianism refuses to go into its reasons, thus signalling that they may be morally indefensible – except

in emergency, itself a matter of definition. In medical ethics, authoritarian "doctor's orders" have given ground to recognition that patients and doctors each have their own kind of *authority*.

KMB

Authority Whatever is held to justify obedience to *power* ("the authorities") or deference to influence ("an authority"). Superior power (of arms or knowledge) may be sufficient to establish temporary, or reinforce traditional, authority. But in the long run, reasons (or authenticity) tend to be demanded; and to be respected, authority should derive from a social consensus or *contract*, based on informed views of what best serves the common good. Authority may be "charismatic, sapiential, or ascribed".

KMB

Authorship of scientific papers is a means whereby an individual's contribution to the work reported is recognised and credited, and through which responsibility can be taken for the findings reported. Increasingly, scientific *research*, especially *clinical research and trials*, is multi-disciplinary and necessarily involves contributions from many people for its conduct and completion. Furthermore, there is explicit and implicit pressure, personally and professionally, for clinicians and scientists to show research productivity, which is most readily measured by authorship of papers. Institutional performance is also now being assessed by publications, measured quantitatively and qualitatively (impact factors, citation analysis), with the objective of determining funding by funding bodies (eg, research assessment exercise).

Authorship is usually determined by the senior contributor, but editors of scientific and *medical journals* and institutional leaders are increasingly requiring it to conform to guidelines (eg, Vancouver guidelines). This is to minimise the risk of *fraud*, *plagiarism*, and the use of "gift authorship" to people who did not contribute to the work, but who may gain from authorship or whose names may confer (sometimes spurious) credibility. Guidelines for authorship vary, and may introduce a level of arbitrariness or discrimination against certain types of contribution. Simply stated, the person should have made a substantive contribution to the work, in its concept, planning, execution, and/or writing. How much is substantive is moot, though it can usually be readily defined in practice. Some have argued that all authors should be able to present and defend the whole of the work, and be willing to take responsibility for it. Yet this may be unrealistic for work that involves several disparate and highly specialised disciplines.

The question of authorship for clinicians who provide the source material for *epidemiological research* or for *clinical research and trials* is a particular difficulty. Arguably, they provide an essential resource of properly defined and characterised patients from which much laboratory or other analytical work may be derived, and without which it could not be done; yet they may not be directly involved in, or able to defend/take responsibility for, the work that is done using that material. In some countries and institutions, heads of departments are automatically given authorship, even if they have had no direct involvement; it can be argued that they provide an essential context for the conduct of the work and have to take ultimate responsibility for what is done under their aegis. While some contributions can be adequately recognised by acknowledgement within the paper or in a listing of collaborators, this may be insufficient to meet the needs of the contributors or institutions for external recognition. Increased awareness of these tensions

and the debate around authorship have probably reduced abuse, but there is a dynamic tension between a variety of sometimes conflicting imperatives.

AJP

Autonomy Literally "self-rule", autonomy is, in summary, the capacity to make deliberated or reasoned decisions for oneself and to act on the basis of such decisions. It has at least three components, the abilities to think for oneself, to make decisions for oneself, and to act for oneself on the basis of such autonomous thought and decision. Respect for people's autonomy is an important moral principle or value, to be found in a wide variety of moral theories, as diverse as *utilitarianism* and the deontological philosophy of Immanuel Kant. It is always qualified by the requirement of equal respect for the autonomy of everyone potentially affected by such respect.

Respect for autonomy, especially of their patients, is one of the *prima facie* "four principles" that it is widely agreed those involved in health care need to consider. It grounds such ethical concerns as the prima facie obligations to obtain *informed consent* from patients before doing things to them; not to deceive patients; to keep promises; and (at least in part) the obligation to maintain *confidentiality*.

Problems arising in the context of respect for autonomy include: conflict with other moral concerns; and questions about the proper *scope* of application of respect for autonomy, especially in the contexts of care of children (at what stage in their development do children become adequately autonomous to have their decisions respected even if others believe that these decisions are not in their best interests?); of severely mentally ill patients and of elderly patients with senile dementia (what degree of

19

mental impairment renders patients inadequately autonomous to have their remaining autonomy respected when their decisions for themselves are regarded as not being in their own best interests?); and also in the context of emergency medicine, where severe shock, pain, distress and impaired consciousness are often encountered and may severely impair patients' autonomy.

See also: Adolescence; beneficence; child, status of; decision-making capacity; justice; Kantian ethics; non-maleficence; order of preferences; paternalism; scope; self-determination; truthtelling.

RG

Autopsy An autopsy (literally, seeing for oneself) also known as a "post-mortem examination" is an examination carried out by doctors on a body after death to determine as accurately as possible the actual cause of death and any other conditions contributing to the patient's demise.

When death is thought to be due to unnatural causes (including *suicide*) or to *violence* (homicide or accidents) or through medical mishaps, the autopsy will be officially instructed by independent legal officials (in Scotland by the Procurator Fiscal and elsewhere in the UK by HM coroner). Jurisdiction over the body is retained until the completion of the legal investigation.

In deaths from natural causes when there is a desire to discover the exact cause of death or to assess disease progression and efficacy of treatment, the decedent's next of kin may be asked to consent to an autopsy which is then performed by hospital pathologists.

Any autopsy involves dissection of all body cavities and collection of body fluid and tissue samples for analysis and laboratory study. A reconstruction of the body takes place before its final release for disposal.

AB

Autopsy, requesting permission for A sensitive task that often falls to relatively junior medical staff. Apart from coroner's cases, this may be to clarify cause of death or to advance knowledge, comprising a form of medical *audit* or *clinical research*. Sometimes a limited examination may be permitted or samples can be taken through small skin punctures. However, full or limited examinations may be contrary to religious or cultural traditions (eg, some Buddhists and gypsies), which must be respected.

AJP

Aversion therapy *See* Behaviour therapy.

B

Bad news, breaking It is unethical to make assumptions about what patients should be told when they are found to have a life-threatening and/or severely disabling condition. Patients who perceive that they were given too much or too little information about their illness will fare worse psychologically than those who perceive the information as adequate to their needs. Many patients are already aware of their predicament. The task then is to confirm that they are correct. When patients have little or no awareness the task is to establish and respond to their needs for information, and then to elicit and try to resolve their concerns.

See also: Empowerment; hope; truthtelling.

PM

Balint Movement This is an approach to general medical practice, named after its initiator, the Hungarian-born psychoanalyst Michael Balint. The ideas were tested in a series of research seminars where difficulties between doctors and patients were the starting point. Balint developed a critique of standard medical assessments and professional communications, which were to be replaced by listening, understanding the meaning of the presentation, and gaining insight into a "deeper" diagnosis. It remains a particularly valuable approach where a doctor finds herself in a long-term relationship with a patient whose symptoms defy conventional diagnosis but who continues to return for medical help.

Reference
Balint M. *The doctor, his patient and the illness.* London: Pitman Medical, 1957.

RH

Battering is the word applied to patients whose condition has been caused by physical *assault*, frequently by someone who would be expected to be in a position of care. The patient is usually defenceless or dependent (such as at extremes of age or disability) and unable or unwilling to explain the true cause of her injuries. Diagnosis depends on suspicion, objective evidence and challenging the perpetrator. In some cases where there is an ambivalent relationship, the professional must choose between two sorts of potential *harm* – failure to protect the patient versus removing the patient's usual and familiar source of care.

See also: Child abuse; child, status of; disability; violence.

RH

Battery Legal term for wrongfully touching another person, ie without consent.

See also: Assault.

KMB

Behavioural sciences is a description sometimes applied to those disciplines concerned with human behaviour. However, many in these fields believe it is the study of human

knowledge (*attitudes*, beliefs, cognitions, *culture*, etc) rather than behaviour that sets them apart from the so-called natural sciences. Moreover, the term "behaviour" has been criticised for failing to capture the purposive nature of human activity.

DA

Behaviourism In a "hard" sense, the assertion that an account of human behaviour as under the determining control of experienced *reward* and/or *punishment* is a sufficient account; in a "soft" sense, the recognition that the effects of experienced reward and/or punishment form a necessary part of a necessarily more complex account.

References
Cohen D. *JB Watson: the founder of behaviourism: a biography.* London: Routledge and Kegan Paul, 1979.
Skinner BF. *About behaviourism.* London, New York: Knopf/Random House, 1974.

See also: Sufficient/necessary conditions.

BC

Behaviour therapy Originating in *behaviourism* and its study of the effects of reward and punishment in human learning, behaviour therapy now includes such approaches as desensitisation, in which learned anxiety responses are replaced by positive but also learned responses, token economy programmes, which attempt to counter the effects of, eg, prolonged *institutionalisation*, and cognitive behavioural interventions, in which individuals' altered understandings of (aspects of) their lives can reshape their experience of reward and/or punishment.

Many therapists make use of these techniques without subscribing to *behaviourism* in its "hard" version. In practice, ethical questions are concerned with the degree to which clients or patients are treated as subjects with whom the therapist works or objects to be (benevolently) manipulated.

21

Reference
Bergin E, Garfield SL. *Handbook of psychotherapy and behaviour change*. Chichester: John Wiley, 1994.

BC

Beneficence Beneficence literally means "doing good". The moral principle of beneficence is the moral obligation to do good, and is to be found in a wide variety of moral theories. Beneficence grounds the traditional Hippocratic moral obligation of doctors to do good for their patients. Because attempts to benefit others always risk causing *harm*, beneficence must always be considered in the context of *non-maleficence* – the *moral* obligation to avoid causing harm. The two obligations are combined in the traditional Hippocratic moral obligation of doctors to produce net medical benefit with minimal harm. A wide variety of prima facie obligations stem from this obligation. These include: the obligation of medical *competence* (and thus of sound medical education, both before qualification and throughout professional life); the obligation for the profession as a whole to do medical research, so as to establish better methods of producing medical benefits with minimal harm; the obligation to ensure that medical interventions will produce net medical benefit with minimal harm for individual patients (here respect for the *dignity* and *autonomy* of individual patients becomes part of the obligation of beneficence, for conceptions of harm and benefit are idiosyncratic, and what for one patient constitutes benefit for another constitutes harm. For example, many patients who have lost a large amount of *blood* will accept a *blood transfusion* as being highly beneficial; but *Jehovah's Witness* patients will regard blood transfusions as very harmful.) Beneficence also requires assessments of probabilities, both of the anticipated benefits and of the harms risked from medical interventions, and this again requires both a sound medical education and also the carrying out of medical research to establish these probabilities. Problems arising in the context of beneficence include conflict with other moral concerns; the problem of conflicting assessments of benefit and harm; and questions about the *scope* of the obligation of beneficence (to whom is it owed?).

See also: Hippocratic Oath; justice; limits; paternalism.

RG

Benevolence Literally a feeling of being well disposed to others, of wishing them well, benevolence is a different concept from *beneficence* or doing good, which is the primary moral obligation in health care. It is, however, far easier to do good for others if one feels benevolent towards them and thus in health care benevolence to patients or clients is a highly desirable attribute. However, the obligation to produce medical benefits for patients exists quite independently of whether or not health care workers feel benevolent towards them and applies equally to those patients to whom no such feelings are directed.

RG

Bereavement is the loss of someone emotionally close or important and often leads the bereaved to suffer and present physical and psychological symptoms. Such grief may have several phases, including disbelief, searching, anger, and depression. Survivors may feel guilty. Widowers' lives are shortened by grief, which may mimic or lead to other serious physical or psychological illness. Nevertheless, debate remains as to how far health professionals should be concerned with normal life transitions: the ethic of kindness suggests they should, and it would be hard to work in primary care without such a focus.

See also: Death; normality; loss and grief.

RH

Bias A preference for a particular view or for a particular person or group (*prejudice*). Approaching a problem with a one sided inclination, the mind partially made up, is not considered helpful in ethical discussion. Yet while in some roles a person must keep as open a mind as possible, each person will have a particular perspective. Although to prejudge an issue is usually wrong, perhaps the best we can otherwise do is be aware of our own points of view, and their origins and effects, so that we can accommodate the needs of those who see things differently.

Clinicians need to guard against conscious or unconscious bias towards or against a particular patient or group (eg, *heartsink patients* or *homosexuals*). Personal or institutional bias may also be evident in differential application of treatment or access to care, such as differing approaches to men and women with cardiac disease. Bias is a potential confounder in *clinical trials*, where patients or clinicians may have an overt or covert preference or expectation of *outcome*; this is the main rationale for the use of *randomisation* and of *placebos*.

See also: Perspective.

RH/AJP

Bioethics, history of As a professional discipline, medical ethics has existed in one form or another for well over 2000 years. Contemporary bioethics, by contrast, came into existence in a rudimentary way in the 1950s, accelerated in the 1960s, and began to assume worldwide dimensions by the 1970s.

What is the difference between the two fields? The focus of traditional medical ethics was almost exclusively on the professional ethics of the physician and the *doctor–patient relationship*. Bioethics has come to refer to the broader terrain of the life sciences, encompassing medicine, biology, and some aspects of the environmental, population, and social sciences. Where the earlier medical ethics was almost exclusively the domain of physicians (though with some considerable theological interest), bioethics encompasses the work of many disciplines.

The term "bioethics" was apparently first used by the American biologist Van Rensselaer Potter in 1971, though the first book in the new vein of bioethics, *Morals and Medicine*, was published by the theologian Joseph Fletcher in 1954. The great number of medical advances during the 1960s – eg, organ *transplantation, prenatal diagnosis*, kidney *dialysis*, genetic counselling – provided a special impetus to the new field. During that time small groups of professionals and lay people, particularly in Great Britain and the United States, began focusing on the emergent moral problems and organising research and educational initiatives.

By the end of the 1970s, bioethics had spread to all the developed nations of the world, though it was much slower to spread in developing countries. In addition to a variety of private and university efforts, various government agencies and commissions have been formed over the past two decades to help set policy and educate the general public. By the 1990s, bioethics was well established as a strong force in the life sciences and in general policy deliberations.

DC

Biopsychosocial model of illness suggests that there are many factors in the cause or emergence of a medical condition to be taken into account in a full assessment, not just the physical

23

or biological. This may influence the ground to be covered in an ethical as well as a clinical analysis, and may suggest other routes out of an apparent ethical impasse.

See also: Holistic.

RH

Biotechnology may be defined in terms of the applications of advances in genetics from the 1970s. It can be used to cover human as well as animal and plant uses. Some human applications, however, are usually distinguished – eg, gene therapy, genetic screening, genetic testing. One major human use commonly described as biotechnology is in the genetic engineering of new drugs. More commonly, however, biotechnology might be defined as any technique using living organisms or their parts to improve plants or animals or develop microorganisms for specific uses. Animal applications include cloning as a breeding technique, the genetic modification of animals to express human therapeutic materials (eg, insulin) and to produce *xenografts*. The genetic modification of plants has included attempts to enhance preservation (tomatoes), to engineer "natural" insecticides into plants and to engineer in plants an immunity from specific pesticides.

The ethical issues may be specific to the particular use. General concerns have been expressed about tampering with nature, about the effect of general use of biotechnological products on biodiversity, and about intellectual property rights in living matter. Particular concerns include worries about whether the development of techniques for cloning in animals will lead to similar experiments in humans; the effects on animal welfare of genetic modification; the risks to the environment of releasing genetically modified organisms (GMOs); concern about the overuse of pesticides if crops are genetically engineered to resist specific proprietary products; and concern about the monopoly effects of the use of such proprietary products. Against these concerns it has been argued that humans have always tampered with nature (eg, selective breeding); biodiversity has been far more seriously menaced by the introduction of new species into ecosystems; and genetic engineering may offer means to reduce the use of pesticides.

See also: Ecology and medicine; genetics; screening.

DS

Blame (i) Blaming is not necessarily the same as identifying a guilty party, or a morally culpable *act* or *omission*. When things go badly wrong in an institution or in public life, finding someone to blame can relieve others involved of the feeling that they share *responsibility* and encourage the belief that a fresh start is possible (often with unrealistic expectations). Accepting that everyone is equally to blame is psychologically supremely difficult.

(ii) Patients may feel that they are in some way to blame for illness and this, together with *guilt*, may affect their presentation and will need to inform their care. Clinicians may be blamed by patients or relatives for events that occur as a result of disease or its treatment. This may represent *displacement behaviour* for *anger* or distress about the process. Where complications of treatment arise, the issue of *negligence* may arise and may alter the *doctor–patient relationship* and encourage *defensive medicine*; in some jurisdictions, the concept of "no-fault compensation" has been introduced to allow patients to obtain *compensation* without having to prove negligence. The *Patients' Charter* is considered to have encouraged more *complaints* and a more adversarial relationship with clinicians.

See also: Accident; guilt; splitting.

KMB/AJP

Blood and blood transfusion Blood is the extraordinarily versatile fluid that transports essential materials throughout the body and removes waste from the tissues for excretion. Partly because it is readily accessible without harm, it is widely used in testing or *screening* for disease. These may be disorders of blood's many constituents or ones that are reflected, directly or indirectly, by alterations in its constitution; blood is also used for determining an individual's characteristics, such as in blood grouping or tissue typing for transfusion or *transplantation*, or in forensic work and *paternity* testing. In many *cultures* and religions, blood also has a potent symbolism, and may even be a metaphor for identity, and this may influence the perception of its medical use or even limit what clinicians are permitted to do with it. A significant number of infectious organisms can be transmitted by blood, through contact or inoculation, blood-sucking insects, sharing of equipment by injecting drug users, or blood transfusion. Health care workers need routinely to take precautions to avoid occupationally acquired infection, eg through needle-stick injuries.

Patients who lose blood or lack blood constituents may have these replaced by the transfusion of either whole blood or blood constituents. Increasingly it is only a part of blood that is transfused, according to need, to maximise the use of the blood resource and to minimise adverse effects, eg due to allergy, incompatibility, or infection. Red cells, white cells, platelets, whole or fractionated plasma, or concentrates of particular proteins, such as albumin, gammaglobulin (containing antibodies to microorganisms), or Factor VIII can be used. These are the mainstay of treatment for deficiency disorders, such as antibody deficiency or haemophilia, and, by providing passive immunity, are of value in the treatment of serious infections. However, the use of these blood products means the recipient is exposed to blood of many donors, with a concomitant increase in risk of infection. In acute blood or plasma loss, blood transfusion can be avoided or minimised by using plasma expanders. Where cells are used, the blood must be matched to avoid reactions between incompatible blood groups; this requires particular care in the obtaining, labelling and testing of the blood, and in the issuing, checking and administering of the blood transfusion. Some religious groups, such as *Jehovah's Witnesses*, prohibit or limit the use of blood, even in life-threatening situations; this may pose ethical dilemmas, especially if parents refuse to allow their children to receive blood transfusion.

The blood used for transfusion is usually donated by volunteers, although in some circumstances relatives may do so, and in advance of operations the patient may themselves donate blood for short-term storage for their own use (autologous transfusion). Plasma, white cells and platelets can also be obtained in larger quantities by the use of *pheresis* equipment which separates the constituents on line and returns the remainder to the donor. In some settings, donors are paid, but this has often caused problems because it may increase the risk of donations from people at risk of blood-borne disease or people whose poverty may force them to donate when it may be undesirable for their own health. Donors at risk of blood-borne infections (eg, *hepatitis* B and C, *HIV*) are asked to self-defer and are screened for them and for disease to avoid harm to the recipients and themselves; this requires a very high standard from such screening tests, information to donors about what tests will have to be done and their implications, as well as a need for systems to deal with the impact of what may be detected in donors.

See also: Gifts.

AJP

Body Despite its centrality to our existence, the body has excited formal study only in fairly recent times. The body as symbol, however, has a longer history: eg, notions of purity and danger have been inscribed in the way that bodies and their functions have been classified in the past. Moreover, the symbolism of "the king's body" lay at the heart of the constitutional and juridical basis of monarchical societies. No doubt rooted in religious belief and symbolism, the integrity of the king's body represented the integrity of the society. The royal personage was surrounded by ritual and pomp, and the most heinous crime was regicide.

The more mundane body of cells, tissues and organs made its first appearance in the late 18th century. Anatomical books began to describe an underlying structure of systems and microscopic detail; the anatomy room *dissection* and the medical *autopsy* began to subject the body to a close analysis; and the clinical examination became a routine part of everyday medical practice. This discrete and analysable body emerged at the same time as modern Western notions of individualism and no doubt there is a very close connection between ideas such as individuality and *autonomy*, and the perceived analytic separateness of the body. In effect, the symbolic centrality and integrity of the king's body has been translated to the body of "everyman". This means that

the sovereignty of the individual (or consumer, in more market orientated jargon) in modern societies is co-terminous with the inviolability of the body.

The relationship between individuality and the body is also represented in the notion that we both have bodies and are bodies. It therefore becomes possible, at least in part, to begin to separate *identity* from the body; the growth of psychological (and psychiatric) ideas about self during the 20th century provides one example of this possibility – though establishing a formal explanatory link between the psychological and corporal remains a common goal of much of this work, particularly in the field of *mental illness*.

This anatomical body continues to dominate medical thinking and it remains central to the distinction between health and illness. However, the relationship between the individual and the body (to what extent is our identity co-terminous with our body?) lies at the heart of much debate about ownership of the body, eg, as it relates to the legal and ethical problems surrounding spare parts surgery. Yet it seems to be the symbolic body that generates the most interest, particularly in terms of images of the body that pervade modern culture. Eg, body shape has become a central preoccupation of a large number of Western citizens; images of the body, from the pin-up to the idealised man often found in gay literature, are used as means of conveying diverse forms of sexuality; and of course the body still remains a major aesthetic object for many aspects of Western culture.

See also: Culture; eating disorders; transplants.

DA

Bone marrow transplants have an increasing range of indications, including haematological malignancies and certain inherited diseases. Their use raises general ethical issues of *transplantation* (*see transplants*), *benefi-cence/non-maleficence* conflicts, *distri-butive justice*, and patient *autonomy* (especially and frequently with chil-dren). Some new therapies incorpor-ate gene manipulation of stem cells, with the attendant ethical dilemmas.

See also: Genetics.

WP

Boo word A helpful phrase to remind us that some words or concepts in-trinsically contain a pejorative judg-ment (eg, *"abuse"*, *"bureaucracy"*, *"murder"*), and thus arguments con-taining them contain their own circul-arity or bias, and may tell us more about the discussant than the debate. The *Guardian* newspaper frequently uses a set of "irregular verbs" to out-line these, as in the classical cold war triad: "the British keep their ear to the ground, the Americans conduct surveillance, the Russians spy".

RH

Boundaries/limits may be of ethical importance in many ways.

It is often comfortable to be able to state that such and such applies in this case, but not that, although decisions traditionally based on such arbitrary points as "age of consent" in a particu-lar society may be of more interest to gossip columnists or lawyers than thinkers in medical ethics.

More useful are the limits of par-ticular concepts, accepted in normal speech but often stretched to breaking point by philosophers in order to clar-ify the concept. The concept of a per-son, for instance, would have limits – ie is a fetus, a dead body, a beloved budgerigar, a person? Much may flow from the answer. It may be easier to define such a boundary by giving examples of cases that definitely are, and definitely are not such and such, and then examining those that might

or might not be, to decide which side of the line they are.

Concepts may usefully define each other's boundaries or limits: the bal-ance between good and harm is an example, where too much care may become harmful (or one duty may be opposed and limited by another). Such debate may be more productive than finding an artificial weighing system.

Personal boundaries are of major importance to health care workers to prevent exhaustion or inappropriate involvement. A professional must learn she is out of her depth, working too hard, taking on work that is inap-propriate, and so on.

See also: Absolutism; adolescence.

RH

Brain stem death When the brain stem has lost all function the cerebral cortex becomes inactive and the patient also loses the capacity to brea-the and the heart soon stops from lack of oxygen. If mechanical ventilation is established, however, the heart and other organs (except for the brain) can continue to function for many days. If the brain damage is temporary (eg, from drugs or hypothermia) the patient may recover, but if the brain stem is irreversibly out of action then the patient can be declared brain dead. Diagnosis depends on excluding re-coverable causes and establishing ir-reversible structural brain damage (usually a head injury or intracranial haemorrhage), and on demonstrating the absence of all brain stem function. The patient is in deep coma with no cranial nerve reflexes (pupils, facial grimacing, gag reflex); and tests must show that there has been no return of spontaneous respiration. Spinal re-flexes may persist with limbs able to withdraw from a "painful" stimulus. Laboratory tests such as electroence-phalogram (EEG) are not necessary but a strict protocol of bedside tests

27

must be performed by two doctors on two occasions. The time of *death* for legal purposes is when brain death is confirmed – not some later time when the heart stops after discontinuing ventilation.

See also: Persistent vegetative state; unconsciousness.

BJ

Bribery is the use of something, such as money, wrongly to influence an outcome. The line between this and incentives or rewards for special behaviour may be vanishingly thin, and may depend as much on the observer's judgment of the *outcome* and the transparency of the transaction as on the act itself or the agent. Free gifts or trips from pharmaceutical companies may be such a case in point.

See also: Boundaries/limits.

RH

Buddhism The Buddha taught the reality of suffering in our lives: birth, old age, sickness and death cannot just be glossed over. But the path which he taught enables us to free ourselves from the fear and mental disturbance to which they usually give rise. Through conduct which avoids harming others, the practice of meditation and the cultivation of insight, we can gradually liberate ourselves.

The Buddha taught respect for life and for the welfare of all sentient beings. The basis of Buddhist ethics is compassion guided by wisdom rather than a fixed set of rules for behaviour (an exception is the precepts for the daily living of monks and nuns). The Mahayana teachings stress the "transcendent *virtues*": generosity, discipline, patience, effort, meditation, and wisdom. These can be cultivated by practices such as "taking and sending", in which one imagines taking in other peoples' discomfort and disturbed emotions and sending out to

them whatever peacefulness we have attained.[1]

Buddhist practice is seen not only as a preparation for living well, but also for dying well. Dying is seen as a natural part of our journey, and much care is taken to provide a peaceful and supportive atmosphere for the process of dying and for the days immediately following death when some form of consciousness seems to remain. For a discussion of Tibetan Buddhist practice in relation to death and how it differs from Western norms see *The Tibetan Book of Living and Dying*.[2]

From the Buddhist point of view the main task in relating to a sick person is to maintain *openness* and *communication*, not cutting ourselves off emotionally or grasping at possible solutions to their predicament in order to lessen our own distress and embarrassment.

References
1 Chodron P. *Start where you are*. Boston: Shambhala, 1994.
2 Sogyal Rinpoche. *The Tibetan book of living and dying*. London: Rider, 1992.

See also: Religion and philosophy, Eastern; transcultural medicine.

RMB

Bulimia nervosa *See* Eating disorders.

Burdensomeness of treatment To justify the burdensomeness of a treatment, one needs to ask if it is outweighed by the potential benefits. This is best answered by agreement between a competent adult patient and a doctor – although the patient is entitled to refuse, and the doctor not to provide, *treatment* the patient judges too burdensome or the doctor judges clinically inappropriate. When the patient is a child or mentally incompetent, a doctor may be justified in declining to provide treatment which the parents or family request, but the doctor judges disproportionally burdensome, or in providing clinically appropriate treatment which the family judge too burdensome. But none of these disputed courses can be justified (except in emergency) unless the doctor's clinical judgment has been communicated as clearly and effectively as possible and all efforts to reach an agreed solution have failed. A doctor's first duty is to the primary patient's best interests, but when these interests have been served or are unclear, the doctor also has a duty to avoid imposing heavy but avoidable burdens on the patient's family.

See also: Extraordinary and ordinary means.

KMB

Bureaucracy The *management* or government of any system or state by officials, working to the rules set internally by that system and interpreted by the officials, appears to pose problems for democracy and personal autonomous choice. In health care, professional groups respond differently to rules laid down by officials or managers. Although routines and procedures will always be necessary to prevent harms, unimaginative recourse to the rule book cannot be an adequate response to difficult clinical or moral problems. Clinical and moral judgment should spring from, not be imprisoned by, the relevant decision-making frameworks.

See also: Business ethics; National Health Service.

RH

Burnout is a phrase increasingly used to describe the emotional depletion or exhaustion suffered by someone who has had to care for others or another without adequate relief. It acknowledges that positive motivation and emotions (such as altruism, caring, enthusiasm) can be damaged by overuse or overwork, and that the subsequent symptoms are close to psychological illness. Social situations, such

as the Sabbath, and holidays derive from the common intuition that sometimes this tragic destruction of the good should be procedurally prevented.

RH

Business ethics provides a framework or set of standards of behaviour intended to prevent unfair competition or personal gain resulting from business decisions or transactions.

British *National Health Service* (NHS) organisations are now required to have an agreed code of business conduct, covering areas such as *disclosure* of gifts and personal interests. All employees have a responsibility to abide by this code. This follows in the wake of a number of highly publicised cases, chiefly computer system procurements, involving misuse of public funds.

At an organisational level, regulation or *management* of the new healthcare *market* is an attempt to ensure that the "business" of the health service is carried out in an ethical manner. The regulatory framework includes rules and restrictions, such as those on differential pricing, which prevent discounts from being given to purchasers who contract for higher levels of activity. This may be seen by some as putting unreasonable constraints on the effective operation of the competitive market.

The new emphasis on the health service operating as a successful business has encouraged some managers to introduce inappropriate ideas or practices from the private sector, such as "macho management" and the "hire and fire" mentality. This does not reflect the culture of the health service, nor does it make management any more effective. Business managers in the NHS need to have a close understanding of the nature of patient management and care, and therefore of the real ethical dilemmas inherent

29

in clinical practice. Their role is to ensure the most efficient and effective use of *resources*, so that ethical decisions do not by necessity become economic decisions.

See also: Purchasing.

ZW

C

Cadaver (Latin for to fall, to "die") refers to the lifeless body of a human person after the circulation of the blood and respiration has ceased permanently – somatic *death*. Customarily, after ascertaining these findings, the pronouncement of the fact of death is carried out by a medical practitioner, although no statutory instructions exist to this effect.

When body functions are being maintained only artificially in patients in deep and irremediable *unconsciousness, brain stem death* may be pronounced on the basis of diagnostic tests by specialist doctors regulated by nationally agreed *guidelines*.

Once death is pronounced and a medical practitioner can issue an official "death certificate", the manner of the body's disposal is left to the next of kin who can also consent to an *autopsy* and to removal of organs for *transplantation*.

If a death certificate cannot be issued, or the death is one that requires the Procurator Fiscal (in Scotland) or HM Coroner (in the rest of Great Britain) to be informed, the body passes into the jurisdiction of this legal official until such time as investigation is completed: an autopsy can be instructed, the body retained for a lengthy period after death and its disposal limited to burial only.

About 60 per cent of bodies are disposed of by cremation in Britain, a procedure regulated by statute. Before a cremation can proceed certain statutory forms have to be filled in by doctors and these are in turn scrutinised by a designated doctor referred to as the medical referee.

References

Gillett GR. Why let people die? *J Med Ethics* 1986; **12**: 83–6.

Stanley JM. More fiddling with the definition of death? *J Med Ethics* 1987; **13**: 21–2.

AB

Cancer One in five people die of cancer. Cancer is characterised by the uncontrolled growth of cells with the potential to invade locally or to metastasise. Mutations and translocations of genetic material are thought to be the mechanisms behind the development of most cancers. However, only a minority of patients have an inherited risk. Smoking remains the single most important aetiological factor. There has been a stepwise improvement in survival from 5 to 40 per cent throughout this century, with *surgery, radiotherapy,* and *chemotherapy.* New treatments are increasingly more effective with fewer side-effects.

An increasing number of asymptomatic patients are treated for cancer. *Screening* is effective in high-risk groups, detecting tumours at an earlier stage and saving lives. The adjuvant treatment of post-operative patients at high *risk* of relapse decreases the recurrence rate and improves the survival of patients with a number of common tumours, although it presents a dilemma in that some patients, who would have been cured by surgery alone, have to be treated with chemotherapy for the whole group to benefit.

Some interventions have not yet been shown to be cost-effective. As cancer treatments are rapidly evolving further refinements often improve the *cost benefit* ratio, with newer treatments rapidly replacing relatively ineffective or expensive therapies. Short-sightedness in financing treatment and research may be particularly counter-productive in this area.

Some patients miss out on treatments of proven benefit. Too many patients still have limited access to expert therapy. There is a limited number of specialists, treatment is expensive and there is still an outdated prejudice against potentially toxic treatment for vulnerable patients, particularly when the aim is to improve health-related *quality of life*.

Fewer than 5 per cent of cancer patients are treated in *clinical trials*, despite the fact that patients seem keen to be involved. Trials introduce other motives into clinical medicine. Most patients believe that new treatments are better and the pace of new developments can jeopardise the "uncertainty" that validates randomised controlled trials.

Despite the advances, few individuals can be assured of a cure and patients have great difficulty coping with *uncertainty*. There is a much greater awareness of the support needed by patients who are increasingly informed and involved in treatment decisions. In the past paternalistic secrecy has compounded fears surrounding cancer. Though the *doctor–patient relationship* is increasingly marked by openness and co-operation, there is resistance to the consumer-led standard of the American "prudent patient" and a reluctance to be "needlessly cruel" with excessive information for *informed consent*.

See also: Breaking bad news; paternalism; truthtelling.

RTP

Cannabis A recreational *drug*, often considered a "soft" drug, because of the perception that it is (relatively) harmless, and carries a lesser risk of *addiction* and *dependency*. Some communities regard it as integral (eg, Rastafarians) or acceptable (like alcohol or *smoking* tobacco) to their *culture*. It is nevertheless illegal in many jurisdictions and hence may be available from the same sources as "hard" drugs, eg, heroin, cocaine, posing the (perceived) hazard of escalating *drug misuse*. The situation is made more complex since cannabis or its active constituents may have medicinal benefit (anti-emetic, appetite stimulant, euphoric); this has led to moves in the USA to legalise its use on clinical grounds. Some of these are largely based on assertion or anecdote, and may have been used to legitimise pressure for legalisation; since a major route of delivery is by inhalation, it may lead to the apparent paradox of condoning smoking.

See also: Drugs, hard and soft.

AJP

Capital punishment is still used as the ultimate punishment in many countries. The role of doctors in the process presents significant dilemmas for a profession whose usual role is to care for patients and to prevent death. The judicial process should have allowed those with psychiatric disorders to be excluded from such punishment, but doctors may be asked to determine "fitness" for execution. More overt difficulty arises where a doctor may be asked or obliged to conduct the process of execution, for instance by administering a lethal injection or cannulating a vein to allow another to do so. Doctors may be asked to attend executions, either to ensure the criminal does not experience undue suffering or to confirm death. Some regard any of these as an unacceptable distortion of the doctor's professional role and implicitly to be condoning execution.

AJP

Care may refer to looking after another person (whether sick or well), the systems set up to enable people to do so (either for a group, as "community care", or an individual "care package"), or an attitude that promotes welfare or makes concern for well being of major importance. In medicine it is often contrasted with cure, because of a supposed but usually unrealistic aim of professional or patient to eliminate disease or illness once and for all. Enthusiasm for a cure at whatever cost in terms of physical discomfort or distress to the patient is part of the negative medical stereotype, but is sadly all too often still encountered. The best professional interactions will look to combine a good *outcome* with a good *process*: they will be part of effective training to enable the professional, the client, and the system in which they interact all to feel, and be, properly cared for. This is likely to include being approached and communicated with sensitively, used appropriately, paid attention to, treated as a person not just a case, and listened to empathically. It implies the warmth, contact and compassion of the best human responses to those in distress or need, and should include openness and the potential for *reciprocity*.

Modern ethical discourse, by correctly stressing the importance of respect for individual *autonomy*, may appear to promote a model of individual and isolated decision-making, but this is to misunderstand the clear preference of most individuals for satisfactory and warm human contact, and the need in all professional–client interactions for appropriate sharing of *responsibility* and expertise, without which a good and fair outcome is unlikely to be achieved. A supportive approach and environment is always likely to be needed in the anxiety-creating content of illness and health care, even if the professional has to hold herself back in order to allow a patient moral space in which to choose. If over-concern and smothering is inappropriate or unethical, so may be "take it or leave it".

An approach to ethical decisions giving priority to care linked to the virtues of female parenting rather than the drawbacks of *paternalism* has been developed which offers support to caring attitudes and has been especially influential in education and nursing. The questions "What would be a caring thing to do?" or "How would a caring person act?" have helped to give a different perspective to issues such as end of life decisions or *truth telling*. But there is no exclusive prescription here: there may be as many different forms of caring as there are people to give care. Being firm, confronting, or decisive may in some circumstances be the most caring way to act.

Reference

Noddings N. *Caring: a feminine approach to ethics and moral education*. California: University of California Press, 1981.

RH

Carriers are people who, though typically themselves healthy, may pass on disease to others. The two main examples are carriers of *genetic disorders* – eg, cystic fibrosis or females carrying an X-linked recessive gene (eg, for haemophilia); and carriers of infectious organisms – eg, healthy carriers of Salmonella species, *hepatitis* B or C and *HIV*; a notorious example was "Typhoid Mary", a cook who was the source of many cases of typhoid. *Screening* for gene defects and *genetic counselling* can be used to limit the development of genetic disease in the offspring of a carrier. Screening with *contact tracing* or *partner notification* can be used to limit or identify spread of infection.

AJP

Cases Medical ethics has always been grounded in *context*, and the analysis and discussion of cases (and *casuistry* derived from it) demonstrate this commitment. There are dangers, however, that this focus might distort (since someone has to describe or write up the case, and this is often a professional), misrepresent (an anecdote rather than a scientific study), or direct thinking away from principle or policy.

See also: Boundaries/limits.

RH

Case conference This is a term used for a multidisciplinary, often multi-agency meeting to discuss the management of a complex case. It is most often used in relation to child care or *child abuse* cases, or in patients with *mental illness*. Patients or parents, or their representatives, may or may not be present. In some instances, a case conference is formally constituted to make a decision regarding child protection registration and other child care arrangements. Apart from diverse clinical disciplines, case conferences may involve *social workers*, local authority agencies, *voluntary agencies*, the police, and legal professionals.

See also: Child, status of.

AJP

Castration is the removal or destruction of organs of genitalia in either sex by surgical or chemical means. The effects are permanent. It has occasionally been advocated as a therapeutic manoeuvre for sex offenders and the mentally handicapped, aimed at excluding "promiscuous" behaviour, but it is often ineffective and is very hard to justify even if done with permission. Like the debate on sado-masochism, can it be right to inflict major and permanent *harm* by request?

Sex change presents the arguments from a different direction, and removal of the source of sex hormones may be important in the treatment of some cancers. The full consequences of such treatment should be understood by the patient.

RH

Casuistry could be described simply as case ethics. As such, it consists of taking circumstances into account when applying general moral norms to particular *cases*. A good deal of literature on casuistic method and "cases of conscience" appeared from about 1550 to 1650 chiefly – though not exclusively – in Roman Catholic circles, much of it apparently aimed at priests and students for the priesthood who might benefit from guidance on typical cases when dealing with thorny problems in the confessional. In the middle of the seventeenth century, however, Blaise Pascal launched a formidable attack on casuistry, which, he believed, encouraged moral laxity. Since that time, the very word has had a pejorative ring about it, although casuistic method continued to be used for a long time after Pascal's death. It is, of course, easy to imagine how some proponents of casuistry might have used tortured logic and subtle semantics to promote moral laxity. Albert R Jonsen and Stephen Toulmin, however, have pointed out that readers of Pascal's *Provincial Letters* would have done well to distinguish between good and bad casuistry.

A renewed interest in case ethics came about in the second half of the twentieth century, not least as a result of problems occurring in the sphere of medical ethics, where morally relevant contextual details could differ enormously between one case and another. Time and again, it was noted, clinicians found themselves in situations in which there was a clash between two or more *prima facie* duties. Given the complexities of modern medicine, many ethicists see little sense in an approach to medical ethics that is confined to purely abstract principles. On the other hand, some have also noted the inadvisability of relying too heavily on norms concerning case types. They point out that the unique elements of new cases must always be taken into consideration.

Reference

Jonsen AR, Toulmin S. *The abuse of casuistry: a history of moral reasoning.* Berkeley: University of California Press, 1988.

See also: Context.

BHo

Catastrophe Literally an overturning, used (i) of a sudden calamity or an upheaval with unfortunate consequences and (ii) in mathematics to describe discontinuous change in output of a system in spite of continuous input. An extreme and unpredicted disaster should overwhelm neither our capacity to act nor our ability to think through the issues carefully and formulate the best response.

RH

Categorical imperative According to Kant, the basic moral law (acknowledged by the autonomous individual's practical reason) is to act according to principles on which it is rational for everyone to act. Thus one should so act as to treat both others and oneself always as ends, and never as means to ends.

See also: Autonomy; ends and means; Kantian ethics.

KMB

Causation is the relationship between two events or states such that when one occurs the other must occur. Philosophers are interested in the analysis of the phrase "must occur", but scientists are interested in discovering the laws that link events in causal relationships. The problem for medical science is that of the complexity of causal factors, which include the psychological and environmental as well as the biological.

Reference

Chalmers AF. *What is this thing called science?* Milton Keynes: The Open University, 1978.

See also: Chaos theory; epidemiological research; research; scientific method.

RSD

Certification (medical) Health care workers are presumed to be highly dependable and are often asked to certify that certain facts are true, both for medical purposes and in situations beyond medicine. The presumption is of truthfulness.

Illness is an acceptable excuse in society, whereas tiredness or indolence is not, so there is pressure on professionals to be "understanding" and write certificates, which stretch the boundaries of this truthfulness, for a greater good, when bureaucratic rules do not admit of an excuse: for instance, when a working mother must stay home to look after a sick child, or a nervous person does not want to do jury service. It is certainly the case that the "stickler" here can sometimes be accused of doing *harm*, or be of insufficient *advocacy*; and this is a situation challenging the *absolutism* of truth telling. But perhaps the rules should be changed, or a campaign set up to alter them. Whatever position appears to be the correct one, it is reasonable to expect consistency, and that each professional should be able to mark where on the *slippery slope* she would stop, and why.

See also: Bureaucracy.

RH

Chance is the way in which things happen if they are not determined by some form of order or system. The coincidence of a disease and an event may be by chance, even though there may be an inclination to attribute a causal relationship. Chance underlies the concept of *probability*, which is used extensively in *research* to assess the likelihood of an association between, eg, disease and behaviour or attributes. While association does not necessarily imply causation, stronger associations mean that it is less likely to be due to chance; statistical methods are used to assign numerical values to the likelihood that a link did not occur by chance.

AJP

Change is usually understood in the health service optimistically as change for the better. It is loosely used to describe key decisions in an individual's life that may help her to achieve her *potential*, particularly in relation to alterations in life style that may be thought to improve health (who decides this and on what evidence?). It is also the headline word for the imperative in the health service to create or respond to innovation and to make health service work more efficient or effective. People differ in their abilities to take up the challenge. Political rhetoric sometimes seems to imply that there is something desirable in change per se, but this should be demonstrated before it is taken for granted.

Reference
Rogers EM. *Diffusion of innovations*. New York: Free Press, 1983.

RH

Chaos theory is a branch of mathematics that seeks to find order in complex, apparently random systems, based on changes in patterns and sequences. It is a type of *determinism* that can evolve in an unpredictable manner. Applications of chaos theory in medicine include monitoring the spread of infectious diseases, investigation and treatment of cardiac arrhthymias and central nervous system disorders, including epilepsy.

PK/AJP

Chaperone To provide a third person to ensure propriety when a patient (usually of the opposite sex) is to have an intimate examination is seen by some as a vital protection for the patient against abuse, by others as an insurance for the professional against a (misplaced) accusation. It may simply be good manners and good professional practice, but some religions such as Islam in strict interpretation might exclude a man and a woman being alone in any case. Set against these issues are the loss of intimacy and confidentiality, the increased cost, and the practical availability. Since people differ in their judgments about what is intimate, it makes good sense for a chaperone to be offered before an examination, and the choice recorded.

RH

Character The marks engraved on persons as they develop their own moral responses to life's challenges – a process ended only by death or (reducing character to caricature) by pride or despair. Character is educated by learning from mistakes, and sometimes by the questions or example of trusted teachers or peers. A "good judge" of human character, unless silent, is suspect.

KMB

Charity (i) Old English translation of *"agape"*; (ii) occasion or institution of voluntary giving to provide for others in need ("caritas" – Latin for high price of life's necessities). Most modern health care is funded more effectively and efficiently from taxation or insurance. But charitable giving and "charities" have intrinsic moral and social value.

KMB

Chemotherapy is drug treatment that kills dividing cells. The type, combination, dose and frequency of the drugs determine the balance of efficacy and toxicity. Chemotherapy can be given with the hope of curing the patient or prolonging good quality time. Most chemotherapy is given at a dose near to the maximum tolerated dose, although increasingly, hair loss and vomiting are avoidable. When *beneficence* has a narrow therapeutic window, doctors have a *duty of care* to give clear information, particularly about the aims and side-effects of treatment. Patients are increasingly empowered to be involved in decisions about treatment options.

There is good evidence that palliative chemotherapy improves health-related *quality of life*. The fittest patients benefit most. However, treatment can be carefully tailored and monitored to avoid detrimental toxicity.

See also: Cancer.

RTP

Child abuse No coherent theory has yet explained why so many adults wish to harm so many children, when the majority of adults love and respect their children. Globally many more children are subject to slavery, forced labour, prostitution and genital mutilation: acts that result from poverty or the absence of education.

Health care professionals may face ethical problems: (i) in balancing children's needs for protection against their, and their parents', right to privacy; (ii) in maintaining *confidentiality*, and (iii) in deciding where an abused child will be safest.

Reference
Scheper-Hughes, N, ed. *Anthropological perspectives on the treatment and maltreatment of children*. Dordrecht, NL: Reidel, 1987.

See also: Abuse; child, status of.

RN

Childbirth is a normal physiological process. There appears to be a sudden increase in moral status and value of a baby when it is born and enters human society, although it is not entirely clear why this should be so. It is also interesting to note the cross-cultural observation that the first questions when a new member enters society are what the sex is and whether the child is normal. There are occasional severe outcomes of damage and death for mother and baby, some of which can be anticipated during antenatal care. In the UK at present there are professional rivalries over the care of pregnant women between doctors and *midwives* using two different ethical frameworks to inform their argument (the old doctor/patient model and new midwife/client model). Pregnant women and their babies are not best served when this intellectual debate erupts in the form of professional dispute in the antenatal clinics and labour wards.

See also: Autonomy; child, status of the; empowerment; paternalism.

SB

Child psychiatry Children, brought to a child psychiatrist because of the complaints of others, often feel blamed and criticised for their disorder. This limits informed *consent*. When the patient is believed to have been neglected, rejected or physically or sexually abused the child psychiatrist may have to put that child's right for protection above the stated wishes of the patient, of the parents and of the wider family. This alters usual considerations of medical *confidentiality*. Child psychiatry is usually conducted in a multidisciplinary team setting of highly qualified independent practitioners within which roles, leadership and confidentiality have to be judicially negotiated.

See also: Adolescence; child, status of.

CD

Child, status of The last two centuries have seen great changes in the status of children. Before education became widely available, they were often valued as contributors to the family economy from a young age, but such value was moderated by many children dying before adulthood. Education, while adding to their later value as adults, takes away their immediate value to their families, and may reduce the respect and protection they receive as children. In those parts of the world where education is scarce there is often also low life-expectancy with high infant and child death rates, severe poverty and families of large average size, to which children make a significant economic contribution.

To protect the latter children, and to spread more widely the protections offered to children by particular developed countries, the United Nations Convention on the Rights of the Child[1] was adopted in November 1989, and has now been ratified by over three-quarters of the countries in the world. It puts children's *rights* on the same firm footing that international law has given to adults' rights. The convention accords to children established adult rights such as the right to life, but adds the right to family life. The freedoms of association, expression and thought are protected, and a right to both primary and secondary education, while protection from *abuse*, sexual exploitation, direct involvement in armed conflict or abduction or sale are rights to be protected at international as well as national level.

In health care it has been increasingly recognised that children are not just little adults, but have their own spectrum of medical and developmental problems. Recently it has also been recognised that, in some circumstances, children as young as five or six years old have the understanding necessary to take a significant part in decisions about their own health care.

References
1 United Nations. *United Nations Convention on the Rights of the Child*. New York: UN, 1989.
Alderson PA. *Children's consent to surgery*. Buckingham: Open University Press, 1993.

See also: Adolescence; consent; decision making capacity; paternalism.

RN

Chiropractic A method of diagnosis, prevention and treatment which deals primarily with mechanical causes of disturbances of the nervous system and their correction by manipulative means. Consequently it deals with functional disorders (mainly, though not exclusively, musculoskeletal), caring for the human frame in health and disease, with specific manual spinal adjustments or other forms of manipulation as well as various other forms of supportive treatment. Many chiropractors now work closely with their conventional medical colleagues. In the UK, as far as the General Medical Council is concerned, if a medical practitioner refers a patient to a chiropractor then she must do so with a clear diagnosis and must bear responsibility for the chiropractic treatment provided, in spite of the fact that chiropractors are currently seeking statutory recognition and have appropriate professional indemnity to practise.

See also: Complementary medicine.

GL

Choice *See* Autonomy.

Chorionic villus sampling A technique of obtaining a sample of placenta in the first 3 months of pregnancy for *prenatal diagnosis*. Although the risk–benefit equation is different from that of other techniques, the ethical issues are the same. The advantage for pregnant women is that diagnosis (and termination) is performed early.

See also: Abortion; risk–benefit analysis.

SB

Christianity Jesus Christ (1st c CE – Common Era) was a popular healer and moral storyteller, whose reinterpretation of *Judaism* (emphasising intention, forgiveness, love, and justice) led to his crucifixion. That he then rose from the dead is foundational (if variously interpreted) to Christianity. Its ideas and organisation were developed, notably by Paul and Augustine, to incorporate elements of Greek philosophy and Roman order. It became the religion of the Roman Empire and mediaeval Europe, but major splits arose between Eastern (Orthodox) and Western (Catholic), and between Roman Catholic and Protestant (often national) churches. Protestants continued to divide as secular ideas became increasingly influential. Nineteenth century missionary expansion paved the way for new non-European versions of Christianity, ecumenical concern with peace and justice, and spiritual cross fertilization among religions. Christianity is a faith whose worldwide membership continues to grow rapidly.

Practical Christianity includes healing and caring. The churches and individual Christians have played an important part in the provision of health care, although they have sometimes opposed the advance of medical science. Most religious organisations are conservative, and this is also reflected in their approach to medical ethics, notably on *abortion* and *euthanasia*. Christian ethics or moral theology (including casuistry and *agape*istic ethics) provides useful resources for examining such issues; while the pastoral knowledge of clergy and *hospital chaplains* can interpret otherwise unvoiced views. In health care as elsewhere, lay Christians who practise their faith anonymously greatly outnumber those who proclaim that only their own sectarian opinions are "Christian".

See also: Religion and philosophy, Eastern.

KMB

Christian Science Religious movement (USA 19th century) believing in the power of mind over matter and healing through prayer. "Mechanical" forms of medical science (obstetrics, orthopaedics, and oral surgery) are allowed, but medical diagnosis is forbidden or discouraged, and avoided by devout members. Christian Science policy is to support, not reject, families who seek medical care for their sick children.

KMB

Chronic disease presents particular challenges to *patients*, clinicians, *healthcare systems*, and welfare/benefits agencies. By definition chronic diseases are conditions that go on for long periods, cannot be fully treated, and so require *care* not cure. These disorders may continue at the same level of disease/disability, may relapse and remit, show a progressive course, or variations of these. Examples are rheumatic diseases, multiple sclerosis, motor neurone disease, Alzheimer's disease, chronic fatigue syndrome, *AIDS*, diabetes, and schizophrenia. Patients and clinicians need to adopt a *treatment* approach that minimises disease activity, prevents relapses (eg, *prophylaxis*), controls symptoms and develops coping strategies. Such diseases also place considerable burdens on informal carers who provide long term physical and psychological support to the patient. Family and friends may have difficulty dealing with chronic disease, finding it hard to adopt an appropriate role towards the patient over the long term. They may develop behaviour patterns such as distancing or overprotectiveness. This may enhance the impact of disability, accentuating the patient's feelings of isolation or alienation and increasing her sense of *stigma*.

Some clinicians may find chronic disease a constant reminder of their limitations and may also adopt similar attitudes, which will undermine their usefulness. They will need to develop models of care that provide a suitable balance of physical and psychological support, while enabling the patient to adapt and achieve reasonable *quality of life*. Much of this will depend on effective delivery of primary and *community care*, with suitable support from hospitals and specialists in shared care models. Patients may have reduced earning capacity and will be dependent upon welfare systems and benefits, both for their usual needs and additional ones resulting from the illness, exacerbating feelings of dependency. Disease specific *pressure groups*, often set up and run by those affected, may provide valuable practical help, mutual support and advocacy.

By extension the term reminds us that many common conditions have a long term or recurrent pattern, either because of an underlying predisposition in the patient (such as asthma) or emerges during life (such as diabetes) or because it is part of an acceleration of the normal aging process (such as ischaemic heart disease). There is now a move for planned systems of care for such conditions, which anticipate changes in the disease, attempting to ameliorate them, or prevent deterioration. To the operational difficulties of running such programmes for different people with diverse forms of the condition are added the different (and sometimes conflicting) interests of professional groups. One important ethical issue is the clash between a "managed" clinical care system and the patient's need to make decisions and be in control of her own *long term care*, even if this means occasional bouts of "delinquency".

Chronic diseases present policy dilemmas about *resource* allocation, as they require long term allocation of relatively labour intensive care. They may be contrasted unfavourably with those (relatively few) conditions for which cure is feasible. With an aging population, degenerative disease becomes commoner, so resource issues raised by increasing care of the elderly are linked with those of care of chronic diseases. QALYs are an attempt to quantify some of these issues for health policy development.

See also: Fatigue syndromes.

AJP/RH

Circumcision is the operation of removing part or all of the foreskin that covers the glans of the penis. The operation dates back to prehistoric times, but became a religious ritual in Judaism and Islam.

Those who perform circumcision in the Jewish community are usually highly trained but not necessarily medically qualified. Objections have been raised to the operation as unnecessary surgery that probably causes the infant (eight days old in Judaism, older in Islam) considerable distress. There is some move in progressive circles to allow only medically qualified people to perform circumcision, but little pressure to discontinue the ritual. It poses the obvious dilemma between allowing unnecessary and painful procedures and people continuing their own cultural and religious practices.

See also: Mutilation.

JN

Circumcision, female is a procedure ranging from clitoridectomy to infibulation, a more extensive procedure

39

regarded as a form of genital *mutilation*; it is practised in a few countries or ethnic groups. The cultural or social origins are often seen as a reflection of male preferences in sexual practice or in control of female sexuality and are thus widely regarded as unacceptable in Western cultures. The operation is often done by lay operators under non-sterile conditions and on young children, who cannot consent in person, so allowing parents to perpetuate the tradition. In some countries female circumcision is illegal. While the general rejection of the practice is understandable, people from the cultures where it is used may object to interference with their traditions.

See also: Mutilation.

AJP

Claims may have special meaning in insurance practice or in law, but in ethical debate may be useful in the more neutral sense of an assertion, particularly one that states a reason or demands something as due from another (whether this is substantiated or not). This may help to "cool down" discussion where there is more heat than light; for instance, defining a "right" as a "justified claim" then may shift the balance, if the "right" is not accepted, back to the proponent to justify.

References

Campbell A, Higgs R. *In that case*. London: Darton Longman and Todd, 1982.

Toulmin S, Rieke R, Janik A. *An introduction to reasoning*. New York: Macmillan, 1979.

RH

Clarification is sometimes seen as the main issue in any analysis and, while not the prerogative of, may be helped by, philosophy. No one should hesitate to ask for something to be made clear, whether it is in a job interview, a clinical encounter, or an ethical analysis. It should be seen as vital in

discussion, a possible litmus test to reveal humbug. The abilities to obtain it and offer it succinctly are two of the cardinal *virtues* or *skills* in *clinical ethics*.

See also: Role play; videos.

RH

Clinical ethics A form of applied ethics practised in the hospital or health care setting and concerned with actual clinical choices. It may involve a clinical (or hospital) ethics committee, whose functions include ethics policy making, education and case consultation, and/or a clinical ethicist who works alongside staff. Both are familiar in hospitals in North America (where clinical ethicists have accreditation). A few UK hospitals have ethics (as opposed to research ethics) committees.

KMB

Clinical freedom is the right often claimed by doctors to act as they think fit in a clinical situation for which they have responsibility. It is claimed as a means of enshrining: the clinician's unique perspective on the clinical problem she is presented with; the personal and social context in which it occurs; and the desire to exercise her *clinical judgment* and *decision-making* without rigid external constraint. It derives as much from the art of medicine as from the individualisation of its science. It is sometimes regarded as a fundamental and inalienable right in the practice of medicine and regularly features in debates over potential political or other interference. It is not intended to imply a complete lack of external control or *accountability*, but rather that these are provided in more generic terms, according to explicit or implicit codes of behaviour and accepted standards among a clinician's peers, typically through forms of *self regulation*, or legally defined standards, such as support by a substantial body of medical opinion. However, it may be seen by others as allowing a freedom to perform outside or below accepted standards.

A particular example of clinical freedom that is much valued in the UK is the ability of a doctor to prescribe a medicine that she judges to be appropriate, even if it is not a licensed indication for that agent. Recently, the introduction of *guidelines* and purchaser standards, and the purchaser/provider relationship in the financing and commissioning of health care have presented some constraints on clinical freedom, whether in attempting to define treatment norms (sometimes as enshrined in the new dogma of *evidence-based medicine*) or in financial limitations over certain types of treatment, whether regarded as too expensive, of unproven efficacy or as unnecessary.

AJP

Clinical judgment (i) is the attribute exercised by the experienced clinician in resolving a diagnostic or therapeutic dilemma. It derives from a blend of formal training, knowledge acquired from the medical literature and, above all, clinical experience. It is typically used to refer to the "nose" that some clinicians have for the right answer, even though it may be hard to define or articulate its derivation. It refers particularly to the way in which a clinician attempts to resolve an ethical problem, with reference to a "feel" for the issue and experience of similar problems in the past. As an indefinable attribute, and one that is not always justly claimed, it presents a tension with the increasing expectation that clinicians should act according to explicit and definable rules in the practice of medicine, especially if there are major *resource* implications.

AJP

Clinical judgment (ii) In the clinical sense *moral judgment* refers to a situation in which a clinician or another person involved in *healthcare systems* is influenced in decision-making about patient care or *public health* by issues of morality; these may be derived from religious beliefs or a personal view of right and wrong. It may be seen as inappropriate if it confers *bias* or is prejudicial to *equity* of care. It may take the form of implicit or explicit *blame* of people for behaviours that may have contributed to disease or may affect eligibility for treatment, such as refusal to treat *smokers* or the obese. There may be a genuine basis for differing treatment of different patients, but a stated reason may conceal, or be perceived to conceal, a moral judgment. It is generally felt that moral judgments should not influence medical decision-making in the delivery of health care, but should be kept private. However, some clinicians may have a conscientious objection to, eg, therapeutic *abortion* and can exclude themselves. In some cultures, clinicians may be obliged to take account of moral issues. Furthermore, moral judgments may be the basis on which clinicians refuse to participate in, eg, executions or *torture*.

See also: Capital punishment; clinical freedom.

KMB/AJP

Clinical research and trials constitute systematic applied *research* in medicine. Methods range from simple observation and analysis of patients (an interface with medical *audit*), and retrospective or prospective study of clinical events or of laboratory assays on patient groups and *epidemiological research*, to formal clinical trials. A hypothesis is analysed with careful control for the irrelevant variables inevitable in an outbred, free-living population. Statistical analysis based on *probability* is crucial to avoid *chance* associations. Biological plausibility is an essential cross-check against statistically significant findings that are themselves due to chance. Ethical conduct is regulated by international declarations, eg, Helsinki, which provide protection for research subjects, and locally by *research ethics committees*. Clinical research and basic scientific research are complementary and mutually supportive through the generation of hypotheses in one arena and their testing and/or application in the other.

Clinical trials are a formal means of evaluating the safety and efficacy of new interventions, eg, *drugs, vaccines* and *surgery*. They are required for the licensure of drugs by the *pharmaceutical industry* and drug regulatory bodies, and are increasingly used to inform practice *guidelines*. Trials follow extensive preclinical assessment, in laboratory and *animal experiments*, that justifies testing in humans. They are divided into: Phase I studies of *safety*, with only opportunistic and preliminary observations on efficacy; Phase II studies of indicative efficacy and safety; Phase III large-scale clinical efficacy studies, and Phase IV studies that extend evaluation of agents already being used in clinical practice. Initial studies may use healthy *volunteers*. It is necessary to define end-points in advance, not only in terms of the intended clinical benefit, but also in terms of *surrogate markers* that can anticipate it. Their use is critically dependent upon a proven linkage between the marker and the clinical endpoint, in qualitative or quantitative terms.

The patient population must be carefully defined and selected using parameters that limit the risk of false results and maximise likelihood of a definite answer. This may mean excluding some patients, eg, those with advanced disease or at low risk of reaching the end-point, and those receiving non-essential treatments that could be confounding variables, and including sufficient subjects to reach a definitive conclusion (the statistical power). A clinical trial thus necessarily has an element of artifice, excluding some patients. The extent to which extrapolation to such patients is justified is a matter for *clinical judgment* and is a critical issue in the drafting of practice *guidelines*.

Participation by patients and clinicians requires acceptance of the *uncertainty* principles on which the trial is predicated. Yet its very conduct implies that the intervention will improve outcome. This can introduce potential *bias* in patient selection or retention. "Blinding" of patient or both patient and clinician ("double-blind") to the intervention and comparator reduces bias, as does *randomisation*. If no current therapy exists, a *placebo* may be used in the *control group*, whereas if the new intervention is to improve on an existing standard, the latter is the comparator. Proposals for open studies or for patients to be able to choose therapy are driven by an understandable wish to access new agents, especially in advanced disease (eg, *AIDS, cancer*), but may undermine the process of determining the role of the treatment by introducing systematic bias. Compassionate release in parallel with trials can ameliorate this problem. Trials are generally overseen by an independent data and safety monitoring committee that examines the unblinded data for potential safety concerns or the achievement of a clear result, according to predetermined "stopping rules". *Publicity* surrounding trial results and its timing in relation to commercial considerations and drug availability may present significant tensions between the interested parties.

See also: Equipoise; reward.

AJP

Clinical teaching encompasses teaching about clinical medicine in the broadest sense and may be the use of clinical illustrations of basic science material, teaching about clinical topics and individual diseases, or – most commonly – teaching based around a meeting with a patient.

While there is no exact definition, it is most characteristically seen on the ward round, with a student presenting a patient whom she has interviewed and examined (clerked) to the consultant or other member of her team (the firm) in the presence of a group of student colleagues. After the presentation the consultant teaches the group about details of the patient's illness, often using a Socratic approach. The potential ethical pitfalls of this may be revealed by the traditional caricature (which while generally deplored is by no means extinct). The patient was a passive participant in this process, *consent* not usually being sought in a way permitting refusal. The patient was depersonalised and objectified as "clinical material", thus allowing the teaching group to proceed with little thought to the patient's feelings. *Patients* were at risk of being displayed without clothes, or having intimate details of their life and illness discussed by the group. The powerful modelling and brutalising aspects of such activities might be allied with a method of teaching based on the demonstration of knowledge: those who fell short would suffer a "ritual humiliation". The ethical issues here do not need spelling out.

Modern teaching has successfully faced new health and educational philosophies and the new health service : the decline of bed numbers forcing the greater use of outpatients, general practice, and new modes of delivering care such as day care surgery. The patient is no longer passively lying in bed and consent to the process needs active negotiation; in the UK the *Patient's Charter* has to some extent formalised this. Primary care influences have stressed the importance of understanding the patient's own feelings and fears in any consultation, and it is considered good practice to elicit her ideas, concerns, and expectations or knowledge, beliefs, and *attitudes*. There have been attempts actively to recruit the patient as a teacher, valuing her experiences in her own right rather than using them as a substrate for discussion of a disease state. Moves towards more ethical development of student skills have required *students* to learn interviewing methods with actors or specially trained members of the public acting as simulated patients before working with patients. Similarly, examination skills and clinical procedures may be practised first on mannequins and student colleagues. This allows the student to develop confidence in a protected environment as well as protecting the patient from the students' untutored advances. Alongside this patient centred approach to medicine is a student centred approach to learning, focusing on the needs of the learner rather than the omniscience of the teacher.

See also: Medical education; role play; videos.

PBo

Clinical trials *See* Clinical research and trials.

Cloning "Clone" has several different usages. In cell biology it describes a group of cells derived from a single common progenitor cell. In molecular biology it refers to a recombinant vector in a bacterial cell carrying a single foreign DNA sequence. It is also used to describe individuals with the same genotype – eg, monozygotic twins. Artificial cloning of this kind was achieved by transplanting nuclei from an embryo into a number of anucleated recipient eggs of Xenopus. It has been recently found that lambs can be cloned by transplanting nuclei from cell lines that have been established from very early sheep embryos to anucleated eggs, and that the same procedure can be used to obtain viable lambs from cells that have been established from older, more mature embryos; one living lamb has been derived from a cell line that was established from the udder of a six-year-old ewe. These results confirm that the genome does not undergo irreversible modifications and do, of course, raise the issue that cloning of higher organisms and man is now possible.

References

Gurdon, JB. *The control of gene expression during animal development*. Oxford: Oxford University Press, 1974.

Wilmut I *et al*. Viable offspring derived from fetal and adult mammalian cells. *Nature* 1997; **385**: 810–13.

See also: Genetic disorders.

DW

Closure, moral Ethics likes to ask questions, whereas medicine needs answers. This is one of the tensions in any form of applied ethics; at some stage, consideration of different options and arguments will have to stop, and a decision be taken about what should be done. Just as one of the insights of communication skills is that open questions may get more answers, or a greater depth of answer, and closed questions are best used sparingly and only when required, so a better moral outcome might be anticipated if moral closure is prevented until the appropriate moment. When that moment might be could itself be part of a fruitful (and open?) debate.

RH

Codes The medical profession, rather than laying down codes of behaviour, has tended to rely on an ethos of moral *integrity*. However, since the events of World War II the British Medical Association has become a signatory to the International Code of Medical Ethics, and a variety of codes have emerged.

They have been: (a) a response to particular issues, eg, the 1947 Nuremberg Code emerged following Nazi wartime experimentation; (b) designed to meet various purposes, eg, the Declaration of Helsinki (1964 and 1975) on research involving human subjects; the Declaration of Sydney (1968) relating to the determination of the time of death, and the Declaration of Oslo (1970) on therapeutic abortion.

Since 1953 when the International Council of Nurses drew up its first code of ethics a plethora of codes for nurses have been issued. The devolvement of power to the United Kingdom Central Council for Nursing, Midwifery and Health Visiting (UKCC) has led to that body drawing up: (a) a Code of Professional Conduct (latest 1992) for all its practitioners; (b) codes for specific groups (eg, *The Midwife's Code of Practice*, 1994), and (c) codes around specific issues (eg, Standards for the Administration of Medicines, 1992).

Codes clearly have limitations and serve principally to lay down the rights and duties which should underpin professional practice.

References

Burnard P, Chapman CM. *Professional and ethical issues in nursing* (2nd ed). Harrow: Scutari, 1993.

British Medical Association. *Medical ethics today: its practice and philosophy*. London: BMA, 1993.

Thompson IE, Melia KM, Boyd KM. *Nursing ethics* (3rd ed). Edinburgh: Churchill Livingstone, 1994.

See also: Accountability; clinical judgment; clinical trials and research; conscience; doctor–patient relationship; Hippocratic Oath; human rights; incompetence; justification; litigation; malpractice; misconduct; mistakes; moral judgment; negligence; responsibility; statutory bodies.

HM

Coercion (from Latin for to restrain) raises similar ethical issues to *compulsion*. In seeking *consent* to medical *treatment* or participation in *research*, whether the fine line between reasonable persuasion and coercion is crossed depends not just on what is said (the information needed for consent to be valid), but also, inter alia, on how it is presented (eg, which benefits or risks are emphasised, in technical or in lay language, in what tone of voice), by whom (eg, the clinician responsible for the patient's care or for the research project, or an independent clinician), and in what circumstances (eg, whether enough time is allowed for the patient to absorb the information).

KMB

Colleagues/collegiality Colleagues are people bound together by a common bond, such as profession, place or style or work. Through shared values they may provide mutual support. A corollary, and arguably a corresponding duty, is that they help each other by identifying lapses in performance or judgment, whether through the "quiet word" or through referral to a professional body (*self regulation*). Collegiality is the systematic mutual support exercised by colleagues and deriving core values or more literal advice from colleagues. Institutions may be run in a collegial manner by ensuring that their systems, goals and standards are derived from the individuals who comprise them.

See also: Peer pressure.

AJP

Collusion of anonymity is a term introduced by Michael *Balint* and his colleagues to describe the difficulties experienced by a patient and her primary physician when the patient is seen by a series of secondary specialists; it is as if there is tacit agreement for no one to take overall *responsibility* and thus a decision cannot be ascribed to an individual who might be called upon to give reasons or provide explanations. Taken more widely, it can be a criticism of poorly functioning *teams*. It provides a strong justification for empowering both the patient and her primary adviser. In other contexts, the "key worker" principle provides someone who has the responsibility to bring things together and the power to challenge or confront those who are not apparently acting in the patient's best interest.

Reference

Balint M. *The doctor, his patient and the illness*. London: Pitman Medical Publishing, 1964.

See also: Balint Movement; empowerment; teamwork.

RH

Coma *See* Persistent vegetative state; unconsciousness.

Commercial interests In response to cost control imperatives, commercial *market* forces have been introduced into the US medical care system and many other systems in the industrialised world; they now dominate the insurance and delivery of care in the private sector. Government financed insurance is also turning to the market. Health care in the USA is becoming an enormous, investor owned industry. The full impact of this development remains to be assessed but it is already clear that while competitive commercial markets can control spending on health services, serious concerns exist about access, quality, community services, and the loss of professional values. Assuming commercialisation survives, more government regulation will almost certainly be required to protect the public interest.

45

Reference
Relman AS. The impact of market forces on the physician–patient relationship. *J R Soc Med* 1994; **87**, 22 [Supp]: 22–5.

See also: Business ethics; National Health Service.

ASR

Commitment may be seen as a key virtue for anyone offering any but the shortest term care for patients, and a marker of an important professional boundary. The professional makes an implicit promise to a patient to provide appropriate care, unless requested not to do so, in a way that takes account of their being persons with a relationship. Within this relationship, the professional distance must be appropriate and regularly reviewed. It is possible to be too closely committed, as well as too distant.

The term is also often used in relation to the amount of work undertaken by a professional, which may be crucial for her mental health.

See also: Boundaries/limits; covenant; promise keeping.

RH

Communication Medical care must be based on an accurate identification and understanding of all the patient's current problems. Otherwise, important problems may remain hidden and hinder physical and psychological recovery. Doctors and nurses have to guard against their tendency selectively to respond to cues about physical problems (such as pain) in preference to cues about psychological problems (such as depression). They also tend to assume that there is only one main problem and then make no effort to screen for others.

In exploring a patient's problems the patient may become distressed. It is unethical either to stop exploration or to insist on further exploration without first negotiating with the patient whether she wishes to proceed or to change the topic. Using open directive questions "How has the operation affected you?", questions with a psychological focus: "How did you feel when you learned it was multiple sclerosis?", clarification "You say it upset you, in what way?", empathy "No wonder you felt so angry", and educated guesses "You seem terrified of a relapse", promotes patient disclosure of key concerns. However, medical and nurse training do not always ensure that doctors and nurses acquire these skills. Consequently they often use behaviours that block *disclosure*.

They do this because they fear that probing will unleash strong emotions and they will not be able to contain these, in which case the patient will then be harmed psychologically. They also fear that establishing the reality of patients' predicaments will bring them, the doctors and nurses themselves, too close to suffering and loss. This, in turn, might jeopardise their own professional functioning and emotional survival, especially if they lack practical and psychological support from colleagues.

It is unethical to expect doctors and nurses to communicate effectively unless their training equips them with the necessary communication skills and strategies, gives them the confidence to use these, and convinces them of their value both for patients and for themselves. Practical and psychological support must also be available.

See also: Doctor–patient relationship.

PM

Communitarianism A political theory or movement advocating a middle way between collectivism (eg, fascism, Soviet communism) and laissez faire liberalism. It emphasises the public as well as private good, the *responsibilities* as well as the *rights* of individuals, and policies based on *consensus* rather than ideology or *compromise*. Its advocacy of family interests and community values has implications for both *distributive justice* and individual *autonomy* in health care.

KMB

Community care The theory of community care is derived from the belief that many people are better cared for in their own homes or in the community, rather than in institutional settings. This belief is often fortified by moral objections to the long-term *institutionalisation* of those in need of care.

Fundamental changes in the organisation of health services in Britain and of local authority social service departments were incorporated in the *National Health Service* (NHS) and Community Care Act of 1991, by which health authorities and general practitioners holding their own budgets acquired responsibility for providing for all those in their care, whether with appropriate support at home, or in NHS or independent hospitals and nursing homes. The care manager for social services has a parallel duty to arrange and review care packages that are means tested. *Responsibility* is therefore divided between the health and social service agencies.

Although substantial resources were made available from public funds, it soon became clear that the demand for services and the costs of meeting increasingly complex needs exceeded official predictions.

Since meeting the criteria of eligibility does not of itself guarantee access to services, care managers are confronted with the knowledge that only those with the highest risk assessment are likely to receive the service they need.

Since the implementation of the Act agencies have attempted to plan services jointly to enable people to remain in their own homes for as long as possible. The most contentious issue has been raised by those with long-term mental health problems, many of whom have not been able to adapt to living in a community which cannot offer them an adequate level of support, and who are often perceived as posing a threat to themselves and the public.

It was anticipated that much of the funding for home care by the primary team would be released by savings made by the closure of beds as patients came to spend less time in hospital. Ethical concerns centred from the beginning on whether support services in the community would in fact be in place before such beds were closed.

See also: Mental illness.

EMJ

Compassion Literally, "suffering with" (not "feeling sorry for"); attributed to Buddha, Allah, and Christ. A doctor or nurse either devoid of, or regularly overwhelmed by compassion, is dysfunctional. "Suffering with" can motivate and inform, but can also oppose and inhibit meaningful action to relieve suffering. Timing and tolerance guide discrimination.

KMB

Compensation is what one receives in return for a job done, but is increasingly seen in the narrow sense of the payment to be given to anyone injured or harmed by professional *negligence*. The cost of justice brings issues of reality to fine ideals, but at the same time puts ethics into the realm of the courts, where precedent and different forms of bias may enter.

See also: Litigation.

RH

Competence has both medical and legal interpretations. For doctors competence means the ability of patients to understand and take decisions upon any aspect of their health care. A competent person must give fully informed consent before any medical procedure is undertaken. Refusal to accept *treatment* that the doctor considers to be necessary does not imply any lack of competence. In emergency the doctor may still act (without consent) providing it is in the best interests of the patient. The law defines competence in children by chronological age. The English courts are increasingly allowing doctors to judge when competence has been attained.

See also: Autonomy; consent; decision-making capacity; incompetence.

JSH

Competence to practise Doctors must ensure that they are competent to practise the specific medical procedures they undertake both regularly and infrequently. This will usually involve training. Inexperience offers no legal protection against unsatisfactory performance. In the UK the Royal Colleges now require career grade doctors to participate in continuing professional development. This may involve individual study or further training, both individually and with others. The *General Medical Council* (GMC) now has procedures requiring unsatisfactory doctors to submit themselves to performance assessment and, if necessary, retraining.

See also: Burnout; Disciplinary Procedures; experts and expertise; incompetent professionals; malpractice; misconduct; peer pressure; peer review; reasonable person standard.

JSH

Complaints from patients are significant ways of addressing performance, competence and *accountability* – when *litigation* for *negligence* does not arise. Patients are entitled to receive explanations, *apologies*, and assurances that defects will be remedied.

Only a relatively small number of complaints proceed to litigation.

An ideal complaints procedure should embrace the basic concepts of sympathy, speed, openness, a willingness to right wrongs and fairness to both sides, virtues often sacrificed to cumbersome bureaucracy in the past. New arrangements in the UK from April 1996 are aimed at resolving patients' concerns and giving detailed explanations through local resolution and independent review procedures. Disciplinary proceedings are entirely separate.

Reference

NHS Executive. Complaints; guidance on implementations of the NHS Complaints Procedure. London: NHSE, 1996.

PH

Complementary medicine is an umbrella term used to describe many differing and often unrelated therapies. The British Medical Association (BMA) report, *Complementary Medicine: New Approaches to Good Practice*, published in 1993, used the term "unconventional therapies" rather than complementary medicine. These therapies were defined as: "Those forms of treatment which are not widely used by the orthodox health care professions, and the skills of which are not taught as part of an undergraduate curriculum of orthodox medical and paramedical courses". The therapies include *acupuncture*, Alexander technique, aromatherapy, Bach flower remedies, *chiropractic*, clinical ecology, crystal therapy, healing, herbalism, *homoeopathy*, hypnotherapy, iridology, kinesiology, massage, nutritional medicine, *osteopathy*, radionics, reflexology, and Shiatsu.

Most of the disciplines within complementary medicine have their own diagnostic system which leads directly to specific therapeutic interventions. The "major" complementary therapies both in terms of widespread use, scientific evidence and coherence include acupuncture, chiropractic, clinical ecology, herbalism, homoeopathy, osteopathy, and nutritional medicine. Conventional doctors are becoming increasingly interested in a variety of complementary medical therapies. In the UK over a third of general practitioners practise some form of complementary medicine and over three-quarters regularly refer patients for treatment. The services of both medical and non-medically qualified practitioners of complementary medicine are now widely available within *primary care* and the divisions between these two areas of medicine are becoming increasingly blurred; for instance, acupuncture is now available in almost all pain clinics and is a recognised physiotherapy treatment.

It is historically self-evident that the alternatives of yesterday are becoming the conventions of today. This has largely come about through patient demand, but it is clear that as further research emerges and conventional and complementary medical practitioners learn how to work more closely, increasing integration will occur between these two previously antagonistic areas of medical intervention.

GL

Complexity is a major problem in ethical thinking, where principles and policies may not easily be outlined, unless through simplification. There are strong moves to reverse the process by acknowledging both the need to see judgments in *context*, and to unpack all aspects of particular issues by looking at the different *perspectives* of the relevant people and systems. *Routines* and simple solutions may be important, but may sometimes create ethical problems in themselves; at the very least, there is a human need for an individual's complexity to be

acknowledged, even if it then has to be laid aside for good reasons.

RH

Compliance is the extent to which patients follow specific advice from a clinician, often applied to the willingness to take *prescribed* medication. It is an indicator of the success of the *doctor–patient relationship* and the patient's understanding and acceptance of the clinician's advice. It is affected by the patient's acceptance of her disease and the need to treat it, and by actual or perceived adverse effects. *Empowerment* of patients and prescribing only those interventions that the patient accepts should enhance compliance.

AJP

Complicity Literally, this is the condition of being an accomplice, and is the description of the position faced by someone whose *role* necessarily but unwittingly gives them knowledge of an immoral act, or whose skill is required to prevent further *harm* once such an act is committed, and who thereby by her involvement and social position appears to confer approval or blessing on the situation when otherwise she might be expected to oppose it or expose it. A health care worker might find herself in such a position during a consultation (the dilemma of *confidentiality*), or by being involved in *war, capital punishment* or *torture*. Being a health care professional confers no immunity in these cases from the judgments of law or of history, but no one should doubt how much *courage* is required to take a personal moral stand and follow the dictates of one's own *conscience*.

See also: Boundaries; limits; quietism; whistleblowing.

RH

Compromise – leaving aside the sense of placing oneself in peril ("found

49

in compromising circumstances") – is the aim of reaching agreement where two or more persons or arguments clash. It may be seen as a major aim in clinical ethics. "To agree to disagree" may be satisfactory in arguments, but where action has to be taken, this luxury may no longer be affordable. Several steps can be outlined. First comes an acknowledgment of a *conflict*, and a *clarification* of the issues: then viewing the problem from everyone's perspective and reviewing evidence or competing arguments; and finally finding a way through which provides for key priorities for each party. Understanding the emotions that underlie points of view may be important. Negotiating skills can be learnt. Those who have a reputation for compromise and *pragmatism* risk leaving others confused (at best) and feeling deceived (at the worst) and there may be some issues which should be considered absolute, ie, boundaries not to be crossed under any circumstances. Doctors killing or sleeping with patients would be examples offered by some.

RH

Compulsion (from Latin for to drive) may be (a) external, using physical force, or (b) internal and psychological, when the drive to do something is not easily amenable to *reasoning* or control. Health care professionals may find themselves (a) having to compel patients (not) to take action, in order to prevent possibly greater harm (such as restraining the wildly psychotic or suicidal), while (b) acknowledging drives (including that to help others) in themselves, which may be poorly understood. *Voluntary* action by emotionally self-aware rational persons is an ethical ideal to strive for, but not always possible to achieve in practice. A classic question (Ulysses and the Sirens) is whether

people who enslave, or impose external contraints (compulsion) upon themselves when they believe they will not otherwise be able to resist (compelling) temptations, are acting freely.

KMB/RH

Compulsory testing and treatment
Under most circumstances a person can be subject to medical examination, investigations and *treatment* only with that person's consent. This follows from the principle of respect for *autonomy*, and is protected by the legal concept of battery (see also *assault*). Patients unable to give *consent* (for example, because they are comatose) are normally treated on the basis of what is in their best interests.

However, the question sometimes arises as to whether a person should undergo medical investigation or treatment compulsorily. There are two kinds of justification for this: firstly, when the investigation or treatment is in the best interests of the person herself; secondly, when it is in the interests of other people.

With regard to the first justification, it is well established, in common law, that a competent adult can refuse even life-saving treatment: respect for autonomy trumps concern for the person's best interests. However, *competence* comes in degrees, and deciding when a less than fully competent person's refusal of treatment should be respected can be a problem. The Mental Health Act (MHA) (1983) allows for compulsory detention, assessment and treatment of a person suffering from a "mental disorder" in order to improve the person's health, or for the safety of others. The major justification for these compulsory powers is that the patient is not competent. The MHA does not explicitly use the concept of competence.

The second justification for compulsory testing and treatment is for the good of other people. This is the sole justification for the Public Health (Control of Diseases) Act 1984 which allows magistrates to order a patient to be removed to hospital and to submit to medical examination if she is suspected of being a carrier of a *notifiable disease* (such as cholera).

See also: Beneficence; carriers.

TH

Computers in medicine have highlighted the need to balance an increasing need for information in delivery, documentation, and assessment of health care with the requirement to protect medical *confidentiality*. Although few issues are uniquely raised by use of computers, the greater potential for misuse of data by unauthorised persons than with conventional notes have emphasised the need for controls, in particular data security and access issues. Some control is provided by the *Data Protection Act*, but additional measures are increasingly necessary, especially as health data are used for *purchasing* and with proposals to develop national databases. Many consider that encryption of personal health data is a necessity. Patients increasingly see clinicians entering data on to computer during consultations and may be wary about providing information that would normally have been more overtly restricted to the clinical encounter; such perceptions may subtly alter the *doctor–patient relationship*.

Computers have also been used to assist with diagnosis, but with limited success to date in replacing clinician-based analysis; this may reflect an insufficient understanding of the way in which clinicians sift information relating to diagnosis, against a background of published data or analysis and their own experience. Computer-based systems have had more success in *triage* and assessment of probability

of recovery in critically ill patients, though their use has been regarded with suspicion when applied to decisions regarding withdrawal of treatment.

See also: Treatment.

AJP

Concrete vs abstract This is one of the important polarities in clinical reasoning, and those who find the other type of thinking difficult may try to reject the insights. Nevertheless, both are necessary for good clinical ethics, and the test bed of theory remains practice.

RH

Condom A device placed over the erect penis or inside the vagina, to prevent contact between genital secretions in sexual intercourse, as a prophylactic against *sexually transmitted disease* and in *contraception*. Their efficacy is partial and is critically dependent upon their regular and correct use and application throughout intercourse. It is also dependent upon manufacturers' quality assurance schemes and regulatory standards. The role of condoms in reducing the risk of *HIV* infection has increased their use, but some religious leaders oppose this owing to the contraceptive effect. Personal or cultural objections and limited accessibility may also reduce their utility in some settings.

See also: AIDS.

AJP

Confidentiality is a vital part of the understanding on which the *doctor–patient relationship* is based and is a central ethical pillar of clinical practice among all health professionals. It results from the fact that, in order to enable the clinician to provide care effectively, the *patient* may need to

51

reveal sensitive aspects of her personal life. These and her medical circumstances, which could lead to disadvantage, *stigma* or *discrimination* if known to others, must not be divulged to third parties without the patient's explicit *consent*. A duty of confidentiality is not only enshrined in professional tradition, as in the law and the church, but is also set out in international *codes* and in duties regulated by statute through the *General Medical Council* and other professional bodies. The duty extends to others in the *multidisciplinary team, nursing, paramedical professions,* management and clerical staff. The professional ethic may be taken for granted by the patient, but she may wish to establish an understanding with a clinician before revealing everything or may seek explicit confirmation of the clinician's duties and clarify any limits to confidentiality.

Teamwork requires the sharing of information, but some have felt that sharing secrets within a team makes nonsense of the concept of confidentiality, particularly where agency or generic staff not involved in setting up or reviewing team procedures are involved. It is likely that few patients understand how many people, in complex cases, need to know about their condition. In addition, some paramedical workers feel that they should not reveal to the doctor information acquired at the peripheries of their working life (such as a receptionist who sees an epileptic friend driving when she shouldn't be). Both teaching and learning and support or supervision (formal and informal) may entail the sharing of information normally regarded as confidential: some supportive professional interchanges verge on gossip. Family medicine poses a particular set of dilemmas. These are areas where every person needs a clear idea about the ethical limits and practice of sharing information.

A potential difficulty in maintaining confidentiality arises where information is revealed in a clinical encounter that is relevant to the personal health or welfare of another or to the *public health*. The clinician may then experience a conflict over the duty of confidentiality and a duty to warn, eg if the patient reveals an intention to harm others, or actions that would have that effect. There are additional tensions if the clinician is also responsible for the care of the third party (eg, a spouse or partner). The clinician may also have statutory public health duties to report a patient's condition, eg *notifiable diseases*. Particular difficulties arise in regard to HIV infection and *AIDS* and in some psychiatric conditions leading to violence against or harm to others; the duty of confidentiality towards children under 16 seeking *contraception* and *abortion* who do not wish their parents to be informed has engendered some discussion. In most circumstances the clinician may be able to negotiate with the patient a way for her to remove or minimise *risk* to others. However, if the patient refuses or is unable to do so, some clinicians will feel obliged to breach confidentiality. If so, they are obliged to inform the patient of this. The GMC outlines specific circumstances in which a doctor may breach confidentiality. However, such breaches, if they are known to have occurred or be likely to occur, may mean that patients will withhold information that is relevant to their own health or that of others.

Individual clinicians, according to their conscience and guided by statute and ethical training, will vary in the limits they apply to confidentiality. It is probably unrealistic to aim for absolute confidentiality, though some will aspire to it. Some professional groups are obliged by statute or codes of practice to apply stricter rules of confidentiality, including those working with *sexually transmitted diseases* and in *occupational health*. Clinicians involved in reporting *clinical research* findings may need to take care not to identify patients inadvertently or in such a way as to allow deductive disclosure. Similarly, *publicity* about medical matters requires clinicians to safeguard personal health information; issues can be debated effectively without personal identifiers. In some instances, patients will not only seek confidentiality but anonymity, eg in sexually transmitted disease clinics remote from their social milieu. Medical insurance is a contract voluntarily taken on by patients which will necessitate disclosure of health information for the policy to remain valid.

New tensions have arisen regarding patient confidentiality in arrangements for *purchasing* health care, and in hospital and other health service information systems. Names of patients are not usually essential for the former. Release of personal health information should be based on a careful assessment of "need to know". Retention of such information is covered by the *Data Protection Act*, which requires that the purpose of collecting and storage of data be defined. The more people who have access to such information, the greater the risk of inadvertent breaches of confidentiality. All staff who deal with such information should have employment terms and conditions that specifically require them to observe confidentiality, especially if they are not bound by a professional code.

Organisational confidentiality is increasingly being required of health care staff, not only in relation to patient details, but also in regard to contracts, finance and other corporate issues, in *trusts* eg. If staff feel that this places unacceptable constraints on them when they consider that policy or practice is against the patients'

or the public interest, *whistleblowing* may be an option. These issues emphasise the need to develop codes of *business ethics* appropriate to organisations involved in health care.

See also: Child, status of; computers; forensic psychiatry; insurance, medical.

AJP/RH

Conflict is often the origin of important ethical issues. Some would see it as vital and enduring, as part of "the way that Nature works". Avoiding it at all costs will entail, usually, continuous *compromise*, which would be unacceptable to most; on the other hand, conflict in itself can cause major harm.

See also: Trade off.

RH

Conflicts of interest Physicians are expected to put the medical needs of their patients above all other considerations. Conflicts of interest arise in clinical practice when practitioners become involved in arrangements that introduce other considerations that are potentially incompatible with the best interests of patients. A conflict of interest is not an action, but a situation that can adversely influence action. Even if they do not actually lead to unethical actions, conflicts of interest are inherently problematic because they weaken professional standards and undermine trust.

The adverse factors in clinical conflicts of interest are of two general types. The first are financial incentives, such as those that may induce a physician to prescribe a particular drug or device, recommend a procedure or refer a patient to a particular medical facility. The second are financial disincentives or restrictive contractual agreements that may reduce services by encouraging the physician to limit her choice to certain treatments or drugs, by discouraging her from referring to specialists or admitting patients to hospitals or by encouraging her to restrict the time she spends with patients. Both types of factors militate against patients' interests because they predispose physicians to behave in ways not consistent with their best professional judgment.

Conflicts of interest in medical practice are ubiquitous and often of only minor significance but they should be eliminated or avoided as far as possible. Particularly worrisome are those conflicts of interest likely to harm patients or add substantial costs, incommensurate with benefits.

Disclosure is a necessary but usually insufficient remedy because patients are often unable to evaluate the significance of the disclosure or act on it. Professional *self-regulation* would be the ideal solution but is often lacking because physicians are not immune to the seductions of financial gain or to the pressures of the medical market place. Most observers have therefore concluded that control by government and professional organisations is needed. In the USA many laws, regulations, and professional codes of conduct are being promulgated to address this problem.

References
Rodwin MA. *Medicine, money, and morals: physicians' conflicts of interest.* New York and Oxford: Oxford University Press, 1993.
Thompson, DF. Understanding financial conflicts of interest. *N Engl J Med* 1993; **329**: 573–6.

ASR

Congenital malformations are primary anatomical defects in newborns which produce abnormal function, eg, cleft lip. Forty per cent are multiple and 20% recognised by chromosomal analysis, eg, Down's syndrome.

Antenatal diagnosis may involve techniques which carry definable risks to the fetus; anomaly screening may show unexpected abnormalities whose management, eg, termination, poses ethical dilemmas.

In infants with multiple malformations ethical difficulties arise in connection with decisions to start, withhold or withdraw treatment. These require careful considerations of prognosis, the infant's best interests, burdens/benefits of *treatment*, and the family's cultural and religious preferences.

In older children the ascertainable wishes of the child, if of sufficient maturity, understanding and experience, should carry substantial weight in *decision-making*.

See also: Burdensomeness of treatment.

VL

Conscience Literally, "knowing together" – coming to a judgment by examining severally, together and in context, all known sides of a moral question. Some regard conscience as the voice of God or a moral sense one should always obey (even when religion teaches that it is in error). Others reduce conscience to psychological or social conditioning, citing cultural differences in its judgments. These differences vitiate claims that the same act can be right or wrong in all circumstances. But the activity of conscience itself (examining, unifying, judging) is universal; and (arguably) it is capable of unifying a growing circle of morally relevant factors with increasing sensitivity and impartiality.

KMB

Conscientious objection When a significant minority (usually religious) objects in principle to a legally required or permitted practice, the *law* may make limited exemptions. Conscripts with principled objections may be excused from fighting, but not other wartime national service. Doctors (and other staff) with conscientious objections to *abortion* may refuse to participate in medical, surgical or (possibly) administrative procedures required for termination of pregnancy: but they have a duty to provide impartial *counselling*, speedy referral and any required treatment incidental to termination or necessary to preserve the pregnant woman's life or health. Abortion, however, is an exception to the normal rule that doctors are not permitted to refuse to treat certain categories of patients or to refuse to offer forms of treatment that are within their competence.

KMB

Consciousness We all know about consciousness, but it defies simple definition. It is the entirety of subjective experience – the state of awareness of sensations, of oneself, of one's memories, thoughts, emotions, and intentions. Consciousness provides us with a private account of the world around us and of the causes of our own actions. That account includes a "first-person" sense of *self*, of other selves, of *choice* and intentions, and of moral constraints on personal action.

Historically and religiously, the conscious mind has been equated with the concept of a spiritual soul, traditionally thought to exist separate from the physical *body* and capable of survival after death. René Descartes (1596–1650) identified the pineal body within the brain (actually a hormone gland involved in regulating bodily rhythms) as the interface between the mechanistic functions of the nervous system and the separate, spiritual soul. He imagined that the soul could move the pineal body to intervene in brain mechanisms, so as to exercise choice and intended action (downward causation).

Modern neuroscience offers the prospect of understanding completely how the brain functions without reference to the dualistic notion of a separate, spiritual influence. Indeed, most of what the human brain does (the "computational" processing of sensory information and of motor output, learning, control of bodily function, and so on) never enters consciousness. In his book *The Astonishing Hypothesis*, Francis Crick argues that consciousness itself will be explained by science. However, because of the private nature of the evidence, the process by which activity in circuits of nerve cells might generate *subjective* experience remains deeply mysterious. David Chalmers calls this the "hard problem" of consciousness, which might depend on a hitherto unrecognised fundamental property of information-processing systems. Mathematician Roger Penrose suggests that consciousness reflects quantum mechanical interactions between nerve cells.

Reductionists argue that all our actions are essentially the result of causal processes in the closed physical system of the brain, which is determined by our genetic make-up and the rich influences of personal experience. But if the subjective feeling of intended action (free will) is illusory, the notion of personal *responsibility*, on which legal systems and the structure of society are built, must also be revised.

Moral attitudes towards other people and even animals are predicated on the presumption that they too are sentient, ie conscious of sensations and emotions such as pleasure and *pain*. Ethical debates about *abortion*, mercy killing and experimentation on animals all hinge on the question of whether others are conscious, highlighting a deep dilemma – that it is impossible to know the content of other minds.

See also: Euthanasia; genetics; moral agency; persons and personhood; spirituality.

CB

Consensus on medical issues may be implicit, arising from internalised standards of clinical practice based on experience and evidence, or explicit, in the form of consensus statements or *guidelines* set out after formal consideration by relevant *experts* representing a range of opinions and brought together for the purpose. Consensus statements may be viewed as guidance for less expert clinicians or as a standard of care expected by patients and/or purchasers of health care; they may also be used as a responsible body of medical opinion in legal cases. They should not constrain legitimate diversity of practice (*clinical freedom*) based on *clinical judgment* exercised in particular cases.

See also: Purchasing.

AJP

Consent The ethical principle that every person has a right to *self determination* is reflected in *law* through the concept of consent. Thus, the law of consent is of the utmost importance in medical law because it is the mechanism by which the law protects and preserves a patient's bodily integrity and ultimately the right to decide what is to happen to her. In general, medical *treatment* may only lawfully be undertaken with a patient's consent. A doctor who acts without a patient's consent risks criminal prosecution for *assault* or more likely, being sued for damages in the tort of *battery*. Exceptionally, medical treatment may be given without consent where the patient is unable to consent, eg, if the patient is unconscious and an *emergency* occurs or where the patient is permanently (or even temporarily) unable to consent through mental disorder or disability and treatment is reasonably necessary in that patient's best interests.[1]

Consent may be expressly given where the patient explicitly agrees to what is proposed by the doctor or it may be implied from the circumstances or the patient's conduct where it may reasonably be inferred that the patient does, or would, agree to what is proposed. The law does not require a patient's consent to take any particular form although it is common in the hospital context for a consent form to be used. A signed consent form is only evidence (and is not conclusive proof) that a patient has given consent to a treatment. It is the reality of the patient's consent that is the concern of the law.[2]

A legally valid consent (or refusal) of medical treatment requires three elements: (a) the patient must be *competent* to consent (or refuse) treatment; (b) the consent (or refusal) must be based upon adequate information; and (c) the consent (or refusal) must be voluntarily given.

A patient will be competent to give (or refuse) consent if she is capable of understanding what is involved in broad terms in the medical treatment, including the procedure itself, its consequences, and the consequences of non-treatment. In law, the issue is whether the patient is competent to make the particular decision: hence a patient may be competent to make some, but not other, decisions.

An adult patient (one who has attained the age of 18) will be presumed to be competent to understand a medical procedure unless there is good reason to doubt it, eg, if she is mentally disordered, mentally disabled, or affected by external factors such as drugs or alcohol. In such cases the patient will be competent to consent only if she is capable of "comprehending and retaining treatment information", "believing it" and "weighing it in the balance to arrive at a choice".[3] Thus, a patient who denies her medical condition exists or the likelihood of its outcome (eg, that she will die without treatment) or who is compelled to refuse treatment in either case because of her mental disorder, will not, in law, be competent to make a decision concerning her treatment.[4] It is important to notice, however, that a patient is not incompetent to make a decision about her medical treatment merely because her decision seems irrational or the reasons for it are unknown.[5] Hence, a decision based upon a patient's religious beliefs must be respected as a valid decision even if the patient's choice is to die rather than be treated: eg, a *Jehovah's witness* refusal of a *blood transfusion*.[6]

The position of a child is somewhat different. If a child is aged between 16 and 18 she will be presumed to have the capacity to consent to medical treatment to the same extent as an adult.[7]

A child under the age of 16 will be able to consent to medical treatment providing she is sufficiently mature and intelligent to be able to understand what is involved in the treatment.[8] Thus, a child's capacity to consent will, in practice, depend upon the individual child and the nature of the medical treatment, in particular its complexity and seriousness. A child may be capable of understanding what is involved in some *procedures*, eg, setting a broken arm, but insufficiently mature to understand others, eg, a heart by-pass operation.

If a child is not able to understand, and is therefore in law incompetent to make a decision about her medical treatment, then the power to consent is that of the parents or others with parental responsibility (a local authority if the child is in care). The parents' consent will be legally valid if it is exercised in the "best interests" of the child. The court, if asked, may also make a decision in relation to a child under its inherent jurisdiction or the Children Act 1989 and will also always act in the child's "best interests".

A recent controversial development in the law has established that while a competent child may consent to medical treatment, the child's refusal will not necessarily be valid. A parent (or other with parental responsibility) or the court may give a valid consent to medical treatment notwithstanding the child's refusal. It may be that the parents (and possibly also the court) may only do so if the child's life is threatened or the treatment is necessary to avoid serious permanent harm to the child.[9]

For a consent to be valid, a patient must understand in broad terms the basic nature and purpose of the medical procedure.[10] In other words, a doctor has a legal obligation to volunteer sufficient information to the patient so that the patient understands what is being done, why it is being done and what its likely consequences will be. It is not necessary, however, that a patient should be aware of the inherent risks in a medical procedure or any alternative procedures to it in order for the patient's consent to be legally valid. A doctor will only have a legal duty to volunteer this further information if it would be negligent (unreasonable) not to do so. Also, a patient's apparent consent will be invalid if it is induced through *fraud* or misrepresentation as to the nature of the medical procedure.[11]

References
1 *Re F (A Mental Patient: Sterilisation)* [1990] 2 A.C. 1 (H.L.).
2 *Chatterton v Gerson* [1981] Q.B. 432 (Bristow J.).
3 *Re C (Adult: Refusal of Medical Treatment)* [1994] 1 All E.R. 819 (Thorpe J.).
4 Kennedy I, Grubb A. *Medical law* (2nd ed). London: Butterworths, 1994: 135–48.
5 *Sidaway v. Bethlem Royal Hospital Governors* [1985] A.C. 871 at 904–5 per Lord Templeman.
6 *Re T (Adult: Refusal of Treatment)* [1992] 4 All E.R. 649 (C.A.).
7 Family Law Reform Act 1969, s. 8(1).
8 *Gillick v. West Norfolk and Wisbech A.H.A.* [1986] A.C. 112 (H.L.).
9 *Re W (A Minor) (Refusal of Treatment)* [1992] 4 All E.R. 33 (C.A.).
10 *Chatterton v Gerson* [1981] Q.B. 432 (Bristow J.).

11 *Sidaway v Bethlem Royal Hospital Governors*
[1985] Q.B. 524 (C.A.).

See also: Child, status of; duress; informed
consent; mental illness; negligence.

AG

Consequentialism Moral theories
(notably utilitarianism) maintaining
that the results of actions (or of rules
for action) are what matter. However,
certain questions arise: which consequences (likely, possible or remote),
for whom (individuals, populations,
environment), and on whose evaluation, should be weighed, by what
means and by whom? Practical problems include unintended side-effects
and focusing on the measurable.

KMB

Consistency In logic a group of statements is consistent if they could all
be true together; and a system of logic
is consistent if it does not yield both
a formula and its negation. More
loosely, someone may be called inconsistent if either she claims to believe
P on Monday and not-P on Tuesday,
or claims to hold principle P but does
not act in terms of it. But there is
nothing logically inconsistent in these
cases.

See also: Logic and logical reasoning; multidisciplinary teams; teamwork.

RSD

Consultation, ethics of In spite of our
interest in the ethics of new technology, or of *public health* decisions,
the encounter between *patient*/poten-
tial patient and health care professional remains the centre of medical
work and the source of most moral
interest or concern. Issues to be considered include *power*, the relationship, *confidentiality, promise keeping,
honesty* and so on, but may be represented by apparently small items such
as what a person is called, how
greeted and dealt with, dress and

cleanliness, and so on. Modern practice likes to be patient-centred, but
analysis of consultations suggests that
this is much easier in theory than
in practice, even when it involves a
balanced meeting between personal
and professional expertise and experiences. Nevertheless such an approach
is clearly a key to modern standards
of good practice.

See also: Autonomy.

Reference
Tuckett D et al. *Meetings between experts*. London:
Tavistock, 1985.

RH

Consumerism Since the birth of the
generalist consumer movement in the
1960s, a patient led consumer movement in health care has gradually
evolved. Many health care professionals see this as detrimental to high
standards, regarding their professional judgment as better than any
service users' perception in judging
the quality of care. But consumerism
in health care can be seen as a welcome antidote to *paternalism*, and to
the indiscriminate use of patients as
research fodder.

See also: Autonomy; empowerment;
Patients' Charter.

JN

Contact tracing is systematic follow-
up of contacts of infectious disease,
such as tuberculosis and some *sexually
transmitted diseases*. The objective is to
notify and to screen such contacts in
case they have unknowingly acquired
infection, for their own benefit and
as part of infectious disease control.
Contact information is given by the
index case so tracing procedures must
avoid breach of *confidentiality*, especially where the infection carries
social *stigma*. It is done by specialist
staff, eg, tuberculosis visitors and
health advisers, the latter using contact slips that advise contacts to go to

a sexually transmitted disease clinic and that carry a code specifying the condition to the clinicians.

See also: Screening.

AJP

Context reminds us that ethical decisions are not made in vacuo, and that a principle has to be expressed in practice. Some modern thinkers, especially women philosophers, remind us that whether a decision is good may well depend on its context. Both medicine and law are used to thinking about specific cases. Nevertheless there is concern about *situation ethics*: to be moral, a decision has to be universalisable in some sense. So an individual context is one pole (and hitherto a somewhat undervalued one) in ethical analysis, which must move between the particular and the general.

See also: Casuistry; complexity.

Reference
Nussbaum M. *Love's knowledge*. New York: Oxford University Press, 1992.

RH

Contingent/necessary Literally, "touching/unyielding" – the distinction between what may and what must happen, exist or be true. What is necessarily true cannot be denied without self-contradiction. Most "facts" about the world are contingent – true, in so far as they are congruent with knowledge systematised by abstraction from direct experience.

KMB

Continuity of care is considered vital in caring for any long term illness and increasingly it is realised that few conditions are completely "one off".

See also: Chronic disease; long term care.

RH

Contraception This is action to prevent pregnancy. Usually it implies regular sexual intercourse without risking conception, although "abstention" is reported by some couples as their contraceptive method.

A contraceptive method should be effective, unobtrusive, fully reversible, and have no adverse effect on health. The more biologically potent a contraceptive agent, the more effective it may be but the greater the possibility of some adverse effect or of irreversibility. These designed methods may also be less obtrusive.

Some methods are obtainable only through doctors or specialist nurses. These tend to be the more powerful methods and the aim of the prescriber is to limit harm by evaluating risk factors in the circumstances or lifestyle of the user.

Contraceptive methods not requiring medical intervention are: *condoms*, interrupting sex before ejaculation ("withdrawal"), timing sex according to ovulation time ("*natural family planning*"), and prolonging breast feeding. Where there is no health care, these are widely used, although condom supply needs an effective distribution system. There are also folk methods, with similar actions, specific to certain communities.

Ethical points in contraception are that people should have: good access to information and services; no *coercion*; fully *informed consent* before prescription (of an oral contraceptive) or a procedure (fitting an intrauterine device, giving an injection, inserting an implant), and methods should be discontinued if consent is withdrawn. Services should be focused on groups finding most difficulty in gaining information: young people, the disabled, ethnic minorities, and refugees.

For contraception to be fully and practically effective, any scheme of provision needs supporting with services for *sterilisation* and early termination of unplanned pregnancy.

Major interest has centred on the extent of contraceptive use in economically deprived and developing

59

communities. Evidence suggests that people usually wish to make good use of contraception and the main problems are those of information, provision, and distribution.

Moral objections to contraception usually come from one of two directions. The first sees the sexual act as indissolubly connected with reproduction. Any intrusion here is thus a cheapening or perversion of both (and against God's purposes, in, for instance, traditional Roman Catholic thinking). The second sees the power (economic and political) in family size, and is suspicious that the motives behind any external attempt to limit population growth are aimed against the value, or values, of the group as a whole. However, individuals, such as mothers, usually see clearly the personal, family and economic benefits of restricted family size (or each child being wanted); and the view of sex as a human good in itself is now widespread.

See also: Abortion; abortion – ethical aspects.

JAM

Contract Literally, "a drawing together" – of two parties in a legal, financial or moral agreement, each promising to do or provide something that the other wants or needs. (A provider undertakes to supply specified health services to a purchaser who undertakes to pay a specified amount for them; a patient promises to comply with a regimen which the doctor prescribing it promises to monitor.) A contract normally is more limited in scope (a mutual bargain or quid pro quo) than a *covenant*.

KMB

Control groups are used in *clinical research and trials* and in *epidemiological research* to control for irrelevant variables in testing the primary hypothesis. They should be chosen to minimise differences from the test group, in particular for known confounding variables. These will vary according to the study, but may include demographic factors such as gender, race and age as well as study-specific variables such as severity of disease and other therapies. In clinical trials, controls receive the current standard of care and, where appropriate through use of *placebos* and *randomisation*, provide the standard for comparison with the test therapy.

AJP

Cooperation and competition are issues for modern health care, even if obscured in a unified service. Even though the basis of medicine is the individual consultation, much subsequent work is that of a team. Yet there will be bound to be different approaches and points of view within a team: where there is unacknowledged competition, *teamwork* may be undermined. In the broader health service, right wing reforms have suggested that competition between providers is not only useful, but essential, to prevent inefficiency. The counter argument is that *resources* are spent on keeping up with the competition ("If St Maggie's has a helicopter, then we must have one too") rather than dealing with the priorities of the local population. Watch this space.

See also: National Health Service.

RH

Corporate values Modern *business ethics* has suggested that, since every group has to decide about its *priorities*, and that these derive from the values expressed by an organisation, it is best that these be overt and discussed. This may be a step forward, but only if these values can be called upon, enacted, and, if necessary, challenged or redebated should circumstances require.

See also: Colleagues/collegiality; institutions.

RH

Cosmetic surgery is a branch of surgery dedicated to changing the outward appearance of individuals for whom this is a perceived *disability*. It uses the techniques of plastic surgery, but is usually not done in response to injuries but to perceived shape or the changes created by lifestyle. Ethical questions centre round whether this work calls justifiably on the resources of a health service, what should be done about people's apparently distorted views of themselves, and the role of the professionals in correcting such apparent distortions, viz. societal views of *gender* or *race* that might mistakenly move items such as a round tummy or a dark skin into the pathological.

See also: Congenital malformations; priorities.

RH

Cost–benefit analysis attempts to provide a balance-sheet of the costs (losses) and benefits (gains) to society over time, all expressed in today's money terms, of investing in a particular service. A summary statistic, the "benefit–cost ratio", is calculated which, if greater than 1, indicates that the benefits outweigh the costs.

Reference
Robinson R. Cost–benefit analysis. *BMJ* 1993;
    307: 924–6.

See also: Health economics; QALYs.

MP

Cost containment means action to restrict the cost of health services. Virtually all payers for medical services, whether public or private, take measures to contain costs. These measures have become increasingly firm and sophisticated since 1980, when the main payers recognised that, unless they acted, health expenditures would continue to rise at a rate that could cause them severe funding problems. The fewer the payers, the easier it is to set expenditure limits, provided you are sufficiently determined. The record of the UK *National Health Service* from this point of view is strong, relying mainly on global budgets and capitation. Other countries use other means. Cost containment is inevitable. Ethically, however, those who set the expenditure limits must take responsibility for the implications in terms of the range and quality of services that the money will buy. There are also ethical dilemmas for the clinician if (as in the NHS) the clinician plays key roles in the rationing process.

See also: Health care systems; purchasing.

RJM

Counselling is a form of helping others, related to, but to be distinguished from, *psychotherapy*. Like the latter, counselling uses as its only method listening and responding to the other, but most forms of psychotherapy are more probing or analytical in approach. The boundary between the two is not, however, absolute, since some counselling methods draw heavily on psychotherapeutic theory, in particular theories of unconscious motivation. Traditionally counselling was regarded as advisory in nature ("giving counsel"), but in recent times this has been replaced by an emphasis on non-directiveness and "client centredness". In this approach, which originates from the client centred therapy of Carl Rogers, the counsellor is primarily a listener, reflecting back to the client what is communicated in a way which enables the client to find her own solution. Thus the counselling skills required are empathetic listening, a warm but non-possessive approach to people and an accepting, non-judgmental attitude. Alternative counselling approaches allow a more active role to the counsellor, but there is wide agreement that the personal qualities of the counsellor are central to effective helping.

In health care settings counselling is often episodic and informal, rather than set within the traditional "fifty minute hour" in a private office. Frequently it is provided as part of medical or nursing care and few doctors or nurses have specific training in counselling skills. Thus a number of ethical issues arise. First, there may be a confusion of roles: a doctor committed to a specific form of treatment may be unable to offer genuinely disinterested help to the person, uncertain of what is the best choice for her. Second, a doctor or nurse may lack the skills required to help a person in an emotional crisis (eg, after the loss of a child). Referral to appropriate help is an ethical imperative in these circumstances. Finally, the essentially open-ended nature of counselling may be inappropriate when the doctor or nurse has a duty to third parties – an obvious example is suspected *child abuse*. Despite these difficulties, the provision of at least basic counselling training to all health professionals would enhance the quality of health care they provide. Ill-health does not divide neatly into biological and psychological packages.

References

Egan J. *The skilled helper*. Monterey: Books-Cole, 1975.
Rogers CR. *On becoming a person*. London: Constable, 1981.

See also: Doctor–patient relationship; stress.

AVC

Counterarguments Arguments that oppose a position, claim or argument. Response to counterarguments is an important component of ethical reasoning, either by providing reasoned support for an ethical position, claim or argument, or by leading to modification or abandonment of those ethical positions, claims or arguments that cannot withstand sound counterarguments.

RG

Counterintuitive Going against an intuition. In the context of ethics, a position, claim or argument that goes against a feeling or intuition about what is good or bad, right or wrong, or what ought or ought not to be done. While *moral* intuitions are important components of the moral life, they themselves require ethical scrutiny, for they may be wrong.

RG

Courage is a *virtue* greatly regarded in the past, where heroism was always seen positively. There has been a tendency to eclipse this recently in a more sensitive age. However, the nasty realities of long term diseases are not necessarily all relieved by modern treatments; while pressure on professionals from all quarters appears to be mounting. So the courage to persevere throughout difficulties, or to speak out in defence of what one knows to be right, has returned to its key position in the life of patient and professional.

See also: Chronic disease; heroes.

RH

Covenant Sometimes used in contrast with *"contract"*, covenant stresses an open-ended *commitment* to the other without a careful assessment of personal gain. According to May, it epitomises the professional relationship in medicine, since it provides a foundation for *trust*.[1] However, it may also encourage paternalistic and possessive attitudes towards patients and lead to *burnout*. A balance between contract and covenant seems necessary.

References

1 May WF. *The physician's covenant.* Philadelphia: Westminster Press: 1983; ch.4.

Campbell AV. *Moderated love.* London: SPCK, 1984: 102–4.

See also: Paternalism.

AVC

CPR *See* Resuscitation.

Criminal behaviour is defined by legal classification which, in the UK, is enacted in law by parliament. Certain acts and omissions may be criminal at one time but not at another, and in one society and not in another, eg, homosexual acts committed in private by male persons over the age of 21 years prior to the Sexual Offences Act, 1967. The primary characteristics of criminal acts are that they are generally considered a public wrong and/ or a moral wrong. Criminal proceedings differ from civil proceedings in that they can result in the imposition of punishment accompanied by the judgment of community condemnation. Criminological theory is traditionally influenced by two contrasting concepts: classicism, emphasising free will and portraying crimes as the outcomes of voluntary actions based on rational calculation; positivism, portraying crime as behaviour into which an individual has been propelled by factors beyond her control. Early positivists emphasised individual characteristics of the criminal but later research concentrated on social and environmental influences. These contrasting viewpoints lead to different approaches to crime control and the processing of criminals through the justice system. Increasing the personal cost of crime to the criminal through deterrent sentencing, or making criminal activities more difficult, are both influenced by the view that criminal behaviour is the outcome of rational decision-making. Where criminal behaviour is perceived to be the outcome of individual psychopathology

a rehabilitative sentence might be considered more appropriate. Similarly, if it is seen as the outcome of an adverse social environment, then it is argued that closer political attention is required to social conditions than to crime control.

See also: Forensic psychiatry; imprisonment; police.

JC

Critical care *See* Intensive care.

Culture When culture refers to human society it is generally taken by social anthropologists to mean the sum of a society's distinctive creative achievements as well as the characteristics of its normative beliefs governing the relationships between individuals. The culture of a society or a distinctive group within it is usually embedded in a set of religious beliefs or dominated by a secular, materialist outlook. It may place great value on youth and enterprise or on age and wisdom. It may stress *tradition* and continuity and the importance of stability in social relations, or the desirability of flexibility and acceptance of *change* defined as progress.

The concept has proved to be useful in considering ethical issues arising in the practice of medicine. Those who wish to innovate with proven, more effective procedures to promote health or prevent illness have often found opposition from those they wished to help. This is sometimes described as "cultural lag". The projected improvements clash with some treasured customs or beliefs to which the society or group clings. Before condemning out of hand those who resist change, however, there is a moral obligation on the part of the innovator to ask whether it is legitimate to persuade individuals to give up practices or beliefs that they value and are an intrinsic part of their culture. It is never appropriate to attribute

63

resistance to stupidity or malevolence.

It is often valuable to contemplate critically too the culture of present-day medicine. It is affected by the cultural climate of the society in which it exists.[1] Professional bodies develop their own cultural milieu. It can be defensive and resistant to change emanating from innovators from inside or outside its ranks. It may place too much value on loyalty to colleagues and too little on the *welfare* of patients in situations where the two can conflict. Equally, because the culture of modern medicine places a high value on scientific discovery it can be dismissive of scruples from those who want to consider more thoroughly problems that may arise from its implementation.

Reference
1 Payer L. *Medicine and culture*. London: Gollancz, 1989.

See also: Colleagues/collegiality.

MJ

D

Data protection Under the Data Protection Act, there is statutory provision to ensure the *confidentiality* of mechanically processed data. The purposes for which such data are held have to be registered with the Data Protection Registrar; and in law that limits their legitimate use, and thus access to them. The protection so given is applicable to mechanically processed data in general. Personal health information is thus included, but only to the extent that it is mechanically processed. The bulk of personal health information is still held manually, so it is not protected in this particular way, but relies for its confidentiality on guidance given from the health department.

DB

Death From earliest records the traditional view, enshrined in religious and commonsense beliefs, was that death occurred with the last breath of life. This view predates scientific medicine but is nevertheless overlaid with a moral and practical requirement to uphold a distinction between duties to the living and duties to the dead.

The word "death" has many applications: civilisations die, communities die, and people die. While civilisations and communities may regenerate, the death of a person is an irreversible state involving a fundamental physical transformation. Many religions depict death as the separation of the eternal soul from the body, and some philosophers see it as the loss of personal identity, but the actual determination of death is a practical matter involving an observable physical change in the person concerned. Thus doctors have sought to identify a stage in the dying process when essential integrating functions have ceased. What counts as essential will depend upon the significance of *consciousness* and the ability to breathe.

Developments in *resuscitation* technology and organ *transplantation* have led to a reappraisal of cardio-centric notions of death in favour of brain-related criteria[1]. As the brain is irreplaceable and essential to integrated functioning, brain death definitions have been accepted by medical authorities throughout the developed world.

Yet the definition of brain death has given rise to ethical disputes. Those who equate irreversible loss of psychological continuity with death emphasise loss of the capacity for thought, speech, observation and meaningful interaction with other beings and the environment. Practical tests would require evidence of loss of higher brain functions, such as the cerebral cortex. Opponents argue that patients lacking in mental function but capable of breathing unaided would be candidates for burial, cremation or organ *donation*. For many this is morally repugnant. This problem is avoided in whole brain or brain stem formulations of death, which require loss of both mental and physical features of integrated life, including loss of respiration and irreversible loss of the capacity for consciousness.[2]

References

1 Lamb D. What is Death?. In: Gillon R, Lloyd A, eds. *Principles of health care ethics*. Chichester: Wiley, 1994: 1027–40.
2 Pallis C, Harley D. *ABC of brain stem death* (2nd ed). London: BMJ Publishing Group, 1996.

See also: Brain stem death; persistent vegetative state; unconsciousness.

DL

Decent minimum of health care is a concept in resource allocation that defines a "bottom line" below which health care provision should not humanely go. There may be situations where this could not apply, such as battle, and there remains a persistent conflict between policies that advance this basic line and those that leave it where it is and advance only in chosen areas.

RH

Deception In *treatment* this may be morally justifiable if a patient's *decision-making capacity* is known (not just presumed) to be, in relevant respects and at the relevant time, sufficiently impaired to make deception the only way of avoiding her being harmed. Avoiding *harm* or disturbance to other patients (except in emergencies, a resource issue) is insufficient reason.

In *research*, deception may be proposed in some psychological studies or because, eg, a *placebo* cannot be disguised. This contravenes the requirements of *informed consent*, unless subjects are warned that they may be deceived, which may invalidate the research design. Some believe that such research is never permissible. Others argue that it may be justifiable if the deception is sufficiently trivial and/or the potential findings sufficiently beneficial.

See also: Lying; truthtelling.

KMB

Decision-making capacity (DMC) The capacity to understand relevant information ("explained in broad terms and simple language"), to consider its implications in the light of one's own *values* and to come to a communicable decision. DMC may be partial or fluctuating, *communication* may be non-verbal, and the decision may be to let another person decide. Conscious patients should be presumed to possess DMC. If in doubt, the test (to be decided on the balance of probabilities) is not the patient's status ("patient" or "too young/old"), or the decision's outcome (whether it would "be made by a person of ordinary *prudence*") – but whether the "individual is able, at the time when a particular decision has to be made, to understand its nature and effects". Legal tests of decision-making capacity for some purposes – eg making a will – can be more stringent than those for consenting to or refusing medical treatment.

References

British Medical Association and the Law Society. *Assessment of mental capacity. Guidance for doctors and lawyers*. London: BMA, 1995.
Law Commission. *Mental incapacity*. London: HMSO, 1995.

See also: Competence; consent; substituted judgment.

KMB

Declarations are statements of principle, reflecting consensus, shared values, and professional solidarity. They remind practitioners of acknowledged professional obligations but

65

seldom seek to justify positions adopted; these being held as self-evident. Declarations of commonly held ethical principles flourished in the post-war period but are less representative of current analytical approaches to medical ethics. Awareness of changing relationships, multicultural values and potential conflict between ethical principles has stimulated demand for *dialectic* rather than declaratory formulas. Some moralists deprecate the diminishing emphasis on traditional ethical certainties and declarations.

See also: Codes; ethical debates, methods of; guidelines; principles.

ASo

Default decisions are made, in effect, passively by the failure to make a positive decision. Eg, failure to instigate a specific therapy provides the default of allowing matters to take their course, without formally deciding so to do. It could be argued that it is an abrogation of *responsibility* and that failure to make a decision when the situation demands it amounts to culpability. Awareness of what would occur by default if a decision is not made should enable a clinician to decide positively whether or not to act.

AJP

Defensive medicine is the investigation or treatment of patients based solely on fear of potential *litigation* and not on actual clinical need. The clinician is acting on perceived personal risk from legal redress, whether by the patient, third parties or the state, rather than in the best interests of the patient. Ironically, it could even put the patient at additional risk; it is often assumed "only" to increase financial burden to the patient, third party payer or the state. Arguably, if the clinician is at legitimate risk of litigation, then what is done is not defensive but is simply conforming with established standards of clinical practice. If so, the risk of defensive medicine is only present when legal precedent or statute, or perceptions about them, force clinicians to act against their *clinical judgment* and that of a responsible body of medical opinion. Where there are duties to two individuals, such as in the care of mother and *fetus*, defensive medicine is especially likely to be promoted. The practice of defensive medicine is often said to be a feature of the medico-legal context of the USA.

AJP

Dementia is a syndrome of acquired global impairment of cognitive function. It occurs most commonly among older people and the two commonest forms are senile dementia of Alzheimer type and vascular dementia, which are progressive. Non-progressive dementia may follow brain damage due to trauma or anoxia.

The earliest feature of progressive dementia is usually a memory defect but reasoning, speech, and *personality* are also affected. These impairments raise practical legal issues relating to testamentary capacity and *power of attorney*, but the central ethical issue is that of personhood. Is a demented person the same person she used to be viewed through the veils of amnesia, loss of reasoning power and impairment of speech, or has the disease changed the person rather than merely the *personality*? This issue is of particular relevance to the morality of implementing *advance directives*. The doctor's responsibility is to the patient, not to the perhaps different person that patient may once have been.

Ethical issues also arise in trying to obtain *informed consent* to medical or nursing care from a demented patient apparently unable to understand or answer the relevant questions. A common specific problem is that a demented patient is not eating enough; should a nasogastric or a gastrostomy tube be inserted? It is not proper for family members to bear full responsibility for such decisions as their motives may be complex and they may in later years bear a sense of guilt or anxiety over the choice they made.

In some instances difficulties in communication with demented patients may arise from their impairment of memory rather than speech or reasoning; such patients forget the question and what they wished to say in response before they have finished saying it. Short questions and attending particularly to the early part of a patient's response may improve communication. Unfortunately, memory defects prevent patients from comparing present with past states, and their responses are often inconsistent.

See also: Force feeding; hydration; nutrition; persons and personhood.

GE

Denial is an important defence mechanism. It enables individuals to protect themselves against an intolerable threat, eg, a life-threatening *disease* such as *cancer*. It should be respected despite the difficulties it might cause unless its continuance seriously hinders clinical management and/or compromises the family's adaptation.

It is unethical to confront it aggressively because this will connect individuals with intolerable *pain*. However, it is worth trying to break denial in two ways: first, by asking individuals to consider aspects of their illness experience that are inconsistent with their view of the diagnosis; second, by checking if there is ever a moment when they doubt that things are going to work out.

PM

Dental ethics Dentistry is a self-governing profession. In the UK general guidelines on what constitutes both ethical behaviour and serious professional misconduct are issued by its regulatory body, the General Dental Council.[1] Individual dentists have obligations to their patients, their profession, and the community;[2] and can obtain further guidance on ethical issues relating to all practical matters from the British Dental Association[3,4] and other sources.[5]

Similar general ethical principles as apply in other areas of medicine underlie both the individual dentist–patient relationship and the overall provision of oral health services. Such principles include the patient's right to give informed *consent*, the dentist's duty of care to patients, and the duty of *confidentiality*.

However, certain issues are particularly important in the dental context. First, certain factors in dental services provision – such as working patterns, isolation, changing disease levels, and *National Health Service* (NHS) payment methods – have the potential to encourage unethical practice; although rare, when this happens it must be curbed. Consequently, eg, failure to keep abreast of current good practice is censured. Fee-for-item payment methods could theoretically foster overprescription, while capitation payments could encourage underprescription and lead to difficulties in children with high disease levels obtaining care. Such consequences would obviously be unethical, and disciplinary measures could (and do) follow. Normally, however, such problems are overcome by a combination of good practice, continuing education, peer review, and official monitoring.

Second, in some dental situations there is inherent conflict between the general ethical principles that apply. Eg: (a) Individually, potential conflict

67

exists between the *HIV*-infected patient's right to confidentiality, and the interests of the dentist, her staff, and other patients. Normally, however, the patient's rights are paramount unless there is a serious risk to society. A combination of good clinical practice as to *infection control* and a general recognition of the duty of confidentiality in enabling the dentist to be informed fully about the patient's clinical situation, enabling most effective delivery of relevant care, usually suffices. (b) The profession's community obligations should motivate it to promote water *fluoridation*. This is desirable in utilitarian terms; but conflict arises between the rights of anti-fluoridationists and of those who potentially will benefit from freedom from pain and disease.

References

1 General Dental Council. *Professional conduct and fitness of practise*. London: GDC, May 1994.
2 Federation Dentaire Internationale. *International principles of ethics for the dental profession*. FDI, revised 1986 (reprinted in 3 below).
3 British Dental Association. *Ethical and legal obligations of dental practitioners*. Advice sheet B1. BDA, 1988.
4 British Dental Association. *Consent to treatment*. Advice sheet B6. BDA, 1993.
5 Seear J, Walters L. *Law and ethics in dentistry* (3rd ed) Oxford: Wright, Butterworth-Heinemann, 1991.

See also: Utilitarianism.

JBr, CSc

Deontology From Greek for "what is due". Theories of *rights* and duties, or of what is absolutely right and wrong (as opposed to relatively good and bad) to do. Modern (notably *Kantian*) deontology is based on unconditional respect for persons (or other forms of life) and may require doing what is right regardless of the consequences. But deontology can derive from other religious, ideological or moral imperatives, including the *duty* always to weigh up the consequences of any proposed action.

KMB

Dependency relates to the condition of relying on something or some person for certain needs to be fulfilled. A degree of dependence is necessary for a person to assume the role of a sick person, allowing her to receive care and empathy from others and facilitating a sense of security.

In clinical practice the term "high dependency" is used to denote a need for highly specialised care for critically ill or injured patients from trained staff with technical expertise within the confines of a designated unit.

Dependence on substances is to be differentiated from *addiction* in that it is characterised by emotional withdrawal symptoms when a practice or ingestion of a substance is abruptly terminated, while addiction is marked by physical symptoms.

See also: Autonomy; illness behaviour; intensive care; order of preferences.

HM

Depression is a long-term and intense alteration in mood or affect, characterised by misery and withdrawal, and accompanied by physical symptoms (eg, sleep disturbance, poor appetite) and, variably in different cultures, typical changes in behaviour or facial expression. It is seen as a *mental illness* when it is not understandable just as sadness or as a "normal" reaction (such as *bereavement*). It may come with or be precipitated by other physical or mental illness, but may appear out of the blue. Its importance lies in its prevalence, consequences to the individual and society, and the possibility of *suicide*. It is often treatable or preventable, but many health workers are poor detectors of it.

It is of utmost importance also in medical ethics. It may reduce communication and practical IQ and so alter a person's judgment or actions.

The distinction between sadness and depression may be hard to make. Suicide is a tragedy without parallel. Debate surrounds the extent to which, or point at which, depression justifies intervention against a person's wishes, and when it is of such a degree as to render her decisions invalid. There is also disagreement as to whether it is always bad, and justifies medical (or pharmacological) intervention, or whether it is, though painful, an appropriate state preparatory to other change – the therapist's "breakthrough" as against "breakdown". Great sensitivity and care is required to create the right balance, but *courage* may be required in taking decisive steps when there is real and preventable *risk*.

RH

Desert What someone deserves (literally, earns by service) – as a result of her actions or her status. Since ascriptions of status or of responsibility for actions are often morally contestable or difficult to justify, desert is an inappropriate criterion for the *microallocation* of health care *resources*.

See also: Bias; merit.

KMB

Detachment is a stage in normal psychological development (from the parent figure(s)), but also is considered a desirable stance in professional conduct in health care. Involvement (or overinvolvement) by the professional in the concerns of the patient is considered by some to be undesirable and even harmful. There is clearly an appropriate moral *distance*, but patients are more frequently harmed by a doctor's apparent lack of interest than the reverse. And, as Howard Brody has pointed out: "The cemetery is not filled with the corpses of patients who died because their overinvolved physicians became irrational and ineffective."

Reference
Brody H. *The healer's power*. New Haven, Conn: Yale University Press, 1992.

RH

Determinism Theories that privilege an observer's or third-person view of actions as the effect of causes over direct first-person experience of existential choice. Philosophically, these two perspectives are not necessarily incompatible. *Chance* and *complexity* (eg, in physics or *genetics*) make psychological fatalism no more scientifically than morally justified.

See also: Existentialism.

KMB

Developing world As generally used, the term "developing world" is-outdated and nearly useless, except for those who believe that economics defines life. In most settings, "developing world" is a modern way of saying "third world", perhaps minus some of its colonialist overtones. "Developing world" lumps together poor countries with poorly functioning infrastructures; thus, nations as enormously different as Bangladesh, Indonesia, Angola, Peru and Algeria are considered alike. More recently, the United Nations Development Program (UNDP) has designed a "human development index" which, by joining many measures of social, political and economic life, creates a composite and more satisfying scale for describing each nation's societal "development". Nevertheless, new terminology, based on new approaches to describing human development which respect societal diversity (such as a blend of traditional indices with measures of realisation of international *human rights* norms) could usefully replace the term "developing world".

JMa

Diagnosis related groups (DRGs) were initially developed by Robert

Fetter and John Thompson at Yale University, as a means of differentiating medical activities for purposes of comparing quality, utilisation, and costs. Before that time, unit costs were often calculated on the basis of patient days or outpatient visits – obviously inadequate definitions since, eg, the cost for the actual day of a transplant operation is very different from the cost on the day of discharge, and there are also great differences in terms of expense between one medical condition and another. Thompson and Fetter used what might now (following Oregon),[1] be termed diagnosis treatment pairs as the key to better differentiation – in other words a condition linked with whether it was treated surgically or medically, and then adjusted for age, comorbidity, and complications. They then grouped these pairs into some 500 clusters, based on ICD codes, to describe the totality of hospital output. The US government, which was seeking ways to measure hospital activity for Medicare reimbursement purposes, then seized on the DRG methodology. Basically what they did was to pay a fixed amount per specific DRG to each hospital, leaving the latter to make a profit or loss on the transaction, rather than reimburse that hospital's costs. Many other governments, including France, Australia (at the state level) and Korea, have since adopted DRG reimbursement. What it does not do, however, is provide any incentive to curtail admission, unlike capitation or global budgets. In the UK[2] there has been considerable interest in DRGs for purposes of managing clinical activity within hospitals, but little use has been made of them for hospital reimbursement. The *National Health Service* has developed its own variant of DRGs, called Health Related Groups (HRGs) and there is a National Case Mix Office at Winchester working on them.

References
1 Honigsbaum F. *Who shall live? Who shall die?* – Oregon's health financing proposals. London: King's Fund, 1991.
2 Bardsley M, Cole J, Jenkins L. *DRGs and health care: the management of case mix.* London: King's Fund, 1987.

See also: Purchasing.

RJM

Dialectic From Greek, "pick out", "discuss a question". The use of reason and speech to seek the truth by examining all relevant arguments, beginning from the familiar, known or probable. It exposes contradictions, either in assumptions and arguments (Socrates) or inherent in mind or matter, where possible reconciling them (Hegel, Marx, Asian religious philosophy).

KMB

Dialysis replaces kidney function on an acute or long-term basis. Being costly and not universally available its use raises issues of *distributive justice*, especially as renal failure occurs more frequently in the elderly and in non-Caucasian populations. With severely ill patients the ethics of futility arise, with conflict between the principles of *beneficence* and *non-maleficence*. Selection for long-term dialysis may involve physician bias and ill patients may have impaired volitional *autonomy* at its initiation. There is a moral hazard of future suffering and especially the ethical dilemma of discontinuing therapy, either at the initiation of physician, patient or patient's advocates.

WP

Difference in terms of class, *race*, *age*, and so on is sometimes seen as a threat, and it definitely affects relationships between people. However, these are usually not morally valid distinctions, and would be considered wrong and contrary to *justice* in a health care system, the more so if they affected outcome. There is evidence that professionals are often not conscious of their actions here (eg, when GPs spend more time with middle class than lower class patients); self-assessment is part of the work of a reflective practitioner. Difference is valuable, and should be valued in a multidisciplinary group or society. Whether it is or not may be a measure of that group's maturity.

RH

Difficult patients If the professional–patient relationship means anything at all it will also mean that both sides have likes and dislikes, even if these have to be overcome. The doctor who treats all patients alike is yet to be born, and one hopes never will be. However, some patients with greater anxiety, a particular past, more complex problems, or abrasive personalities become difficult to deal with. These have been labelled as *"heartsink"* or *"thick file"* cases in general practice for obvious reasons. With some notable exceptions, however, this usually comes from an individual professional's perspective, or may be a product of the system. Heartsink or difficult doctors make heartsink or difficult patients. Starting again with a full assessment, especially of the patient's anxieties or experiences, may show a way through. But if none is found, a patient deserves to have her difficulties resolved by being offered different professionals. As Tom Main pointed out, the really difficult patients are usually health professionals, their children, or their spouses. Sometimes these patients frustrate their professional carers so much that the latter behave primitively and start to become punitive.

Reference
Main T. *The ailment and other psychoanalytic essays.* London: Free Association Press, 1989.

See also: Doctor–patient relationship.

RH

Dignity may be something to be stood on in a ward round, but is morally important at times when patients need to receive intimate examinations or when professionals become involved in a process that would normally be personal and private. There need to be procedural safeguards for people at risk. There is a particular concern that dying patients, whose prognosis cannot be altered, are subjected to continuing professional interference because it is hard to "pull out", and so they may die overmedicated or with tubes in situ, when the position could be made less medical and human dignity restored.

RH

Dirty hands debate There is no doubt that dirt harbours disease, but in the moral context the phrase expresses the problem of moral *pragmatism*. To be effective, particularly in *politics*, may involve a choice between two evils. Philosophers approach this in different ways. Thomas Nagel has witnessed impartiality as providing the legitimation, as in, for instance, the violence we sometimes allow to a state in contrast to an individual. Corruption is real and smelly; but both Machiavelli and Hobbes have pointed out the folly of total moral isolation. Modern life prefers to consider *humour, compromise,* or careful extrication as showing a way through the ethical minefield.

Reference
Coady CAJ. "Politics and the problem of dirty hands" in Singer (ed), *A companion to ethics.* Oxford: Blackwell, 1991.

RH

Disability In recent years the meaning conventionally given to the term "disability" has been challenged by disabled people. Theorists such as Michael Oliver and Jenny Morris[1,2] emphasise the role that social restrictions play in disabling individuals, and reject approaches which solely

71

focus on the medical condition of disabled people. They distinguish between an "impairment", which is the functional limitation within the individual caused by a physical or mental disorder, and a "disability", which is the loss or limitation of opportunities imposed on people with impairments by social and environmental factors.

Thus, eg, a person with a spinal injury may be unable to walk (her impairment), but the degree to which this restricts her life activities will be determined by the design of buildings and by social *stigma* which combine to exclude and segregate people who use wheelchairs (their disability).

Disabled writers assert that disability needs to be seen as part of the broader fabric of human experience, part of a continuum ranging from a super-fit athlete through an older person with the physical constraints seen as normal for her age group (a touch of arthritis, perhaps, or a slight loss of hearing) to a person who is labelled as 'disabled'.

While acknowledging that some impairments inevitably entail physical pain or fatigue, the way in which a disability is perceived as a personal tragedy is challenged, and the processes by which disabled people are turned into objects of pity or charity are rejected.

Hand in hand with this emphasis on the social construction of disability, the dominant role of the medical profession in managing disability has also been questioned. While no one doubts the importance of medicine in the control and alleviation of impairments, the power that doctors exert over disabled people's lives is being challenged. If the barriers created by the social environment are more important than an individual's impairment in determining that person's ability to function, it follows that it is inappropriate for doctors to determine employment capacity, educational provision or the allocation of financial benefits (all areas in which doctors currently play a powerful role).

References
1 Oliver M. *The politics of disablement.* London: Macmillan, 1990.
2 Morris J. *Pride against prejudice, transforming attitudes to disability.* London: Women's Press, 1991.

CG

Disadvantage A neutral word is needed to describe circumstances that prevent people gaining all they could from life (in contrast with resources or privileges enjoyed by most others), in order to prevent such people being further damaged by a negative label. Since ill health is a major disadvantage, most health professionals struggle to provide equitable health care, disregarding other disadvantages: but such evidence as there is suggests that this is more difficult to deliver in practice – such as when lower-class patients receive less consulting time than middle-class patients.

RH

Disappointment is probably one of the least understood, yet low key, negative emotions which link with other factors in a person to create the circumstances for the onset of illness. It can be seen as a potent form of loss event, usually unrecognised as such, where aims are no longer attainable or hopes are dashed. The rejected Victorian suitor is the classic case: and was probably better understood, and less medicalised, in his time than our own.

RH

Disciplinary procedures Compliance with established standards of conduct and performance is encouraged by the implementation of investigatory and disciplinary procedures in cases where those standards are contravened. Disciplinary procedures may be invoked for three types of failure: personal misconduct; professional misconduct; and inadequate professional competence.

Health professionals may be subject to disciplinary processes by the *statutory body* for their profession or by their employing authority, both of which issue guidance clarifying the forms of *misconduct* that attract penalties. Disciplinary processes invoked by employers can result in censure or dismissal from employment but those of the statutory bodies can restrict or remove health professionals' ability to practise by removing them from the register of approved practitioners.

See also: Competence; General Medical Council; incompetent professionals; misconduct; self regulation.

ASo

Discipline has the common meaning of "instruction" but appears in medicine in several forms. It indicates the special interest, area of skill or expertise of a professional, usually with academic overtones. It covers the public requirement to police professional behaviour in order to detect those whose standards fall below those required, and it also indicates the action taken when a professional is found in breach of those requirements and is admonished, punished or removed from the professional roll.

RH

Disclosure is the duty on the clinician to inform the *patient* of her diagnosis, (eg, *cancer*), and of the *risks* associated with it and its *treatment*. It is a necessary precondition for informed *consent*, ethically and legally. The main concern is how far disclosure should go and what discretion a clinician has in limiting it to avoid causing undue fear or distress. This turns on the patient's situation and *decision-making capacity* as well as the level of risk. While telling the truth is vital to the *doctor–patient relationship* and to empowering the patient, there is also a need to avoid harm from discussing unlikely complications. Striking the right balance is often as much a matter of *clinical judgment* as one of legal precedent. There are also issues to do with the extent of disclosure to, eg, relatives and partners, in the absence of formal consent to this by the patient: for instance, where the patient presents in coma or another state where she is unable to make her wishes known, but where a decision is needed. Cultural factors may play a part, as do changing expectations, with society moving away from acceptance of *paternalism*.

See also: Empowerment; truthtelling.

AJP

Discrimination A professional response must involve discerning the differences between situations or problems, which may be aided by certain classifications or categorisations. However, when this distinction is made without the backing of reasonably objective assessment, or involves social or personal *bias*, a disadvantaged client or patient may be further harmed. Positive discrimination denotes the attempt to correct *disadvantage* by providing more for those who appear to have less.

See also: Prejudice.

RH

Disease *See* Health, illness and disease, concepts of.

Disinterest should be distinguished from lack of interest; it implies not lack of concern, but *impartiality*.

RH

Displacement When direct expression of an impulse or reaction to events is felt to be unacceptable, its emotional force may be displaced immediately or later on to another subject or object. Having a sense of proportion when finding oneself doing this or finding oneself on the receiving end of another person's displaced anger, often helps to avoid turning a resolvable mundane crisis into a dramatic moral dilemma.

See also: Displacement behaviour.

KMB

Displacement behaviour When an emotion goes unrecognised it may be incorrectly attributed to a different source or person by an individual and that individual's reactions may show displacement behaviour, for instance, a professional in an unhappy personal relationship may displace her anger on to other staff at work or on to patients. *Somatisation* may be a particular case within, rather than between, individuals.

RH

Dissection To understand human anatomy, dissection of a body (*cadaver*) is an essential part of a doctor's training. Following the Anatomy Act of 1984, all cadavers for dissection are bequeathed in their own lifetime for benefit of medical education and scientific understanding. Each medical school has an approved HMIA Licensed Anatomist responsible for acceptance, embalming, dissection, and eventual burial, or cremation. Although at first to many students often frightening and slightly distasteful, the dissection of a human cadaver is a formative experience, and also serves as a part of the psychological preparation for medical practice. It acts as a discussion point for pathological processes, dying and death itself. Students often use the experience to develop means of dealing with conflicting emotions engendered by the situation and of showing respect.

Reference
Druce M, Johnson MH. *Clinical anatomy* 1994; **7**: 42–9.

PA/AJP

Distance, moral Professional tasks differ from personal ones, and a different emotional and moral distance from a social one is appropriate in the professional–patient relationship. It is likely that this will change in differing tasks in health care, and will need regular review and adjustment. The level of involvement has been compared to a reader's involvement with fiction, but professionals may sometimes need to view from two "positions" at the same time. Having conflicting roles may be particularly problematic, such as being a *fundholder* making general *resource* allocation decisions at the same time as having to be the advocate for a particular *patient*. It is undeniable that physical distance alters moral compunction either way: Jesus Christ's injunction was to love your neighbour; but "out of sight is out of mind". It is said that the problem is solved by surgeons with towels, and by psychiatrists with diagnostic labels.

See also: Doctor–patient relationship; veil of ignorance; proximity.

RH

Distributive justice *See* Justice.

DNA fingerprinting/profiling Within every body cell, with the exception of red blood cells, a dense accumulation of the intracellular constituents (known as the "nucleus") is found. This nucleus consists of the complex organic chemical, deoxyribonucleic acid (DNA) which functions as the repository for all the templates (genes) required for the construction of every protein in the body.

Each DNA molecule comprises several hundred sub-units or "base pairs" which are made up from the four bases: thymidine, adenine, guanine, and cytosine. The specific sequence in which these bases occurs is permanent, is replicated identically in every cell and is inherited equally from both parents; it is absolutely unique to every individual except in identical (monozygotic) twins.

DNA can be extracted artificially from the nuclei of living, shed or dead cells and after splicing it into smaller fragments (through using enzymes) it can be layered on to a gel and fragments ranked by size through their movement in an electrical field (electrophoresis); different fragments can be specifically identified by markers known as "probes", prepared artificially, and on to which a radioactive or fluorescent label is attached.

Different bands of fragments – resembling in their appearance and display a "bar code" – can thus be produced and photographed: the "DNA fingerprint" or "DNA profile". These profiles can be compared with others obtained from other individuals whose DNA was extracted and treated similarly, and also with random "data bases" derived from samples of the local population.

By counting the number of matching bands in two profiles, the likelihood, the statistical odds that both samples came from the same individual, can be calculated. Recent controversy has arisen regarding the adequacy of these calculations for members of ethnic minority groups, for which limited population data may be available.

When only small amounts of DNA are extractable, a laboratory technique known as polymerase chain reaction (PCR) allows DNA amplification to an amount that can be subjected to the full procedure.

See also: Genetics; paternity.

AB

DNR orders or Do Not Resuscitate orders, are instructions that a patient should not receive cardiopulmonary *resuscitation* (CPR) in the event that she suffers a cardiorespiratory arrest, usually in hospital. They are an example of witholding *treatment*, where the patient's prognosis is such that attempting resuscitation would be futile and inappropriate. The ability to resuscitate patients who have a prospect of survival means that staff may consider it obligatory to perform CPR in a patient who arrests unless there is a written DNR order by the responsible consultant, releasing them from that obligation. DNR orders should, if possible, have been discussed prior to a crisis with the patient, her *next of kin*, or other *proxy*. They do not necessarily exclude other active treatment measures.

AJP

Doctor–patient relationship This is considered to be a paradigm for most professional–client/user relationships in the health service, and is of importance both because of its *healing* (and harming) potential and because there are key differences between relationships in this context and similar ones elsewhere: for instance, although it partakes of elements of friendship and of a commercial relationship, neither adequately covers the necessities or nuances of the clinical encounter. It may be considered sui generis (unique) because of the *power* gradient between an ill patient who cannot assess herself completely, and who is unlikely to have the range of knowledge of the doctor but who, crucially, also is impelled to regress by internal (psychological) and external (contextual) forces, and a professional who may be tempted to take over in a mode of *paternalism* and who may have been attracted to a helping role because this style of work suited him. The health of this relationship depends on the *attitudes* of those involved; the importance of these is accentuated by the strong bond[1] which may develop and which remains a great force for healing and support (in some incurable conditions, or some branches of medicine, arguably the only force available). The emotional *distance* between the individuals in such encounters therefore needs to be correct and requires regular adjustment to avoid the opposing problems of under-involvement (*arrogance* etc) and *dependency*.

The ethical issues of this relationship are central to medical ethics, even if sometimes overshadowed by the perplexities caused by the wonders of scientific progress. The question "What should I do" is almost never asked in isolation, and is really "What should I do in this context and relationship" and yet the aspect of *mutuality* in these questions has been poorly developed in some thinking. There may be some who correctly criticise healthcare workers for paying too little attention to *public health* and *evidence-based medicine*, but excellent achievements for patients in these spheres will usually be destroyed by poor interactions with professionals. The need to examine critically and constructively the ethics of healthcare relationships is with us for all time.

Reference
Downie R. The doctor–patient relationship. In: Gillon R, Lloyd A, eds. *Principles of health care ethics*. Chichester: John Wiley, 1994

See also: Autonomy; communication; confidentiality; contract; courage; placebo; symbolism; treatment; trustworthiness.

RH

Donation To donate is freely to transfer title of some thing to another. One cannot legitimately donate what one does not own, and items one donates have the status of property. The common association of altruism with donation can be misleading; one may express residual altruism in the act of sale. Non-voluntary donation, eg,
cadaver donation where the "donor" has made no bequest, is a fiction.

See also: Blood and blood transfusion; sale of organs; transplantation.

CAE

Double effect The principle of double effect permits an act which is foreseen to have both good and bad effects, provided: the act itself is good or at least indifferent; the good effect is the reason for acting; the good effect is not caused by the bad effect; a proportionate reason exists for causing the bad effect, eg, morphine for pain may shorten life.

Reference
Gula M. *Reason informed by faith: foundations of Catholic morality*. New York: Paulist Press, 1989: 265–82.

BHo

DRGs *See* Diagnosis related groups.

Drug misuse or abuse occurs when a person uses a drug in a non-therapeutic way to obtain pleasure or an altered mental state. They may be taken by mouth, by injection, or inhalation. The distinction between drug misuse and recreational use is strongly determined by cultural and social mores: thus alcohol is widely regarded as a social custom; cannabis is regarded in some societies similarly, but in most as a "soft" drug; opiates, which were quite widely used in Eastern societies and considered acceptable in some Western societies in the past, are now generally regarded as "hard" drugs of abuse; cocaine, LSD, amphetamines, ecstasy and other drugs are generally regarded as drugs of abuse. The different approaches to drugs in part reflect their capacity to lead to harm and particularly *addiction*, most notably in respect of opiates and cocaine; but alcohol, which undoubtedly can lead to *dependency*, is a notable anomaly. Drug dependency clinics help addicted patients to come off drugs and to cope with initial withdrawal symptoms. They also offer long term strategies for coping without drugs and programmes of maintenance on safer drugs (eg, methadone). Harm minimisation has become a specific goal in the light of *AIDS*. Opiates are the most potent form of pain control in clinical practice, but their use is often tempered by concerns, which are often exaggerated, of fear of inducing dependency. Injecting drug misuse, where needles, syringes, and other materials are shared with others, whether through necessity or as part of the culture of drug misuse, is associated with the spread of serious blood-borne infections, including *hepatitis* viruses B and C and *HIV*.

AJP

Drugs are chemical entities used in *treatment* and form a major part of medical practice. They may be specific therapies for particular conditions or may serve to control symptoms. They are generally developed and produced by the *pharmaceutical industry* under (inter-)national regulation to ensure *safety* and, to varying degrees in different jurisdictions, efficacy. Drug safety and efficacy are generally determined after a period of preclinical evaluation, including *animal experimentation*, through *clinical trials*. Many can be prescribed only by doctors and be dispensed by *pharmacists*, but simple and well-established drugs may be available directly to patients over the counter. The prescription of some drugs may be restricted to certain specialists. Dangerous drugs, mainly opiates, are subjected to strict controls of prescription and storage, to avoid *drug misuse* and *addiction*. Patients may have the expectation that a doctor will prescribe a drug for a clinical problem, even if there is no effective agent for their condition; this

may lead to overprescribing or to the use of *placebos*.

See also: Prescribing.

AJP

Drugs, hard and soft The traditional distinction between hard and soft drugs is increasingly unclear and redundant. A recreational drug is any chemical substance which is taken to achieve, through physiological modification, a psychological and behavioural effect which is valued and enjoyed by the taker. Many such drugs produce *dependence* and may lead to deleterious physical and behavioural changes which also generate a *public health* risk and social problems.

See also: Cannabis; drug misuse; addiction.

AT

Dualism A tendency to explain things in terms of two basic and opposed categories, particularly common in Western religious and scientific thinking. The separation of body and mind in philosophy and medicine raises questions about how the physical and psychological are related; but also about relating that distinction to one between objective or scientific knowledge of mental phenomena, and the subject's own personal or existential knowledge – from which, it can be argued, scientific knowledge itself ultimately derives.

KMB

Due process is the observation of equitable rules in legal or quasi-legal inquiries, allowing the accused a means of appropriate defence against misguided, false or malicious accusation, eg, through the revealing of the evidence on which accusation is based and an opportunity to challenge it. Due process must also safeguard the *whistleblower* and should not inhibit reporting of lapses in professional

77

standards. In some recent cases of suspected scientific *fraud*, the accused have been denied due process, damaging their reputations and denying them access to grant funding before they had seen the case against them or had a chance to respond.

AJP

Duress For a patient's *consent* to be legally valid it must be *voluntary*. Thus, it must be freely given without duress, ie, without *coercion*, pressure or undue influence. Whether a patient's consent is voluntary is a question of degree and will depend upon the individual circumstances of each case. Where there is a danger of pressure, coercion, or undue influence, the court will be alive to that risk in determining whether the patient's consent is in fact freely given, eg, if the patient is a *prisoner*[1] or may be acting under the influence of members of a religious sect.[2] The *law* does not prohibit a patient seeking advice from others or others seeking to persuade the patient of what decision she should make providing this does not overbear the independence of the patient's decision. In deciding whether the will of a patient is overborne, the law will take account of the patient's condition, eg, whether she is tired, in pain, depressed, or under the influence of drugs. Also, the law will have regard to the relationship between the "persuader" and the patient, eg, the influence of parents or spouses is more likely to affect the patient's decision.[2]

References
1 *Freeman* v *Home Office No 2* (1984) QB 524 (CA).
2 *Re T (Adult: Refusal of Treatment)* (1992) 4 All ER 649 (CA).

See also: Decision-making capacity.

AG

Duty What is due or owed to others, either because they have *rights* which should be respected, or by virtue of particular relationships, eg, *Hippo-cratic Oath*, duties of gratitude to teachers, *non-maleficence*, and *confidentiality* to patients. In *Kantian ethics*, duty is central, based on respect for persons and a universal "do as you would be done by" principle: but others question whether absolute submission to this "Stern daughter of the voice of God" (Wordsworth: "Ode to Duty") represents a realistic view of human nature. More recent duty-based (or *deontological*) ethical theories acknowledge that *prima facie* duties can conflict, and that in such circumstances there may be no general decision procedure for prioritising them.

References
Paton HJ. *The moral law: Kant's groundwork of the metaphysic of morals.* London: Hutchinson, 1948.
Ross WD. *The right and the good.* Oxford: Clarendon Press, 1930.

KMB

Duty of care is an expression used, often in legal context, as a reminder about one of the key professional duties from which much may flow, once a professional takes on a patient. It would, for instance, prevent a doctor stopping work at the end of her shift if she was in the middle of a clinical task; or would require her to keep her knowledge and skills up to date. This duty is usually seen as owed to patients, but could be argued as being owed to others, such as relatives or even to oneself. It could loosely be seen as equating with the principle of *beneficence*, in that it usually implies positive action, although the law relates to it through negligence and the harm of failing to avert *harm*. The standards in English law are assumed to be those of the ordinary skilled professional in whichever branch she finds herself (Bolam judgment).

Reference
Brazier M. *Medicine, patients and the law.* London: Penguin, 1987.

See also: Negligence.

RH

E

Eastern philosophy *See* Religion and philosophy, Eastern.

Eating disorders Anorexia nervosa is a mental illness, with risks of extreme psychological and physical harm to the sufferer as a result of starvation and the means used to achieve it. A major part of the clinical picture includes the protestation that nothing is wrong in the face of severe emaciation. Without treatment sufferers risk long term physical damage, eg, through stunted growth, osteoporosis, and impaired reproductive function – and ultimately death. The dangerousness of the condition may justify extreme measures to maintain nutrition, such as assisted feeding.

Starvation also leads to significant psychiatric morbidity, in particular *depression* and obsessive compulsive disorder, and it may be difficult to treat these conditions without restoration of weight. At a low body mass (measure of weight) cognition may be impaired too, interfering with the ability of a sufferer to understand the seriousness of her condition, and to give consent to treatment.[1] Determining the ability to give *consent* to treatment and to refuse it can be difficult. In the UK the Mental Health Act may be used to detain patients against their will.

Linked with this is the fact that the condition usually develops in childhood and *adolescence*. As *minors* whose psychological development has been interrupted, patients often lack maturity of judgment. The Children Act may be used to invoke the authority to act in a child's best interests. For patients with an early onset, involvement of the family improves outcome, suggesting the need to understand the illness in a family context.

In an older age group, the sufferers' children may have disturbed eating patterns and growth curves, raising the question of whether artificial means of reproduction are appropriate in patients with anorexia nervosa.

Unlike other *mental illnesses*, the meaning and explanation of the behaviour are not alien to our culture. Explanations have, however, varied over time and place from, eg, vague abdominal distress in the past to the drive for thinness in contemporary life, and lie on the border between overvalued ideas, obsessional thoughts, and delusions. Changes in the psychopathology reflect changes in culture but in general food refusal is a powerful communication, as exemplified by fasting saints, hunger artists, and hunger strikers. Current societal pressures towards thinness, and ambivalence about an adult female shape, apparently derive from what are, to some, male dominated ideas in, eg, the media.

Other eating disorders, in particular bulimia nervosa, are increasingly common, as are minor versions of eating/fasting cycles and eating-then-vomiting among young women which makes disordered eating patterns almost a "normal" variant of behaviour.

An issue for clinicians is the assessment of patients requesting surgery who consider themselves overweight or the wrong shape. In some cases *cosmetic surgery* is no longer provided by the National Health Service and may be excluded by private health insurance.

Reference
1 Treasure J, Szmukler G. Medical complications of anorexia nervosa. In: *Handbook of eating disorders*. Szmukler G, C Dare C, Treasure J, (eds). Chichester: John Wiley, 1995.

See also: Child, status of; families.

RK/JLT

Eclectic In the general sense, deriving a view that combines the best from several different sources as opposed to working according to one particular set of principles or processes. Most clinical practice is eclectic by nature; eclecticism is espoused by some schools of psychiatry.

RH/AJP

Ecology The study of plant and animal communities, which vary greatly in complexity: the vast boreal forests of Canada and Russia may comprise four tree species, a tropical rain forest 200. Biologists stress the delicate mutual interdependence within a community. Everything is connected and it is impossible to change one thing only. Human beings used to live in just such natural balance with their environment. No longer: hence the term is employed by environmentalists concerned with human impact on natural systems. Eliminating particular plants or animals, introducing foreign species or pathogens can all have serious and sometimes irreversible effects on natural communities. The use of antibiotics or antiviral drugs in humans or animal husbandry may alter the ecology with potential of future hazard, as may the use of hormones in animals.

See also: Generations, rights of future.

AM

Ecology and medicine The actions towards patients of doctors and nurses, however well intentioned, have always the potential for *harm*, but until recently this harm would be considered to be restricted to those within that interaction. However, the increasingly powerful treatments in the hands of doctors may be capable of significantly and permanently altering the environment more generally. Some, such as the possible effect of excreted hormones on altering the fertility of fish, or the CFCs in inhalers damaging the ozone layer, are probably of minor significance compared with the effects of industry (including the pharmaceutical industry). However, these ecological "side effects" need to be noted, while greater attention is paid to the potential disasters awaiting mankind from multiple antibiotic resistance, or to the animal population from gene manipulation. These issues place particular responsibilities on all who promote, develop, or use biomedicine.

The massive growth in human population threatens to outstrip the earth's *resources* but also to destroy much of the diversity and beauty which are its key features. This raises problems for those who wish to argue that placing something in the category "human" makes it precious to the point where its destruction is immoral or its disappearance is to be prevented in every way possible (such as in the *abortion* or PVS debate). It also brings a further aspect into any debate about *infertility* and its "treatment". The Gaia hypothesis of James Lovelock proposes another way of looking at this problem. This suggests that all living things on this planet should be thought of as part of a single living being. To survive, this being needs feedback systems that ensure the conditions of the environment that support its life are maintained. Humankind has a key role in maintaining that global environment but might expect that, if this responsibility is not upheld, the earth itself might use other methods to reduce the destructive effects of humans, by reducing population through plagues, reduced fertility, and so on.

Reference

Lovelock J. *The ages of Gaia*. Oxford: Oxford University Press, 1988.

See also: Genetics.

RH

Economics *See* Health economics.

Effectiveness and efficiency are terms used in *health economics* to distinguish between (a) what a medical activity achieves (its effect) and (b) whether or not an equal or better effect can be achieved at the same or less cost in terms of effort or *resources* (efficiency). In traditional Aristotelean logic, the efficient cause is what makes something happen, as opposed to the material cause (what it is made of, the material), the formal cause (what it is, the plan or idea of it) and the final cause (what it is for, its purpose). A medical intervention or policy may be effective without being efficient, or again may be effective and efficient for some patients only at the cost of depriving others of the opportunity of equal consideration of their needs ("opportunity cost"). Medical effectiveness and economic efficiency alone are insufficient to determine morally appropriate interventions or policies: it is also important to take into account the broader social and symbolic purposes, or final ends, of medicine and health care.

References

Campbell AV. *Medicine, health and justice: the problem of priorities.* Edinburgh: Churchill Livingstone, 1978.
Cochrane AL. *Effectiveness and efficiency: random reflections on the health service.* London: Nuffield Provincial Hospitals Trust, 1972.

KMB

Egoism In everyday usage, selfishness; in ethics, the view that people either do, or ought to, act in their own self-interest – as opposed to *altruism* (self-disregarding concern for others' interests). But people can act against their own *self interest* for non-altruistic reasons (eg, resentment, revenge); and if everyone espoused ethical egoism, the social life needed to achieve their ends would not be possible. Enlightened or long-term self-interest suggests that a degree of altruism is necessary, probably for survival and certainly for happiness.

KMB

Elderly *See* Age and aging; geriatric medicine.

Elective ventilation *See* Intensive care; transplants.

Electroconvulsive therapy (ECT) involves the passage of electricity through the head in order to induce a synchronised cerebral discharge and hence a seizure. It is the fit and not the electricity per se that is thought to be beneficial. Electroconvulsive therapy was introduced in the late 1930s. Nowadays it is delivered under general *anaesthesia* with a muscle relaxant. It is used chiefly in the treatment of depressive psychosis but may have a role in mania and acute schizophrenia.

Electroconvulsive therapy is controversial for five reasons. First, as an unequivocally physical treatment it occupies a pivotal position in debate about the nature of *mental illness*. Second, the ambiguous term "shock" treatment leads to misunderstanding about the aim of the intervention. It refers to the electricity rather than any wish to disturb the recipient. Third, it is an uncongenial treatment compared with *psychotherapy* or taking tablets. Fourth, it is associated with some side-effects, particularly problems with memory. Lastly, until the 1980s ideas of the efficacy of ECT were based more upon clinical tradition than *clinical research* evidence. This has now been rectified by the positive results of double-blind controlled trials. Furthermore, evidence suggests that memory problems are transient, although a few patients may have more lasting impairment. Nevertheless, ECT remains at the centre of dispute for the reasons outlined above.

Many people receiving ECT have an impaired ability to give truly *informed consent*. In the UK, a competent person can give written consent to receive ECT even when she is detained under the Mental Health Act 1983. However, ECT without such consent requires that the patient be assessed by an independent psychiatrist appointed by the Mental Health Act Commission. In emergency, treatment may be started before the second opinion is obtained.

Wide controversy has led ECT effectively to be banned in some countries. Too often debates about ECT are ill-informed and ideological. Decisions made on this basis are themselves ethically questionable. The balance of *risk* and advantage associated with ECT seems comparable with many other treatments that provoke far less dispute.

RLP

Elegance Reasoning in mathematics or logic can be assessed not just for its validity but also for its elegance. In other words, reasoning can have an aesthetic dimension, which is thought of in terms of conceptual economy or simplicity.

See also: Logic and logical care.

RSD

Embarassment is a minor form of shame which is socially useful and cohesive, and enables people who differ or who notice unacceptable thoughts or desires to direct their gaze elsewhere, and continue to live together in a civilised way. However, it is an important emotion in health care, where it may prevent open discussion of an important topic or physical examination in circumstances where it might ideally be required. It fuels the needs for *confidentiality* and *privacy,* and for making a physical examination feel safe by use, for instance, of a *chaperone* or consulting a professional of the same sex.

RH

Embryo research Although research on the previable human fetus has been condoned and can be carried out legally under strict *guidelines* this has been very limited. However, the advent of fertilisation of the human egg in vitro and its widespread use as a treatment for the alleviation of human infertility (*in vitro fertilisation* – IVF), has allowed greater access to scientists to the preimplantation human embryo. Public concern over the monitoring and type of this research led to the inclusion of specific clauses within the Human Fertilisation and Embryology Act (1990) whereby research on the human preimplantation embryo beyond 14 days is a criminal offence, save under licence and within the following categories: (a) promoting advances in the treatment of infertility; (b) increasing knowledge about the causes of congenital diseases; (c) increasing knowledge about the causes of miscarriages; (d) developing more effective techniques of contraception; (e) developing methods for detecting the presence of gene or chromosome abnormalities in embryos before implantation; and that these data cannot be acquired by other means (eg, animal models).

Reference
The Polkinghorne Committee. *The Polkinghorne report: Review of the guidance on the research use of fetuses and fetal material.* London: HMSO, CM 762, 1989.

See also: Embryo therapy; fetus and embryo; GIFT; infertility; pre-embryo.

PBr

Embryo therapy The ability to identify the molecular faults that produce specific inherited defects and the ability to diagnose these errors by prenatal testing either in the fetus, using *amniocentesis* or *chorionic villus sampling,* or in the preimplantation embryo, by biopsy of single cells while still in culture during the first five days following fertilisation in vitro: this has raised the tantalising possibility of injecting specific segments of genes into the cells of the developing embryo to try and correct these errors. In contrast to gene therapy used in children or adults, where the genes may be incorporated into specific somatic tissues in the hope of correcting the abnormality therein (eg, to replace the production of dystrophin in the muscle in Duchenne muscular dystrophy), if injected into the developing embryo the effects of these new inserts would be carried on through the generations as they would also be incorporated into the germ cells of the embryo which would give rise to its gametes (sperm or eggs). Hence the controversy about applying the principles of gene therapy to the early embryo.

See also: Embryo research; genetic disorders; genetics; pre-embryo.

PBr

Embryo transfer The procedure by which human preimplantation embryo(s), usually generated by *in vitro fertilisation (IVF)*, are introduced to the uterus in the hope of achieving a pregnancy. UK law allows the transfer of a maximum of three embryos in a single treatment, with concomitant risk of multiple pregnancy.

See also: Embryo research; GIFT; infertility; reproduction; surrogacy.

VNB

Emergency Ethical difficulties arise frequently in emergencies and are the more difficult to deal with because the decision has to be arrived at immediately. Particular issues that need to be addressed in individual patients are: the decision to begin *resuscitation*; the decision to terminate resuscitation; the potential for infection of the rescuer; the problem of *informed consent* to use particular techniques; the right of loved ones to observe the resuscitation attempt; the morality of permitting trainees to practise certain techniques, eg, tracheal intubation on patients who have not responded to resuscitation; the problem of diverting precious but limited *resources*

to resuscitative efforts of one individual in a mass casualty situation.

The decision to begin resuscitation will depend on the patient's immediate and long term prognosis, the patient's own wishes, and her presumed ability to cope with *disability* of one form or another. It should not be influenced by doctor pride. An ethical resuscitation policy should be drawn up in every hospital to ensure that these factors are complied with.

The decision to terminate resuscitation will depend on the time for response by the emergency medical services, the interval between cardiac arrest and the application of Basic Life Support (BLS), and the interval between the application of BLS and the arrival of Advanced Life Support (ALS) facilities designed to restart a spontaneous circulation. Evidence of cardiac or cerebral damage and knowledge of the potential prognosis and underlying disease process influence the decision. Resuscitation attempts should be prolonged in patients with hypothermia or who have ingested sedative drugs. Young children often tolerate periods of hypoxia.

Infection of the rescuer can be minimised by protective apparel but there is no protection against needlestick injuries. There appears to be no evidence of *HIV* transmission from mouth to mouth ventilation.

Certain countries require informed consent to be obtained before new equipment can be used. This provides a considerable hindrance to progress in resuscitation techniques.

The right of loved ones to be with their partner, child or parent during the resuscitative process is a matter of debate. There is a large body of opinion in favour of this but that viewpoint must be balanced against the added stress placed on the rescuer and the potential for abhorrence as the resuscitative process becomes more and more *invasive*.

Further ethical decisions that may need to be considered as an emergency: *blood transfusion* in the exsanguinating unconscious *Jehovah's Witness*; blood transfusion in the exsanguinating child of a Jehovah's Witness; artificial ventilation in the high cervical spinal cord injury; resuscitation of the patient who has made multiple *suicide* attempts.

See also: Child, status of; intensive care.

PJFB

Emergency, concept of Within health care an emergency usually indicates a sudden and pressing need that requires an instant and decisive response: without such a response there might be loss of life or a serious injury. But it is defined by what might or is feared to be about to happen (whereas a *catastrophe* has already occurred), so this perhaps of all the descriptive categories in medicine is most obviously a social or individual construct. Each person or group could be said to have their own sets of fears or signs that predict disaster. For instance, one early teenager may know that the appearance of blood from her vagina is her first menstrual period, whereas another may know that all blood loss is serious and she may bleed to death unless she seeks medical help at once. In response to this variation professionals sometimes discuss "real" emergencies, by which they appear to mean situations where biomedicine predicts a high chance of serious harm and usually includes the concept that a medical intervention may prevent that harm (the seriously drunk, though at great risk, are certainly seldom admitted to hospital and may be ejected from a casualty department or medical practice). Individual and group concepts of an emergency are greatly affected by what has happened before. Anxiety may be heightened by media accounts of disasters elsewhere. Healthcare planning for emergency units and *out of hours work* is therefore difficult: a morally satisfactory response must include paying attention to individuals' judgments while being prepared to enter into dialogue and if appropriate educate sensitively those whose ideas are plainly incorrect or judgment faulty.

RH

Emotion Ideas are informed by facts but moved by emotions. Emotions are triggered by current events (not always clearly perceived), arise from the past (memory), and can overwhelm the future. Reason ignores emotions at its peril, but acknowledging them, it may guide, and gain support from them. Not all emotions are agitated: some are settled or creative. In medical ethics, clinicians may often be right to suspect philosophical clarity leading to *counterintuitive* conclusions, but wrong always to trust gut feelings or the heart's reasons, which may be reflex if not reflected on. Emotions were formerly called passions, the subject not acting but being acted upon. In patients (same root), emotions can provoke physiological changes and precipitate critical events. But emotional chemistry is more difficult to measure and control than physical, demanding of clinicians not just scientific but also self-knowledge, derived from impartial (and where necessary self-forgiving) observation of their own reactions to everyday events. Critical moments (moral dilemmas or difficult duties such as breaking *bad news*) can create perplexity, in which "there is a portion of fear which predisposes the mind to anger . . . the first defence of weak minds is to recriminate" (Coleridge). Against this, medical education cannot ensure but can encourage personal growth, while many relevant communication skills and techniques are teachable.

KMB

Emotivist A 20th-century philosophical argument: moral views arise directly from the emotions, are neither true nor false, and expressing them is essentially a way of trying to persuade others to share our feelings. This devaluation of reason in ethics has been widely criticised, but it enlarges on something recognisable.

KMB

Empathy is the ability to enter into someone else's frame of reference and experience her experiences imaginatively as one's own, perhaps in order to understand that person's point of view or to support her by sharing what she is going through. It differs from sympathy in that the latter implies pity, but empathy, though focused upon the other person positively, is not judgmental either way. It is seen as key to *counselling* (especially as expounded by Carl Rogers) and to sensitive health care. It may provide insights into ethical problems at an interpersonal level; for instance, when a competent chooser appears to be making an irrational or even repugnant choice, or where there seems to be a moral or decision-making impasse.

See also: Compassion.

RH

Empowerment of patients enables them to participate actively in decision-making. It is achieved by an effective *doctor–patient relationship*, in which the patient is fully informed about the nature of her disease, understands the disease and its prognosis, and is encouraged to make her own choice about therapy. The giving of information and explanation of options can be verbal and/or written, but should be at a level and in language that is appropriate to her educational background and culture. It is increasingly used in clinical practice, instead of the *paternalism* of the past.

The ethos of empowerment is especially well developed in obstetric and *AIDS* care. It can avoid ethical dilemmas that result from clinicians inappropriately taking decisions that properly belong to the patient and that can be resolved only with a knowledge of her own personal philosophy or inclination, and where the strictly medical issues are evenly balanced. Empowerment enables the patient to take greater responsibility for her own disease management, enhancing *compliance* and more effective use of *resources*. Patients may elect to use *complementary medicine* or seek other sources of advice about their disease and its management. Empowerment also allows the patient explicitly to ask the clinician to make the decision, so it does not force her to make choices she feels unable to make.

See also: Decision-making capacity; treatment.

AJP

Ends and means An end is the aim or goal of action – either enjoyment of the action itself (eg, making music), or what the action produces, which again may be either an end in itself (eg, a painting), or a means to an end (eg, a tool). Persons are always ends, never means (*Kant*); good ends may not justify evil means.

KMB

Ensoulment When the fetus becomes a human or rational soul (after being first a vegetative, then an animal soul). "Soul" is the organising principle of life, not necessarily a thing. Ensoulment takes place later for mediaeval than for modern Catholic thought: the older view, which more closely recapitulates the stages of evolution, allows a *moral* distinction between early and late *abortion*.

KMB

Epidemiological research is a form of *clinical research* that utilises data on populations or groups of subjects or patients, using *probability* and statistical methodologies to assess associations between defined factors and disease risk. It can be hypothesis-generating or -testing. It endeavours to control for individual variability and for extraneous variables to the hypothesis under test, and to identify interactions between variables and hierarchies of different variables. It uses retrospective or prospective surveillance methodologies and specific tools, such as case control studies, where cases are matched with controls, or meta-analysis, where the results of several studies are combined to enhance their statistical power.

See also: Evidence-based medicine.

AJP

Epilepsy is a neurological disease that typically demonstrates itself by recurrent episodes of sudden loss of consciousness or convulsive seizures. The underlying causes and degree of brain abnormality vary, but the moral issues lie in the relative unpredictability of the attacks, their devastating effects (because the person loses consciousness or control) and the fact that the sufferer is unaware of what she is doing or its effect on others in the environment. The patient thus suffers not only from the physical effects of the seizures (physical injuries and neurological after-effects) but also from the knowledge that her person is no longer under her control. This creates a sense of shame in the person, and has given the condition a *stigma* in society in general which seems totally out of proportion to the medical events. The sufferer may become isolated, or may fear such and help to create it. Since many fits come without warning to a wide-awake person an epileptic may not be allowed to undertake ordinary tasks open to everybody else. For instance, it would usually create an absolute and life-long exclusion from public service vehicle driving, and from private vehicle driving until the fits were controlled completely for a satisfactory number of years, and this might mean, should an employee be discovered to be epileptic, that she might lose her job or be excluded from a particular workplace. Because of the stigma and the epileptic's unconsciousness during the attacks the sufferer may attempt to hide the condition or fail to appreciate its seriousness. The epileptic who fails to stop driving is a classical problem for medical *confidentiality*.

RH

Epistemology From Greek "to know", is the (philosophical) science of knowledge. Do we discover, construct or create knowledge, or a little of each? Where does opinion end and knowledge begin, knowledge end and faith begin? Is what we think we know true because it fits the facts, or because our ideas fit together?

KMB

Equipoise (literally, equally poised or balanced) is a term used in relation to clinical trials and in justification of *randomisation*. It denotes the state of mind of clinicians, individually or collectively, who have no rational preference among the *treatment* options to be compared. A moral dilemma may arise for a clinician who, having say a 60:40 per cent rational preference for one treatment, does not share the collective equipoise of specialists in her field, and is invited to recruit patients for whom she is responsible to be randomised in a trial which may ultimately justify her own preference, especially when her preferred treatment is available only to patients randomised to it in the trial. An important aspect of this and other trials is whether the *patients* or subjects concerned share the clinicians' equipoise regarding the possible burdens (including side-effects) as well as potential benefits of the treatments being compared.

Reference
Lilford RJ, Jackson J. Equipoise and the ethics of randomization. *J R Soc Med*, 1995 **88**: 552–9.

See also: Clinical research and trials.

KMB

Equity a sense of *fairness* appealed to in particular cases when the letter of the *law* is too inflexible or general to express the spirit of natural *justice*. In relation to distributive justice, the notion of fair *discrimination* – treating like cases alike and unlike cases differently.

See also: Cost containment; human rights; resources.

KMB

Ethical May mean either (i) having to do with (the study of) morality ("an ethical question"), or (ii) conforming to recognised standards of practice ("ethical conduct"). Anyone can be immoral: only doctors or others who fail to live up to publicly professed obligations tend to be called "unethical". Pharmaceuticals advertised to doctors but not the general public are termed "ethical" by association.

KMB

Ethical debates, methods of
Although moral issues may properly be detected within a situation that may appear otherwise to be unproblematic, in health care they usually force themselves on to the stage because of some *conflict*, actual or anticipated, and so require discussion. Although some institutions have employed a staff member with philosophical expertise to stimulate, conduct or respond to such discussions, it is usually up to the individual clinicians or patients concerned to conduct the debate.

The aims of ethical discussion could include:

- identification of the issues at stake, whom they affect, and in what way
- further exploration of morally relevant facts together with a reasonable attempt to assess the perspectives and purposes of all involved
- clarification of the concepts and arguments being used
- interaction and dialogue between the various parties to ventilate feelings, share points of view, and make sure everyone feels "heard"
- an analysis or synthesis of different points of view and arguments in order to create a response or way forward.

In the process a number of further questions may need to be asked. These might include whether the person or group who stimulated the debate was actually the one with the problem: who the person or group was whose point of view had been least heard, and what she or they might say; what *roles* individuals were playing, who they were working for, or what "system" they were actually involved in; whether any person or group was distorting the discussion by manipulation, misuse of language, or distortion of concepts and arguments.

The organisation of such debates depends on the circumstances, crucially as to whether they are real and immediate (as in a clinical problem) or theoretical and extendable (as in an educational setting). The first benefits from a willingness of all involved to lay aside special time outside or protected time within the working routine, from attendance of all those involved at a place separate from the normal workplace but familiar enough to feel "safe", and from defined but sensitive leadership that can explain the purposes of the discussion, maintain a good and open process and ensure clearly defined outcomes. The second might use all the current educational techniques, depending on the size and makeup of the group doing the learning. Particularly useful have been found: group role plays, where individuals take a role in a scenario, and then out of role describe their feelings and reasoning; individual or pair work to focus on a case before wider debate; and the requirement to argue from or for a point of view different from the individual's usual one. To divide this work artificially from other reflective forms of professional and personal development would seem to be wasting opportunities.

Reference

Campbell A, Higgs R. *In that case: medical ethics in everyday practice*. London: Darton Longman and Todd, 1982.

RH

Ethical systems Traditional ethical codes (whether of ancient religions or modern professions) derive their authority from custom (in Greek "ethics" comes from "ethos"), or the commands of gods or leaders. Such codes do not necessarily reflect a coherent set of principles, and their various precepts may not be consistent, either internally or with other *codes*. Philosophy is more systematic – either in defending traditional *authority* (eg, by arguing that it embodies self-evident moral intuitions – mediaeval theology; or is required by human frailty – Hobbes) or in constructing more coherent foundations for morality.

Philosophical systems of ethics tend to focus either on achieving what they consider to be good (consequentialist or eudaemonistic systems) or on achieving what they consider to be right (deontological systems).

The highest human good (if such there be, and not simply a variety of different goods) has generally been seen as happiness. This can be interpreted as pleasure (and avoiding pain) – either for the individual, in hedonistic systems, or for everyone (or the greatest number), in *utilitarianism*, both of these systems being consequentialist. Happiness can also be interpreted *eudaemonistically*, as the kind of "human flourishing" that involves realising one's highest ideals, finding the "golden mean" and living in harmony with others and one's own deepest self. Variations on this theme are found in ethical systems from Confucius, Plato and Aristotle, to Jung and modern virtue ethics. A key idea is that being determines action – you do what you are; a good person flourishing has clear moral vision and is disposed to act accordingly. ("Nobody does wrong willingly" – Socrates; "the just man justices" – GM Hopkins). Agapeistic ethics is similar. ("Love God, and what you will, do" – St Augustine.)

Kant's deontological ethical system, based on "the moral law within", has affinities with this, but sees a need to spell out the moral law in axioms with which (because of their clear implications for everyone) it is only reasonable to agree; and on which duties and *rights* can be based. *Reason* had a similar role in Spinoza's system, albeit with a more positive role for the emotions. Agreement on principles and procedures also is central to ethical systems that derive it from the most likely terms of an historical or hypothetical contract among equals (notably today John Rawls's system of *justice* as *fairness*).

In modern *bioethics*, the most familiar ethical system is deontological – the four principles of *beneficence*, *nonmaleficence*, respect for *autonomy* and *justice*. But determining the scope of their application requires recourse to consequentialist or eudaemonistic considerations. In applied ethics generally, each kind of system has valid insights to contribute. So too have sceptics since Hume, and existentialists, when they question the objectivity of all ethical systems. No one ethical system commands universal agreement. But each contributes pertinent questions to the moral spectrum that practical reasoning needs to consider before coming to a judgment.

See also: Agape; consequentialism; deontology; duty; eudaemonia; existentialism; hedonism; Kantian ethics; virtue.

KMB

Ethics committees *See* Research ethics committees; clinical research and trials.

Ethnicity The word derives from the Greek word "ethnos", meaning a nation. Ethnicity refers to the group to which people belong as a result of certain shared characteristics, particularly geographical and ancestral origins, cultural traditions, and languages. The characteristics which define ethnicity are not fixed or easily measured, so ethnicity is imprecise and fluid. Ethnicity differs from race, nationality, religion, and migrant status.

The measurement, or assignment, of ethnicity is problematic.[1] Presently, self-definition of ethnicity is favoured. The result is that the self-assessment changes over time and with context. The currently favoured groupings, eg "White", Indian, Pakistani, hide massive heterogeneity, and this diminishes the value of ethnic categorisation as a means of delivering culturally appropriate health care, and in understanding the causes of ethnic variations in disease.[1,2] The nature of ethnicity, its differentiation from race, and the implications for research have been discussed elsewhere.[1,2] Ethnicity as a concept in health care raises deep ethical issues, which have seldom been aired.

The division of people on the basis of race and ethnicity raises questions about human values, for the consequences of such divisions have been great. Ethical codes have not prevented the disastrous consequences of racism and prejudice. Population growth, travel and rising expectations globally, will require a radical shift in values and stronger application of ethics in the 21st century. Some of the ethical issues in the field of ethnicity and health, based on the framework of *autonomy, non-maleficence, beneficence* and *equity*, will now be focused upon.

Where the ethnicity of the health professional and patient differs, particularly where there are communication difficulties due to language or cultural barriers, *informed consent* is likely to be impaired. This would reduce the autonomy of ethnic minority patients. At a group level, priorities are based on the needs of the ethnic majority, usually by decision-makers belonging to the ethnic majority. A potential danger is that such priorities will be discriminatory or inappropriate and hence, unethical. Eg, the heavy emphasis in the 1970s and 1980s on birth control and tuberculosis as problems of ethnic minority groups, when coronary heart disease was a major killer, may have arisen from such *bias*. Ethical priorities are to involve ethnic minority groups, encourage autonomy, and give due weight to problems both common in, and specific to, ethnic minority groups.

Where there are barriers of understanding arising from ethnic differences between carers and the patient, unintentional harm may result from poor communication. Also, discrimination based on ethnic and racial differences can be the spur to deliberate *harm*, as in Nazi Germany.[3] Usually unintentionally, but sometimes deliberately, the stereotyping and cultural denigration which arises from linking *disease* to *culture* can stigmatise ethnic minority communities as a problem, thus harming their standing in society. Linking disease to culture can lead to unjustified "victim blaming".

There is evidence that ethnic minority groups are not receiving the expected beneficence (good) from their individual or collective interactions with health professionals and health services[2] and with researchers. A beneficent health service would adapt to meet their cultural expectations, eg, examination by a health professional of the same gender as the patient. Have ethnic minority groups benefited from the now voluminous research done on them? If not, were the subjects consenting to participating in *research* without direct benefits to them? Ethical research would inform subjects of the benefits (direct or indirect) they can expect.

Equity is the one ethical principle usually considered in discussions of ethnicity and health. An equitable service would meet equal needs equally but this requires a diversity in the organisation of services, to ensure uniformity in access, utilisation and quality at the point of delivery. This is patently not the case.[2] Eg, in the early 1980s nearly 50 per cent of deaths in men residing in Britain, but born on the Indian subcontinent, were from cardiovascular diseases. Yet, there were no *health education* materials available designed for such men.[4]

In conclusion, the complex concept of ethnicity raises numerous ethical issues, many of key importance in health care. Ethical principles may be in conflict, eg, the desire to do good by improving the health status of ethnic minority groups by changing their cultural autonomy and *freedom*. Ethnic variations pose a challenge to the maintenance of high ethical standards. The implications have yet to be fully explored.

References

1 Senior P, Bhopal RS. Ethnicity as a variable in epidemiological research. *BMJ* 1994; **309**: 327–30.

2 Smaje C. *Health, "race" and ethnicity.* London: King's Fund Institute, 1995.

3 Anonymous. Contemporary lessons from Nazi Germany. *IME bulletin.* 1989; Feb: 13–20.

4 Bhopal RS, Donaldson LJ. Health education for ethnic minorities – current provision and future directions. *Health Educ J* 1988; **47**: 137–40.

See also: Prejudice; racism; silence; stigma; transcultural medicine.

RSB

Eudaemonia Literally from Greek, "blessed with/by a good spirit": for Aristotle the aim and achievement of *wisdom* and virtue. The word has been interpreted variously, in *hedonistic*, ascetic and mystical terms. The traditional translation "happiness" (suggesting luck or "hap") may be less adequate than the modern "human flourishing".

KMB

Eugenics The "science" (Galton 1883) of improving inherited human characteristics. Comparable to cattle breeding, but fallaciously, since value judgments about what humans are good (and to be improved) for, are essentially disputable. Widely influential until discredited by Nazi abuses and growing scientific knowledge of the complexities of human *genetics*; but still alive in propaganda for racist policies and behavioural genetics.

Reference

Soloway RA. *Demography and degeneration.* Chapel Hill: North Carolina University Press, 1990.

KMB

Euthanasia The term euthanasia should be reserved for the "compassion-motivated, deliberate, rapid, and painless termination of the life of someone afflicted with an incurable and progressive disease".[1] It is voluntary if it is performed at the dying person's request or with that person's consent; otherwise it is involuntary. The terms "active" and "passive" euthanasia are ambiguous and should be avoided.

The main arguments against euthanasia are consequentialist and deontological. The strongest of the former include alteration in the *doctor–patient relationship* and reduction in autonomy of society as a whole as dependent people come to view the right to ask for *death* as a duty to do so.[2] The latter argument is that the duty of a doctor is to cure, relieve, and comfort and not deliberately to kill.

Proponents of legalised euthanasia argue that the prominence of *autonomy* in present medical ethics dictates that meaningful patient control must include "decisions regarding the timing, circumstances, and method of death".[3] Autonomy is not, however, the sole nor even the most important ethical principle and must be viewed in balance with other principles. There is no need to move from *paternalism* directly to *consumerism*.

A great many individuals said to be in need of or requesting euthanasia are more in need of explanation and physical or psychological treatment.[4,5] There may, however, remain a small number of psychologically stable patients who feel that their suffering is unbearable and who wish to end their lives by euthanasia. The issue is whether these exceptions should be sacrificed to the principle of not allowing euthanasia.

References
1 Roy D, Lapin C. Regarding euthanasia. *Eur J Palliative Care* 1994; **1**: 57–9.
2 Randall F. Two lawyers and a technician. *Palliative Med* 1993; **7**: 3.
3 Campbell C, Hare J, Matthews P. Conflicts of conscience: hospice and assisted suicide. *Hastings Center Report 25* 1995; **3**: 36–43.
4 Chochinov H *et al*. Desire for death in the terminally ill. *Am J Psychiatry* 1995; **152**: 1185–91.
5 Cole RM. Communicating with people who request euthanasia. *Palliative Med* 1993; **7**: 139–43.

See also: Active/passive distinction; assisted suicide; consequentialism; deontology; slippery slope; treatment.

DO

Evidence-based medicine is a formalisation of current knowledge to define practice and *treatment* norms. It has become something of a mantra in health care planning and is in danger of becoming distorted by misuse or misunderstanding. Essentially it is a way of synthesising knowledge based on formal *clinical research and trials, epidemiological research*, reviews and meta-analysis, clinical experience, and *expertise*. It is systematically appraised and promulgated, eg, in *guidelines*, and then applied in practice, the *outcomes* subjected to continuing *audit* and evaluation. It does not deny the need to adapt this knowledge base to the individual *patient* with *clinical judgment* and should be seen as underpinning rather than negating *clinical freedom*. Informed and conscientious clinicians have long been informally applying evidence-based medicine, without calling it that. It provides a framework for *accountability* of clinical practice and can facilitate *purchasing* decisions. It is also a critical ingredient of continuing *medical education*. However, there are fears that it, or a caricature of it, could impose unreasonable or inappropriate standards, based on incomplete evidence, or that it could become a tool in prioritising or rationing care.

AJP

Evil General synonym for "bad", often divided into natural evil (pain and disease) and moral evil (deliberate wrong doing). The traditional "problem of evil" is: how these bad things can exist in a world conceived as basically good.

Manicheeism posited a bad creating force co-equal with the good one. Christianity blames rather the misuse of free will by created beings, both angelic (the devil) and human.

To account for bad motivations, Freud posited a death wish, a force opposing Eros or Life. Though this idea raises some interesting questions, modern psychologists largely now use the medical model of health and sickness, not considering moral evil separately.

References

Cavendish R. *The powers of evil in western religion magic and folk belief.* London: Routledge and Kegan Paul, 1975.

Freud S. *Civilization and its discontents* [Trans by Joan Riviere]. London: Hogarth Press, 1930.

See also: Blame; choice; Christianity; conscience; criminal behaviour; dualism; guilt; moral judgment; responsibility; sin; suffering.

MM

Evolutionary ethics Herbert Spencer's idea that the direction of evolution is the source of moral value: the good then simply is what evolution demands. Spencer combined JB Lamarck's notion of benign evolution with reliance on competition as its sole mechanism. He coined the phrase "survival of the fittest" and confidently justified social inequality and commercial freedom as evolutionarily necessary.

Though Spencer welcomed Darwin's work and his doctrine is often called "Social Darwinism", his moral conclusions and his Panglossian belief in progress were foreign to Darwin, both being derived essentially from laissez-faire economics.

Despite TH Huxley's opposition, however, these two ideas are still widely associated with the concept of evolution.

References

Hofstadter R. *Social Darwinism in American thought.* New York: Braziller, 1959.

Huxley TH. *Evolution and ethics* [Romanes lecture]. London and New York: Macmillan, 1893.

See also: bioethics, history of; facts v values; self interest.

MM

Existentialism Movement in religion, literature and philosophy (19th century: Kierkegaard, Dostoievsky; 20th century: Sartre, Camus, Jaspers, Buber) arguing that truth is subjective or inter-subjective. We either inauthentically accept conventional half-truths, or authentically choose to give existence our own *meaning* – either by taking responsibility for our creative response to life's "absurdity", or (in Christian existentialism) by making the "leap of faith". Existentialism's emphasis on *choice* and *responsibility* has been influential, and what Jaspers (a psychiatrist) writes about *communication* is relevant to medical ethics.

Reference

Macquarrie J. *Existentialism.* Harmondsworth: Penguin, 1973.

KMB

Exorcism Although exorcism, the practice of expelling evil spirits by means of prayer and the laying on of hands, is little used in mainstream Christian churches, it was clearly a Jewish practice, continued by Christ and his followers in the early Church and was, at one time, part of baptism. It is also practised, in other ways, in other religions.

Exorcism is part of the ministry of healing and in both the Roman Catholic and Anglican Churches is exercised by priests specialising in this ministry and authorised by the bishop. More recently, however, there has been an increase in its use, especially in evangelical and charismatic congregations where a ministry of "deliverance" is practised, with at times, it is reported, dangerous consequences. It has no place in medical practice.

EFS

Experimentation is the process of deliberate (as opposed to observational or opportunistic) test in scientific *research*. It includes laboratory investigation, *animal experiments* and *clinical trials*. Experiments should have defined objectives in testing a hypothesis, use an experimental plan that focuses on that test and allows documentation of effect, and they must be conducted with appropriate oversight (eg, by a *research ethics committee*). Explicit *consent* is required from human subjects where an experiment is being performed, whether exploratory in the context of clinical practice or more formally. Failure to do so on occasion has resulted in the perception that some clinicians use their patients as "guinea pigs".

AJP

Experts and expertise An expert is a person with substantial knowledge, experience and/or skill in a particular domain. The opinion of experts will often be sought on an issue, whether by colleagues in medicine or science, or by legal or other external bodies and the media, when seeking a professional and authoritative view. Because expertise often lies in a relatively narrow sphere, it may be necessary for that opinion then to be put into a wider context. A patient or clinician who has sought an expert opinion may choose to modify or even ignore that opinion, if it does not fit with her own perceptions. Thus a patient may consider what an expert considers a remote risk as one that she herself regards as unacceptable. The patient is in a way the expert on what perspective she takes on an issue, having synthesised expert views. The clinical professions include many specialties and it is increasingly necessary, given the breadth and diversity of medicine, to consult with experts from other specialties. The clinician responsible for the patient's care can then discuss with the patient how to proceed in the light of expert opinion. Expert groups may be constituted to provide advice on issues of policy or practice, eg, in the preparation of *guidelines* or *consensus* statements.

Medical cases that come to the courts or other forms of arbitration may be assessed in the light of expert witnesses, though standards of practice are usually judged on the norm of a responsible body of medical opinion. Some practitioners may put themselves up as experts for legal cases or to the media without necessarily having the requisite expertise. It may be important to establish such a person's credentials, since expertise is arguably a quality that only others can identify.

See also: Authority.

AJP

Exploitation Taking advantage, for one's own (or a third party's) ends, of someone in a weaker position than oneself. Hence, in medical ethics, not only the prohibition of sexual relations with patients, but also the requirement that patient *consent* be fully informed and empowered.

KMB

Extraordinary and ordinary means In discussions about the morality of prolonging life, reference is often made to the maxim that, while ordinary means of preserving life should always be employed, extraordinary means are not obligatory. The distinction to be made here is not between those means that can be described as customary or usual and those that are not. Rather, extraordinary means should be understood as means that do not offer a reasonable chance of success and/or are foreseen to be excessively *burdensome*. Because of the ambiguity, some ethicists prefer other terms, eg, "proportionate" and "disproportionate".

93

Reference

Häring B. *Medical ethics*. Slough: St Paul Publications, 1991: 129–33.

See also: Treatment.

BHo

F

Facts vs values Philosophers have long distinguished facts from values, although there remains disagreement about their relationship. The importance of the distinction for medicine lies in the degree to which a medical judgment is based on fact (and relies on objective and scientifically gathered information and assessment), or an evaluation, both within the accepted medical sphere and beyond. Kennedy showed that many medical diagnoses actually depended on societal judgments and argued that the decisions in those cases should therefore not be made just by doctors. The distinction is further blurred since medicine is no longer seen to be derived from a simple biological model but from a complex *biopsychosocial* (*see biopsychosocial model*) background. Healthcare workers would do well to distinguish which evidence seems factual and which is evaluative (based on personal or societal values). But the complexities of philosophical arguments are probably strictly for academics and the realities of health care often demand that decisions be made on inadequate data. "This one will run and run", to quote learned sources.

Reference

Kennedy I. *The Unmasking of Medicine*. London: Allen and Unwin, 1981.

See also: Society, views in medical ethics.

RH

Fairness Another word for *justice*, especially when those involved freely recognise that each has a "fair share" of the benefits and burdens, or that the arrangements are "fair and square". Recognition of what is "fair" (literally, pleasing to the eye), like *"elegance"* in science, is partly aesthetic. Fairness is an important aspect of John Rawls's contract theory of justice.

Reference

Rawls J. *A theory of justice*. Oxford: Oxford University Press, 1973.

KMB

Faith, bad faith and faithfulness Faith implies trust or confidence, in one's fellows or in God, and a belief in the efficacy of a treatment or the power of a healer is known to be potent and effective in medical care in general. Such *trust* can be abused, and may hold implicit promises: for instance, a *patient* who "has faith" in a doctor is also expressing a view that that professional will continue to respond positively towards her. The professional could be seen, in some sense, to have made an implicit promise to do so, and needs to be faithful to the expectations created. The dilemma is that this response may not come wholeheartedly from the centre of the professional's being, but be part of the *role*, a part "play acted", if you will, and this for thinkers like Sartre would be a supreme example of bad faith, that is, lack of *integrity*.

See also: Promise keeping.

RH

Fallacy A false step in an argument, which seems but is not conclusive. Either the *logic* is invalid or the *rhetoric*, however plausible, confuses or misses the real point. Although from the Latin for "to deceive", in practice often from emotion or ignorance.

KMB

Families The family has been described as a mythological organisation; not because it is a meaningless concept but because it is highly idealised and exerts power over both imagination and emotion. In consequence, the definition varies across societies, over historical time and within subcultures. It has as many definitions as there are people. Historically, lineage has defined the family: a person is emotionally embedded within society by those who are taken to be forebears. Pedigree has become increasingly unimportant. Now the family is mostly regarded as providing a context in which to achieve intimacy and relaxation for adults and nurture for children. The powerful mythology of the family means that any definitions are likely to be considered by some to be oppressive or excluding. The nuclear family (two biological parents living with their biological offspring) remains an ideal in many people's minds, but, in fact, wider and wider configurations of household organisation occur. The nature of parenthood and marriage changes. Social acceptance and public expression of *gender* identity and the changing view of women's place in work modify the structures that people use to gain intimate relationships. Social structures for childcare are extending beyond the family.

Ethnic variation produces multiple forms of family organisation, each of which can be taken as the norm within its own ethnic group.

Despite the diversity and the multiplicity of family structures, the intimate psychological context within which people grow has a profound effect on their sense of identity and belongingness. The emotional security and sanctuary provided by the intimate household for children in the course of development has crucial effects on their future ability to make relationships and to maintain mental health. The familiar and special psychological qualities of the household within which people live as adults contributes to their definition of themselves, their support, nurture, and fulfilment in life.

See also: Child, status of; culture.

CD

Family medicine is often used as loosely equivalent to *general practice*, but should properly refer to the organisation of health care around families or equivalent social groups rather than individuals. It thus takes a particular view of the aims and methods of generalist (as contrasted with specialist) practice or *primary care*, and has been particularly influential in the organisation of such care in the USA. Seeing the family as the prime object of care can be very powerful in the prevention or management of conditions such as infectious disease, and in childhood illness, degenerative or genetic disorders and life events where understanding of interactions within a family group can provide understanding in a way which individual biomedicine cannot. However, such an approach presents of necessity new practical and ethical problems relating to *conflicts* of *values*, *boundaries* and *roles*. How should one view the *adolescent* patient who is leaving the family, or the (perhaps increasing) number of people who prefer a single lifestyle, are in same sex relationships or for whom family interactions remain a negative experience? The extension of the concept to describe the interactions of a team of health care workers may be semantically confusing but may give insight into the dilemmas raised by such work.

Reference

Christie R, Hoffmaster C. *Ethical issues in family medicine*. New York: Oxford University Press, 1986.

See also: Confidentiality; chronic disease; systems theory; teamwork.

RH

Fatigue syndromes Variously termed as chronic or post-viral fatigue syndrome, and also known as ME (myalgic encephalomyelitis), this comprises a group of chronic disorders in which patients experience severe fatigue together with a variety of other neuromuscular and cognitive symptoms that are exacerbated by physical or other activity, and thus greatly constrain what they can do. Although quite common, they remain much misunderstood by the public and doctors. This reflects the diversity of symptoms, sometimes intangible, without evident appearance of ill-health or a definitive diagnostic test. Many patients have psychological symptoms, either as a result of the disease or its chronically disabling impact, or because of the frequent experience that other people, including clinicians, do not believe they are ill. Patients commonly make the diagnosis themselves, after hearing popular accounts, perhaps from friends; this may cause resentment in some doctors. They may be seen as *heartsink patients* or be diagnosed as having primary depressive illness, which is indeed an important differential diagnosis.

There is a bewildering array of theories on pathogenesis and approaches to therapy, ranging from the organic to the psychiatric. The illness is among the best current examples of the polarised mind-body debate. This is often exacerbated by systematic bias in clinical referral pattern. *Advocacy/activism* by self-help groups has done much to raise awareness, but has also provoked some negative responses and led to stereotyping of the syndrome, with undue emphasis on the most severe outcomes. Patients often resort to *complementary medicine* due to failings of conventional medicine. Patients can respond to supportive and focused *counselling*, graded physical rehabilitation programmes, and symptom control. Fatigue syndromes currently present a painful reminder of the limitations of the technological slant in contemporary medicine.

Reference
Royal College of Physicians, Royal College of Psychiatrists, Royal College of General Practitioners. *Chronic fatigue syndrome*. Report of a joint working group: 1996, CR54.

AJP

Fault A human failing (from Latin for "to slip", as in geology). Although fallibility (to err) is human, it is also human to find fault or to *blame*, especially when a fault is attributed to carelessness or habitual inattention. Defining such elusive terms and establishing moral *responsibility* for a fault can be difficult in ethics, but is often crucial in law related to medical *negligence* and *compensation*.

See also: Complaints.

KMB

Felicific *See* Happiness, greatest.

Female sterilisation Aiming at permanent sterility, this is usually carried out surgically. Passage of sperm, eggs or embryos through the Fallopian tubes is prevented by artificially obstructing them. The consequences of the procedure should always be fully understood by the woman beforehand, preferably including a partner – where appropriate – in the preparatory discussion.

See also: Sterilisation.

JAM

Feminism Although there are different forms of feminism, eg, liberal, radical, and ecological, its core characteristic is an acknowledgment that women are discriminated against.

Since sexism pervades the world it therefore pervades the medical world, itself, many feminists would say, a bastion of male power which "has historically been dominated by a male standard of normality".[1]

Feminists would regard any form of medical ethics that does not acknowledge this as inherently sexist and seek to remedy it as hardly ethical at all in that it is perpetuating injustice to half its patients by being part of a system that discriminates against them.

One feminist strand of thought emphasises women's basing of morality in connectedness rather than in *autonomy*. This can be seen as a way of broadening thinking on morality, has implications for the principle of autonomy and challenges health care workers to see their patients in terms of their relationships and their women patients in particular in terms of the responsibility for caring for others that traditionally has been theirs.

Abortion continues to be controversial, with feminists asking why women should need permission from doctors to have abortions. In particular the matter of the humanity of the *fetus*, with the increasing emphasis on fetal, as opposed to maternal rights, is of deep concern to feminists.

There is unease too about the use of reproductive technologies to remedy *infertility* problems. Some feminists argue that societal pressure on women to see themselves as unfulfilled – somehow not "real women" if they don't have children – results in their being driven to desperate lengths to become mothers. Other feminists argue that women are capable of making up their own minds whether they want children and if they have problems conceiving, deciding what, if anything, they are prepared to do to have a child.

Reference
Cook, RJ. Feminism and the four principles. In: Gillon R, Lloyd A, eds. *Principles of health care ethics*. Chichester: John Wiley, 1994: 193–206.

See also: Women's rights.

ALl

Fertility *See* Infertility.

Fetal tissue transplant This involves the use of fetal tissue implanted into patients. The most common indication for this procedure at present is Parkinson's disease in which a fetal brain implant can lead to significant regression of symptoms. The potential use of organs, including the liver, kidney and heart, from fetuses at a more advanced stage of gestation has been postulated. Fetal tissue is less likely to be seen as "foreign" by the immune system.

While there is no doubting the medical benefit from such procedures the question of whose *right* it is to decide whether or not fetal tissue should be used is a difficult one. The rights of the *fetus* should be taken into consideration. Some women, faced with the difficult decision of accepting a termination, derive some comfort from the fact that their fetal tissue may be used for the benefit of others. Difficulties would arise if the practice became widespread and people were moved to conceive simply for the purpose of producing organs for their own use or for the use of close friends or relatives. Conversely, enormous pressure could be put on to individuals to conceive in order to help relatives.

ALo

Fetus and embryo An embryo results from the fertilisation of an oocyte by a spermatazoaon. Strictly speaking, the term embryo is used to describe a conceptus up to 12 weeks of gestation, at which stage it becomes a fetus. In common usage the term fetus is applied to the conceptus at an earlier gestation. The fundamental ethical question with relation to the fetus/embryo is: when does it become a *person*. Some people believe that this occurs at the moment of fertilisation, some when neurological connections are made. In law, it is held that the fetus becomes an individual when it is capable of independent extra-uterine survival. In 1967 when the Abortion

Act became law in Great Britain this watershed occurred at 28 weeks of gestation. Since the mid 1960s there have been a number of significant improvements in perinatal medicine and the limit for legal termination has been decreased to 24 weeks of gestation.

Assisted reproductive technology has created a fresh set of ethical dilemmas for medical and paramedical professionals, concerned with the ownership and storage of embryos created as a result of fertility treatment.

See also: Abortion; viability.

ALo

Fiat (Latin for let it be done) means a highly authoritative and effective command; originally religious, as in "God said 'Let there be light' and there was light"; "fiat mihi", submission to a command, as in the Virgin Mary's "be it unto me according to thy word".

KMB

Fiduciary relationship A relationship of mutual trust or confidence (from the Latin "fido" "I *trust*"); hence *confidentiality*.

KMB

Fidelity A consistent and reliable response to colleagues or to patients is central to the practice of good medicine. It would be unthinkable for a surgeon in an emergency or a GP on a Monday morning, just to declare "she didn't feel like it today". Likewise, since much serious disease is long term, recurrent or chronic (acute illness being often self-limiting per se), a doctor who enters a relationship with a patient should understand the likely length of that relationship and the need for a consistent and faithful management of the condition, as part of the *duty* of (long-term) *care*.

RH

Flourishing *See* Eudaemonia.

Fluoridation Evidence over 50 years has shown that fluoridation is a safe and effective method of preventing dental caries resulting in a large and equitably distributed preventive effect in the population it services.

Fluoridation has been argued to infringe individual *autonomy* but failure to implement it may infringe the equivalent *rights* of those who stand to benefit.

Reference
Harris J. *The ethics of fluoridation.* The British Fluoridation Society, 1989.

RH/CSc

Force feeding The World Medical Association's Declaration of Tokyo (1975) permits *prisoners* to refuse nourishment if the doctor confirms that they are capable of forming an unimpaired judgment.

The capacity to make a decision under common law, requires the ability to receive and retain relevant information and the capacity to believe it. Force feeding could technically be an assault. However, in 1994 the British Court of Appeal upheld the decision of a High Court judge that force feeding was treatment for mental disorder and that the Mental Health Act allowed a person to be fed against her will, irrespective of Common Law capacity.

References
British Medical Association. *Assessing mental capacities.* London: British Medical Association, 1996.
Medical ethics today: its practice and philosophy. London: British Medical Association, 1995.

See also: Eating disorders; mental illness.

VC

Forensic psychiatry is the practice of psychiatry where it comes into contact with the *law*. This is not simply criminal work, but might involve individuals in other work that is connected to the law. In practice, however, the bulk of the work is to do with criminal behaviour in patients with psychological disorder. An increasing number of psychiatric patients are referred to psychiatrists either from courts, *police* or prisons. The psychiatrist is then in the difficult position of being required to give information about the patient to individuals other than medical officers, social workers or lawyers. The ethics of the passage of information is delicate but usually it is clear.

(i) Information to police: Information must never be given to the police about patients under the care of a doctor. Police officers may ask for information where a crime has been committed. However, information concerning a crime should be given to the legal representative of the patient, not directly to the police.

Where an individual is compulsorily detained on a Section of the Mental Health Acts (UK) and is absent without leave from an inpatient unit, the police must be informed: compulsorily detained patients are in hospital by law and are not allowed to leave without the permission of the responsible medical officer; their status is the same as that of *prisoners*. If they are missing the police must be informed. Occasionally the police ask medical and nursing staff to inform them when a patient is being discharged. This information should not be given, as it is entirely confidential. When a patient is discharged from hospital, her Section is also discharged. The patient then becomes informal and the police therefore no longer have any right or reason to know of the patient's whereabouts. It is only when the patient remains on a Section that help from the police may be asked for if she is missing from the unit.

(ii) Courts and probation service: Should a court or a probation officer request a report on a patient, that report may be given with or without the patient's consent. Patients should be advised that they should be legally represented when they are in difficulty with the police. However, the doctor may give a report to a court and/or a probation officer if requested.

(iii) Reporting of serious crime: If patients impart information that concerns their involvement in committing serious crime, ie, *murder, rape* or arson, the responsible medical officer is obliged by law to impart that information to the police. The law of *confidentiality* does not override common law, which requires every citizen to report serious crime. Patients who confess to serious crime should immediately be informed by their doctor that she is duty bound to report it. Clearly, there will be a *conflict* of duty when reporting the crime. However, medical staff have a responsibility to the law of the land, and to individuals who live within the community to keep them safe, as well as a *duty of care* to their patient.

Patients who commit serious crime become a danger within the community and the doctor's role then extends beyond her immediate care to the patient. Reporting serious crime also protects the patient, should she be mentally ill, from continuing to commit serious crime which, in itself, will complicate and disrupt that individual's life and further medical care.

(iv) Evidence in court: If a psychiatrist is asked in court to give sensitive or confidential information about her patient she may refuse to do so. However, if she is directed by the judge to give the information requested, she should do so or she will be in contempt of court.

(v) Child welfare: When a practitioner is concerned about the physical or psychological *wellbeing* of a child, the child's needs have precedence over confidentiality towards any adult involved. Therefore if a doctor is informed that a child is being abused by a parent, and the parent is the informant, the doctor's duty of care is to the child in the first instance and not to the abusing parent, even if the abusing parent is the patient, not the child.

See also: Child abuse; child, status of.

RSi

Forgiveness Literally "giving away", ie, not "holding anything against" someone; hence to say "I forgive but will not forget what you did" is not to forgive. If "to forgive all" requires first "to know all", forgiveness is understandably difficult for humans. But resentment can obscure moral vision by focusing on the other's *faults* rather than on one's own *freedom*; and human flourishing may be possible only in proportion to mutual forgiveness.

KMB

Fostering See Adoption and fostering.

Four principles See Autonomy; beneficence; justice; non-maleficence.

Frameworks Most difficult problems need to be approached in a systematic way, and medical ethics is no exception. The need is for an internalised method of thinking and feeling that will enable an individual to perceive that there is a moral problem, identify it as clearly as possible but in its complexity, and be able to make progress through understanding (empathically and intellectually) and imagination in order to reach some form of conclusion as part of *clinical judgment* or activity. Such a difficult task will require some frameworks of thinking, so as to make reasoning as logical, comprehensive, and explicit as possible.

See also: Empathy.

RH

Fraud in medical *research* came into prominence in 1983. Several instances were reported in this and the following years, principally in the USA but also in Australia, Canada, the UK, and the Nordic countries. In retrospect, however, probably a little research has always been fraudulent. Reports have implicated workers as famous and as diverse as Cyril Burt, Admiral Peary, Heinrich Schliemann, and even Mendel and Newton.

The major types comprise fabrication of data, *plagiarism*, and piracy (stealing ideas). Nevertheless, this list has been extended and hence several countries now prefer to use the term "scientific dishonesty". This also includes *conflict of interest* (professional or commercial), "gift" or "honorary" *authorship*, failure to acknowledge or denigration of previous work, and "massaging" of data (excluding inconvenient results).

The prevalence of fraud is unknown. Some dismiss it as rare, but surveys have shown that over ten years more than a quarter of scientists had encountered an average of 2.5 cases.

Ideas about the cause owe much to the Nobel Prize winner Sir Peter Medawar. Some cases he ascribed to mere deviance, affecting biomedicine no less than the rest of society. Some also were due to the need to have results for publication, given that this is the current benchmark for research grants, tenure, or promotion – while a few were associated with frank mental illness.

But most, Medawar thought, were due to a "Messianic complex" in the fraudster – the conviction that he (and almost all fraudsters have been men) knew the cause of, say, schizophrenia or cancer, and would do anything to save people from developing these, including faking results to prove his case.

Several countries have formed organisations to deal with research fraud. These cover its prevention and the management of a suspected case. The former includes teaching postgraduates about good research practices, and seeing that institutions have policies about data retention, authorship, and supervision of juniors. Management is in three stages: receipt of the complaint by a senior figure (usually the dean or head of the institution); inquiry by 'three wise men' (senior disinterested scientists, one an expert) to see whether there is a case; and investigation, a formal hearing, in which evidence may be tested by cross-examination.

Many of the ethical implications of fraud are self evident. All invented results are a waste of society's finite *resources*; some may even put patients at risk, and the betrayal of colleagues' trust may be devastating. Local *research ethics committees* (or institutional review boards) have a responsibility in prevention. They should, eg, raise questions over applications for an untoward number of research projects from a single source not apparently equipped to do these.

Crucially, moreover, suspected fraud must be managed with *due process*, protecting the rights of both the accused and the "whistleblower" (the complainant, who in many cases has been far more penalised than the miscreant). Above all, all professions have an ethical obligation to set their own standards and to enforce these.

See also: Clinical research and trials; experts and expertise; whistleblowing.

SL

Freedom or liberty, may mean "not bound" (freedom from) or "unimpeded action" (freedom for). "Total freedom" (acting without cause or reason) is psychologically and philosophically problematic. Personal freedom (or free will) in practice is often associated with self-knowledge. Politically, most parties appeal to freedom

(from tyranny, *poverty*, disease; of choice).

See also: Autonomy.

KMB

Friendship has often been used as a model to explain some of the usual facets of a long term *doctor–patient relationship*. However, this may be problematical, because, although a long term patient may become a friend, most medical authorities would advise that friends do not become patients. Also, there may be a need for objectivity in clinical care and a close relationship could create difficulties.

RH

Fundamentalism Any religious (or ideological) movement defending the "fundamentals" of its faith with a literal interpretation of its scriptures or doctrines. Problematical, because such interpretations often involve presuppositions post-dating what they interpret; and paradoxical in religions (eg, *Christianity*) born from protest against literalism – but also populist and powerful, since it is less demanding to subscribe to the letter than live by the spirit of religion.

KMB

Fundholding A voluntary scheme, introduced as part of the *National Health Service* (NHS) reforms of 1991, that gives certain general practitioners an annual budget to purchase defined areas of health care for their patients. The principle is to bring the decisions about the *purchasing* and provision of health care as close to patients as possible. The scheme includes all prescribing, staff, and diagnostic test costs, and has been developed into three types: community, standard, and total fundholding, depending on the amount of community and hospital services included. Savings may

101

be used to improve the services available to patients, *audit*, training, and research and development.

Ethical concerns have focused on the *resources* made available to these practices, and the possible effect of financial considerations influencing decisions in the consultation.

See also: Conflict of interest; general practice; healthcare systems.

TE

Futility is a term used to refer to medical *treatment* that is unlikely to achieve its desired aim, and thus to justify a medical judgment not to provide life prolonging treatment requested by "unrealistic" patients, parents, or relatives. Problems with the concept include the uncertainty of prognosis in individual cases, differing value judgments about probabilities worth chancing, and whose desired aims are to count. While doctors have no obligation to provide treatment they judge futile, careful explanation of the therapeutic options and efforts to reach a joint decision with the patient and/or family are preferable to invoking futility as a *fiat*.

Reference
Weijer C, Elliot C. Pulling the plug on futility. *BMJ* 1995; **310**: 683–4.

See also: Decision-making capacity.

KMB

G

Gatekeeping is a function ascribed particularly to general practitioners in the *National Health Service* in the UK; it serves to point up an important difference between two methods of access to a system of health or social care. A system may be set up either with open access for any who have the ability to purchase its services or who have rights of access – welfare rights – to any services under a state-funded welfare system; or it may be established with a gatekeeper, usually a professional with the discretionary function of sorting out those who have "real" need, or who could benefit most from the services offered. The disadvantage of gatekeeping is that clients may be at the mercy of an individual professional's judgment, and there is a danger of a reverse and cynical definition of *need*, that is, a "genuine" need is defined as something that can be addressed by the current services. (It seems more healthy that the needs people express should constantly challenge the service, as needs will change.) In favour of gatekeeping it could be said that a well-disposed and well-informed generalist can both act as an advocate for the client and can re-shape her request into the most beneficial form. As it is impossible for any system to foresee every person's likely future need or for an individual to understand all that can be offered, the positive interpretation of a gatekeeping role, even with all its attendant risks of *paternalism*, seems important for the primary care section of any health service. But such practitioners should be good practitioners in the broadest sense.

The term gatekeeping has also been applied to a system for checking and filtering referral letters from general practitioners by hospital contracts departments to exclude and refer back those that are outside agreed contracts. This was considered to breach the referring and receiving clinicians' professional duties and has generally been abandoned.

See also: General practice.

RH/AJP

Gender is a system of classification based on sex. The classification may be applied, inter alia, to individuals, behaviours, occupations, objects, clothing, and language. The simplest form of classification involves assignment either to a masculine or feminine gender, based on male and female sex respectively. Assignment to a neutral gender based on intermediate or indeterminate sex may also occur. In modern industrialised societies, there is an overwhelming pressure to classify all individuals as either masculine or feminine, congruent as far as is possible with their male or female genitalia. However, in other societies, and historically, ambiguity of genitalia (whether of developmental or secondary origin) could be accommodated in a third or intersex gender, eg, the berdache (Africa or North America) or Hijra (India). This third gender is generally characterised by distinct attributes and its members assigned special social roles.

The precise attributes used to define the gender of an individual are culturally contingent, varying both historically and with the society in which the individual lives. Certain primary attributes tend to recur and to reflect differences in the biology of males and females, especially their different reproductive roles. These include "feminine" attributes of nurturing, consensuality, emotionality and vulnerability, each expressed primarily within the private domain. "Masculine" attributes include wealth generation, confrontation, domination and control, self-sacrifice and rationality, exercised largely in the public domain. These primary differences are perceived to be associated with gendered differences in personality and in intellectual and affective characteristics. Other attributes are secondary and more idiosyncratic, including styles of clothing and body decoration, language, and permitted or accepted social, religious, cultural and employment activities. However, whilst a society may be highly gendered, in that it seeks to distinguish the two sexes by many criteria, there is in reality a

wide variation among individuals of the same sex in the possession of the gendered attributes and an almost complete overlap between the sexes for many attributes. Thus, most of the gendered structure is built not upon real and absolute sex differences but by the social and cultural elaboration of small or imagined differences. Thus, gender seems to be largely a culturally defined and constructed concept.

Some societies are said to be strongly gendered, in that an individual's sex is the major determinant of what that individual may or may not do socially. Other societies are less strongly gendered, in that features such as age, class/caste or occupation are as or more important than sex in determining what an individual may or may not do. For an individual in any gendered society, the formation of a sense of gender identity as masculine or feminine is important. The formation of a gender identity involves the development of a conceptual framework of what it is to be a man or woman in that society and the clear identification of your place within that framework congruent with your sex. Gender confusion implies the absence of a clear and congruent sense of your position within that framework. An individual's gender identity is manifested in behaviours through which an accepted gender role in society is expressed. It is widely believed, given the strong cultural contingence of gender attributes, that gender is learnt during childhood and is socially reinforced. However, genetic, neural and endocrine contributions to the establishment or reinforcement of a gender identity have also been suggested but not proven.

Given the strong association between gender attributes and reproductive differences, it is not suprising that in gendered societies, such as occur in Europe and its derived cultures, there is assumed to be a strong association between gender identity and sexual preference, a strong masculine gender identity being expected to coincide with a heterosexual attraction to women, for example. While homosexuality may be observed in individuals who experienced gender confusion during and after childhood, many *homosexual* men and women have strong gender identities congruent with their genital sex. Some gender confusion among homosexuals may be a secondary reaction to the perceived social linkage of sexuality and gender in combination with negative reactions to homosexuality. A clear separation of sex, gender and sexual preference may be observed in transsexuals. Transsexuals may be of either sex (male/female) and attracted to either the same or opposite sex erotically (homo-/hetero-sexual), but experience their gender identity as the opposite of their sex.

For doctors who are trained within a gendered society with its general social framework that regards congruence of sex, gender and heterosexuality as the norm and to be expected, absence or ambiguity of congruence can be viewed as pathological. The doctor's own gender can also influence significantly her work with patients and colleagues.

References

Golombok S, Firush R. *Gender development*. Cambridge: Cambridge University Press, 1994.

Ortner SB, Whitehead H. *Sexual meanings*. Cambridge: Cambridge University Press, 1982.

See also: Culture; sex change; sex, determination of.

MHJ

General Medical Council (GMC) as the *statutory body* provides the regulatory mechanism for doctors. Established by the 1858 Medical Act, the GMC: sets standards for medical training; maintains the register of doctors entitled to practise; publishes ethical guidance; and disciplines doctors.

All practising doctors are accountable to the GMC.

See also: Accountability; medical education; professionalism; professional responsibility; self – regulation.

ASo

General practice is a system of health care which responds to the unsorted and immediate needs of individuals as people (in contrast to specialist practice which defines its range of work according to disease type, body system or patient group). It is a major component of *primary care*, being the natural first port of call for those who define themselves as ill, and may contain aspects of *family medicine*. In the UK it is usually delivered from a *practice* by groups or teams of differing size and make-up, responding both to those who walk in (ambulatory care) and those who require *home visits*, as well as providing *out of hours* cover. Some have claimed that it is now the best way of delivering personal, preventive, anticipatory and continuing health care to individuals and families.[1] Its *gatekeeping* function may ensure that self-limiting illness is not unnecessarily investigated and that specialist services are reserved for those who need them most: properly organised, skilled and equipped general practice can respond to the large majority of illness episodes.

Since under normal circumstances the majority of patients presenting do not have a life-threatening disease one task of clinicians in general practice is to educate and reassure, whilst also being alert in order to "marginalise danger" by identifying medically serious conditions (for secondary care if necessary). In this, aims and methods may differ from *hospital medicine*. By virtue of being close to and knowledgeable about the families and social situations of patients, general practice staff can make broad assessments using the *biopsychosocial model*, accept the *uncertainty* of lack of formal diagnosis or closure by using its own *eclectic* categorisations, and gain understanding by focusing as much on the management of the process of individual presentations and *illness behaviour* as on reaching defined outcomes. Some practitioners therefore often proceed by testing hypotheses in several consultations over time, backing up clinical assessment from insights gained in the interaction or from previous encounters rather than by routine laboratory investigations as in the traditional hospital "clerking" model.

The moral problems encountered by users and staff also may differ from those of secondary care because of relationships between patient and professional. Within the team, the aims, methods and *values* of the individuals (which may in turn differ from the overall values of the system or institution), and the many *roles* carried by one individual, all increase the potential for confusion. Eg, the doctor may employ the nurse, who may also be friend, neighbour and (in an isolated practice) patient: the *receptionist* may know more details about a patient's life than the nursing or medical staff because their children play together etc. The professionals may act in the role of advocate, assessor for benefits, agent of a building society, citizen, protector of the children, guardian of the public purse or fund-holding decision-maker, and so on. Distinguishing roles, sorting out who is the person with the moral problem, attending to the person or group least heard, and having insight into the *aims* and *values* of each person or group involved in a dilemma, whilst also being clear about the aims, purposes and values of general practice itself are some of the tasks for a

thinker in this area before she moves on to consider the issues within the usual ethical frameworks. The *complexity* of this work well done makes it amongst the most challenging but rewarding in health care, probably more so for "foxes" than "hedgehogs".[2] To borrow from Jewish humour, it may often be a case of "two GPs, three opinions".

References
1 Royal College of General Practitioners. *The future general practitioner.* Exeter: RCGP, 1989.
2 Berlin I. *The hedgehog and the fox; Russian thinkers.* London: Penguin Books, 1979.

See also: Fundholding; National Health Service.

RH

Generations, rights of future A phrase expressing concern that present human activities are threatening, or at least limiting, the scope of our descendants. It usually refers to the rapid diminution of key resources, eg, fossil fuels, or of natural ecosystems, eg, forests or soils. Such widespread concern is modern. Until recently the earth seemed infinite and human influences minor and transitory. Concern about the rights of future generations may well be regarded as a luxury confined to rich societies, where cynics have been known to riposte: "What did the future ever do for me?"

See also: Ecology.

AM

Generosity indicates a personal nature or attitude that is liberal and prepared to give, in any sense: for instance, people may be generous with money, friendship, their own time, but also in allowing others opportunities or chances to improve themselves. Its opposites would be selfishness and narrow-mindedness. Generosity is important in clinical medicine because it confirms the humanity of a caring interaction, offers space for moral questioning or reframing, and respects individuals' self-rule.

See also: Autonomy; gifts.

RH

Genetic counselling is the process of providing individuals and families who are at risk of, or affected by, a genetic disease with information about the condition, its inheritance and their options. Prior to genetic counselling, an accurate diagnosis must be made using specialist investigations, eg, direct gene tests or chromosome studies.

The ethical basis of genetic counselling is that people must be enabled to make their **own** informed *choice*. Thus two different couples who experience the same genetic condition in their families may choose quite different options as a result of nondirective genetic counselling. This must recognise the clients' emotions and psychological background, and empower them to make decisions based on all the facts as well as their own feelings. Although a person may have a high chance of developing a genetic disorder, she has a right "not to know" or not to seek presymptomatic tests.

Provision of genetic counselling services varies greatly from one country to another. In the UK these are provided by genetic centres staffed by multidisciplinary teams; the emphasis is on a medically oriented service. In contrast, in the USA, genetic counselling is carried out by non-medical counsellors, trained in genetics and counselling techniques. Teamwork is the bedrock of good genetic counselling services.

Reference

Clark A. *Genetic counselling, practice and principles.* London: Routledge, 1994.

See also: Genetics; genetic disorders.

JAR

Genetic disorders There are several different classes of genetic disorders. First, there are some 4000 diseases that are inherited according to Mendelian laws of inheritance. These are due to a single defective gene. Second, there are disorders that result from major abnormalities of chromosomes. Third, there are many common disorders that result from genetic susceptibility to different environmental agents. Because such susceptibilities usually reflect the action of several different genes, these conditions are called "polygenic". Finally, there are acquired conditions such as *cancer* and ageing that seem to result from changes in the genetic constitution occuring spontaneously owing to the action of various mutagens.

Recently, with the advent of molecular biology and recombinant DNA technology, it has been possible to make rapid progress towards an understanding of the cause of many genetic diseases. It is now feasible to isolate human genes, clone them in bacteria, amplify them, determine their DNA base sequence, and transfer them into other cells or animals to study their function. As well as diagnosis and counselling, the "new genetics" is developing techniques for correcting genetic diseases, or gene therapy. This may involve either somatic gene therapy, that is, the injection of genes into body cells other than germ cells, or germ cell therapy, in which genes are inserted into fertilised eggs; genetic information transferred in this way will be expressed in future generations. The new genetics also leads to the identification of genes for susceptibility or resistance to common diseases of middle and old age and play a major role in preventative medicine by defining subgroups of individuals that are particularly sensitive to the effects of environmental damage.

It will soon be possible to identify *carriers* and offer *prenatal diagnosis* by fetal DNA for most common genetic diseases. Several ethical questions arise. Is, eg, *abortion* of a fetus carrying a serious genetic disease acceptable? If it is found that it is more cost-effective to terminate pregnancies carrying serious genetic diseases rather than look after affected children in the community, will pressure be put on parents to undergo this procedure? What do we mean by disease? Although in many western societies few seem to doubt the right of parents to decide not to have children with crippling inherited diseases, there is an increasing tendency to opt for prenatal diagnosis for much milder conditions that are compatible with a normal life span.

Gene therapy is also raising some ethical questions. While somatic gene therapy is no different in principle to organ *transplantation* thoughts are turning to germline therapy. Since in this case genes will be passed on to generations that have had no input into the original decision, new ethical problems will be raised. And given our ability to transfer genes there is increasing concern that this new technology will, in the future, be used for so-called "enhancement therapy", that is, for encouraging traits such as height, musical ability, and other social skills that seem desirable by a potential child's parents. Although there is no evidence that such traits are due to single genes, the possibility remains that it might be possible to enhance certain activities by the insertion of several genes in the long term.

As more is known about the genes involved in the susceptibility to common diseases of middle life, there are fears that our genetic profiles may be made available to employers, life *insurance* companies, and others who may use them as they wish. It is essential that those whose genetic profiles show disease susceptibilities are not disadvantaged. The end result could be a gross inequality of the cost of health insurance and care. Another major concern is the stigmatisation of those with certain traits that are thought to be genetic, homosexuality, psychotic or criminal behaviour, and alcoholism. Although there may be genes involved in these phenotypes there is undoubtedly a major environmental component and it will be many years before the relative roles of nature and nurture are determined.

The other major ethical issue arising from the new genetics is the fear of a resurgence of *eugenics*. Eugenics, which literally means "well-born", first evolved in the UK at the turn of the century from the writings of Francis Galton. Although it was built on a wish for a better and more intelligent society many of its tenets were based on a false idea about the inheritance of intelligence and other beneficial traits. The movement was supported by some of the founders of human genetics, both in Great Britain, and in the USA and elsewhere. It petered out after the Second World War and the discovery of the activities of the Nazi movement in the name of eugenics. It has had a revival with the development of human molecular genetics, the resurgence of the IQ debate, and the socio-biological and biological deterministic movements. New laws have been passed in China to eliminate "inferior births", for example by forbidding those with a hereditary disease from marrying. There are indications in other countries that the principles of the eugenics movement are never far below the surface in thinking about the future of society.

References

Kelves DJ, Hood LR (eds). *Scientific and social issues in the human gene project*. Cambridge, Mass: Harvard University Press, 1992.

Holtzman NA. *Proceed with caution*. Baltimore: Johns Hopkins University Press, 1989.

Weatherall DJ. *The new genetics and clinical practice*. Oxford: Oxford University Press, 1992.

See also: Genetics.

DW

Genetics originated from the study of how biological traits are inherited. Since the pioneering work of Gregorius Mendel around 1850 it has been realised that the physical basis for this inheritance consists of discrete elements called genes. A gene is a segment of DNA, which encodes in its sequence both the structure and the amount of the gene product, which is usually a protein. A particular gene often exists in several different forms, called alleles. The study of the precise structure of genes and of their products is called molecular genetics. Techniques used in this area often involve cutting and joining pieces of DNA of different origin, i.e. genetic engineering or recombinant DNA technology. One of the most publicised achievements of molecular genetics is the successful introduction of functional genes into living cells (gene transfer). Gene transfer into embryonic cells of animals (most commonly mice), with its subsequent germ-line transmission to offspring (transgenic lines), has been used extensively to investigate the expression of genes *in vivo*. A related technique is the inactivation of an individual gene in order to pinpoint conclusively its function (gene targeting or "knockout").

Much progress has been made in mapping how genes are arranged on the 23 pairs of chromosomes that constitute the human *genome* From the medical point of view, genetics has been concerned primarily with inherited disorders which are generally due to changes (mutations) in the germ-cells: but in recent years it has been realised that disease can also arise through similar changes taking place in other cells in the body (somatic mutations). *Cancers* are certainly the most common and important group of conditions arising largely through somatic mutations, although some of the mutations responsible can be inherited as well.

Several aspects of genetics have potential ethical implications.

(i) Knowledge of certain genetic traits may have a profound emotional impact on an individual because they may affect the likelihood of developing a particular disease, or the chance of causing disease in the offspring. Therefore it is imperative that: (a) pertinent tests be carried out only after obtaining *informed consent*, and (b) the wish of the patient to know or not to know the result be respected. For these reasons, testing of children below an age at which they can give meaningful informed consent is a particularly delicate matter, and it is best avoided unless medical intervention at an early age is of the essence.

(ii) Certain allelic forms of certain genes might be associated with early death, leading to denials or difficulties with life and/or health *insurance*. It is understandable that insurance companies must match premiums to risks, but then they ought to make adjustments for favourable as well as unfavourable genes. As far as health cover is concerned, society as a whole should provide it for inherited conditions at least as much as for acquired conditions, since an individual cannot be held responsible for having a certain gene.

(iii) Gene transfer could be used for therapeutic purposes, for instance for treating an inherited blood disease by introducing into bone-marrow cells the normal form of a gene that is mutated and defective in a particular patient (somatic gene therapy). Because any such treatment is highly experimental, it should be subject to all the safeguards – including informed consent – that are mandatory for any new form of treatment. On the other hand, the allegation that this would be a form of "genetic manipulation", unacceptable because against nature, should be rejected, because it is based on tendentious phrasing and/or misconception. Indeed, such treatment would be no more unnatural than using a gene product such as insulin to treat diabetes; and since the gene is introduced only into the bone marrow, it does not entail manipulation of the inherited genome. At the moment somatic gene therapy is limited much more by major technical hurdles than by its risks.

(iv) Since germ-line gene modification is possible in other mammals, it is almost certainly technically possible in humans. This matter is highly controversial. Some argue that if the purpose of the procedure is to prevent a serious disease, there is no a priori reason why it should not be attempted. Others feel that there is a fundamental difference between somatic gene therapy and germ-line gene therapy because the latter is an intervention not just on the individual concerned, but also on subsequent generations. In this respect, germ-line gene therapy *would* differ from any other form of therapy used until now and, if any untoward unexpected side-effects developed, the consequences might be unpredictable. All national and international groups who have considered the matter have concluded that germ-line gene therapy should not be allowed.

See also: Genetic counselling; genetic disorders.

LL

Genome means the entire inherited genetic make-up of each individual. The size of the genome, which consists chemically of DNA, is measured by its number of base pairs (bp): in the human species this is about 3×10^9 arranged into 23 chromosomes of unequal length. It is expected that within a few years most of the genes (estimated number about 100,000) will be mapped, and a significant proportion will be fully sequenced: this massive undertaking is often referred to as the Human Genome Project (HGP). One aspect of the HGP that has ethical implications is that it might be misunderstood to mean that there is such a thing as a "normal" prototype of the human genome. In fact, if the DNA of two random individuals were compared in detail, it is estimated that one would find, on average, one difference in sequence every 1000 bp, ie, as many as one million differences in the entire genome. Thus, there is a vast variability in the human genome, and the variability amongst individuals belonging to the same population is comparable to that among individuals belonging to a different population. Thus, the HGP will help to define genetic differences among individuals and the population (or among populations?), but there is no basis in it for the concept of race.

See also: Genetics.

LL

Geriatric medicine Health care of the elderly, many with multiple pathology and some with impaired *autonomy*, can raise difficult ethical questions – eg, about how actively to investigate or treat, or about what care (residential, nursing home, or hospital) is most appropriate. The relevant criteria are clinical need, efforts to elucidate the patient's wishes and social provisions for care that meet the requirements of *fairness*.

KMB

GIFT stands for Gamete Intrafallopian Transfer. This is a technique for assisted reproduction which was originally devised in order to address the concerns of the Roman Catholic church regarding *in vitro fertilisation* (IVF). Eggs are collected from women following ovarian stimulation. Typically three or four of these eggs are loaded into a transfer catheter together with a suspension of spermatozoa but separated by a micro air bubble. The eggs and spermatozoa are then transferred into the fallopian tube either laparoscopically or trans-cervically where mixing and insemination then occurs.

The technique has become less popular in recent years because it is more expensive than IVF and the results are generally no better than IVF.

ALo

Gifts are sometimes offered to clinicians in gratitude for care received and provide an additional means of individual recognition and *reward*. Recently concern has arisen that they may be used to gain special treatment, perhaps reflecting changes in value systems outside medical and public service traditions. Many health service organisations have introduced guidelines regarding acceptance of gifts, in particular about those that are disproportionate, to avoid personal or corporate culpability, and they may require staff to register any gifts received. Against this, because to exchange gifts and through these express thanks and discharge obligations is a normal human behaviour, to reject gifts may cause distress. In the broader sense, much of health care is based on giving and receiving, whether it is time, attention, blood, a confidential reassurance, sanctuary, or body parts. The giver gives usually without "strings" attached and without expectation of a return, but will expect that the gift is respected, both for itself and the spirit in which it is given, and will neither be wasted nor abused. The morality of giving and receiving is underexplored in medical ethics.

Reference

Titmuss RM. *The gift relationship*. London: Allen and Unwin, 1970.

See also: Gratitude.

AJP/RH

God For theistic religions, the ground of being is by definition undefinable, but not impersonal: knowledge of, but not necessarily about God is possible; myths, metaphors and their inadequacies suggest how. "Playing God" is an incoherent and over-ambitious metaphor, owing more to superstitious fears seeking to set arbitrary limits, than to the religious confidence that scientific curiosity and life and death choices are God-given and thus need to be exercised with loving care.

KMB

Golden Rule "Do unto others as you would be done to by them" – the principle of *reciprocity* taught by, among many others, Confucius, Christ, and Kant. To avoid misinterpretation, it may be necessary to add "if you were in their shoes".

KMB

Good and good enough The search for the good has always been central to philosophical endeavour. In philosophical discussion "goods" refer usually to those entities that we should strive for or value (concepts, virtues, or actions as well as people or things) rather than the current everyday use of consumer products.

In applied ethics, theory often appears to posit some form of "best" action or attitude, or suggest that this elusive creature can be captured by more thought: those at the beginning of clinical practice may share this hope. In reality, dilemmas usually offer at the most a series of unsatisfactory options from which we must choose the least unsatisfactory (least harmful in every sense, least oppressive, etc); and in many cases or situations discussion at whatever level of sophistication is actually only about "getting by", finding a way through which leaves lives and loves intact. Child psychiatry has introduced the "good enough" principle[1] (such as the "good enough parent"), which has been helpful in as much as it enables choosers to steer between the swamp of disgrace or wrongdoing and the frozen heights of anxious inaction, and recognises both the enormous complexity of the factors and field of our choices,[2] and our own necessarily restricted understanding of (and therefore *responsibility* for) the huge range of possible outcomes. Like rowing, life moves forward, while we can only see backwards, and because of this medical ethics struggles to avoid laying *blame* or exacting retribution.

References

1 Winnicott DW. *Playing and reality.* Harmondsworth: Penguin, 1985.
2 Zeldin T. *An intimate history of humanity.* London: Minerva, 1995.

RH

Grace Beauty in motion, or divine assistance: a quality which adds elegance to effort or transfigures the commonplace.

KMB

Gratitude To be thankful for a service is part of normal human currency, and most people are overwhelmingly so when they are restored to full health after a worrying illness. But no professional should expect it as her due.

See also: Gifts.

RH

Greed A voracious appetite for food may present as a clinical problem in patients: a similar appetite for money may distort personal judgment in doctors enough for it to be a recognised "shadow" side of the medical persona.

RH

Grief *See* Loss and grief.

Group work Small groups of up to a dozen or so people are used as the mode of work in treatment and education. In treatment of conditions such as *alcoholism*, problems can be shared between participants and self deception or lack of candour can be challenged. *Confidentiality* and *safety* are group responsibilities. In education, the emphasis is on sharing insights and discovery at a deeper level than rote learning. Group work in ethics can share characteristics of both, since discussion of cases, issues, or ideas enables participants to put forward their own views but make them open to challenge. Group *role play* (with members playing different parts in a problem case) sometimes provides insights that might have been hard to reach through conventional methods.

See also: Silence; support, staff.

RH

Guardianship A guardian is a person who is taking care of a child but is not the legal parent. A parent has parental responsibilities ("meaning all the rights, duties, powers, responsibilities and authority which by law a parent or child has in relation to the child and his property" Section 3, the Children Act 1989 UK). Anyone caring for a child can in an *emergency* act on his or her own initiative and "do what is reasonable in all circumstances of the case for the purpose of safeguarding or promoting the child's welfare" (Section 3, the Children Act 1989). Eg, a teacher is acting as a guardian if she takes an injured child to hospital and signs a consent form on behalf of the parent who is unobtainable. The ethical considerations here would be that the parental *autonomy* is being subsumed and is justified only if reasonable actions were carried out to contact the parent, or failing this another member of the family, and where further delay would be against the child's safety or comfort. The guardian would be expected to act in accordance with the expected wishes of the parents and not to embark deliberately on a course of action that might be known to be contrary to the parents' beliefs. The courts should be involved in the complicated case where a religious belief might make this impossible. The doctors involved must share the responsibility of the guardian in respecting the parents' autonomy, but the child's *welfare* is paramount. Those caring for a child in local authority children's homes, schools, as foster parents, or within the family other than the mother (and father if married) are acting as guardians. It is the responsibility of the local authority to ensure that these people are suitable for such a role and do not put the child at risk. Their right to secrecy is waived in insisting that criminal records are admitted especially when related to crimes against children (especially *child abuse*). Thus again the vulnerability of children is now compensated by placing their welfare at a higher priority than some of the rights of adults, a very different concept from the attitudes of the past.

The more formal term Guardian-ad-litem refers to the person (usually an experienced and specially trained social worker) who is appointed to represent the the child's wishes and interest to courts in family proceedings. The 1989 Children Act stresses that a court making decisions about children "shall have regard in particular to the ascertainable wishes and feelings of the child concerned". This has an important relevance to medical ethics in that doctors may freely share confidential information about their child patients with guardians-ad-litem provided this helps the guardian in interpreting the wishes and feelings of the children. This is difficult in young children but easier with older children who have an increasingly direct say in the proceedings.

There has been a gradual increase in children's autonomy in recent years but at the price of greater stringency over their criminal culpability. This demonstrates the interdependence of rights and responsibilities even in childhood.

See also: Adoption and fostering; child, status of; confidentiality.

GC

Guidelines The term is used in a variety of ways. More important for *bioethics* are the internationally agreed guidelines that have been elaborated, eg, to protect the human subjects of medical research and, more generally, to establish human rights to and in medical treatment. Such guidelines have been prepared by United Nations bodies, of which the World Health Organization has been most active in this field, and by professional organisations such as the World Medical Association.

Second, guidelines represent professional consensus on the treatment of particular diseases.

Third, they may refer to the conclusions of *evidence-based medicine* and be used prescriptively in medical *purchasing* decisions. This last use may raise questions about *clinical freedom*, relations between patients and professionals, and about patient *autonomy*.

DS

Guilt (from Anglo-Saxon "to pay") Feeling of responsibility for having done wrong or caused harm that requires recompense. Courts may determine legal guilt and psychiatry detect pathological guilt, but in ethics attributing and distributing responsibility to and among individuals (eg, in cases of genocide) can be very difficult. Many patients may implicitly or explicitly feel guilt about disease in themselves or others, or about the impact of their disease on others. In some cases this may represent a feeling of guilt about or responsibility for disease (eg, *smoking* and lung *cancer*; *sexually transmitted diseases*); in other cases, it may derive from a perception of disease as a form of punishment, which may have origins in *culture* or religion. Sometimes guilt can itself make people ill.

KMB/AJP

H

Habeas corpus Latin for an action brought to secure the release of a person who is being unlawfully detained. It protects the fundamental right to *liberty*. It could be used to require the release of a patient who was improperly being kept in hospital against her will, eg, outside the terms of the Mental Health Act 1983 or the Public Health (Control of Disease) Act 1984.

JMo

Habit What people automatically do without having to think about it may be good or bad, but no society (or health care system) could function unless there were relatively predictable patterns of behaviour in the population. On the individual level, theoretically the person with true *autonomy* of will could override every habit if she wished to do so, but the perception that we have never yet met such a person suggests that we should develop a more nuanced view of human choosing.

See also: Routines.

RH

Happiness, greatest *Utilitarianism* claims that we should aim to produce "the greatest happiness of the greatest number". Does this mean maximising the average happiness of everyone, or the total amount of happiness, which may be greater if a minority do not share it? Is happiness to be calculated in terms of the quantity or the quality of pleasures, or alternatively in terms

of the satisfaction of people's preferences, which do not always put happiness first? Might it not be more realistic to settle for the minimisation of pain? Is what matters most the effects of one's individual acts, rules of conduct, or way of life as a whole? Such questions led to the modification of Bentham's original "felicific calculus" (calculus of happiness) by Mill, Sidgwick, and others, but as an ideal the intuitive appeal of greatest happiness continues to influence much popular and medical thinking, and to be robustly defended by hedonistic, preference, act, rule, way-of-life and other utilitarian philosophers.

Reference
Sprigge, TLS. *The rational foundations of ethics.* London: Routledge, 1988.

See also: Hedonism.

KMB

Harm Whatever is bad for someone is harmful and nothing is harmful unless it is bad for the one harmed; thus harm is intrinsically a (negatively) evaluative concept. The question of whose evaluation should be determinative is contentious. Subjectivist accounts state that harm is necessarily a subjective matter, with the evaluation of the person potentially harmed being determinative. Objectivist accounts state that harm is objective, its existence and evaluation being possible quite independently of, or even in opposition to, the beliefs and evaluations of the one potentially harmed. As evidence, subjectivists might cite examples of differing personal responses to a proposed medical *treatment*. Thus one person may regard the effects of treatment for mild overactivity of the thyroid gland as beneficial (the patient's metabolism is slowed down by such treatment), for another such effects may be neutral, while for a third they may be perceived as positively harmful, greatly

113

interfering, eg, with this patient's creative ability. Objectivists might respond by arguing that the harms and benefits for each patient might well be different because of their different contexts, idiosyncratic responses and their individual perceptions of those harms and benefits, but that the harms and benefits involved were none the less objective: for in each case the badness or harmfulness for the person concerned was an objective fact, and existed independently of whether or not the person agreed or perceived this to be the case.

Sometimes disagreements between objectivists and subjectivists are based on mutual misunderstanding. Thus the objectivist may be stating that the physical effects of a given treatment are objective facts (eg, the physical changes of an altered metabolic rate are objective facts and can be discovered and measured whether or not the patient is aware of them or agrees that they exist). The subjectivist can agree but state that none the less, whether those objective changes are harmful or not is necessarily a subjective matter, determinable at least in part only by the subject who is affected by them. Whatever the philosophical truth of the matter, it is now widely agreed that, at the very least, health care workers must have very strong reasons to disregard the evaluations of patients themselves about the harmfulness of proposed or actual interventions – for quite apart from harm/benefit considerations, health professionals also have a duty to respect the *autonomy* of their patients or clients.

See also: Beneficence; non-maleficence.

RG

Healing (a) the physical regeneration of injured body tissue; (b) (more broadly) the overcoming of trauma and the restoration of the wholeness of the person. In its broader sense healing is sometimes contrasted with cure. Thus a dying or disabled person may be healed psychologically or spiritually, though not necessarily physically changed. Healers practise a range of therapies including prayer, anointing, laying on of hands, massage, meditation, and *counselling*. There is debate about the claims to physical effects made by some healers, though the *placebo* effect is well known in scientific medicine. The ethical issue is that of *veracity* – are people given false hopes or alternative ways of coping with ill-health?

Reference
Pattison S. *Alive and kicking*. London: SCM Press, 1989.

See also: Care vs. cure; health, illness and disease – concepts of; potential; spiritual healing.

AVC

Healthcare systems Strictly, a healthcare system could be any organisation that comprises a number of hospitals or other providers of health services working collaboratively. Thus, eg, the Veterans' Administration, which has traditionally owned and run hospitals and other health services all over the USA for those who have served in the American armed forces, or (also in the USA) the Indian Health System. Conceptually, such a system could be public or private, for profit or non-profit.

The World Health Organization has recently promoted the concept of the District Health System, to emphasise the need in all countries, whether poor or rich, for all the health services (however owned) within a given geographic area to work together for the local population, and in particular for hospitals to support *primary care* practitioners.

At the national level, the term is used to describe a country's health services, whether or not they actually fall within a single unified system.

Hence people speak loosely of the Swedish, German, French, Japanese, or American healthcare system, disregarding the fact that the last of these has no homogeneity: whatever its merits, it is certainly not a single entity. The British *National Health Service* is relatively unusual in being in this sense a unified healthcare system.

Systems are enormously varied, but they tend to fall into families, according to the method of finance (eg, tax based, or financed by public insurance, or direct pay), the form of ownership and management (eg, public or private) and the degree of centralisation or decentralisation that prevails. In very general terms, systems fall into a spectrum ranging from large, relatively centralised, publicly owned and managed systems like the NHS at one end to heterogeneous, decentralised, mixed ownership and financing non-systems, like the USA, at the other. Each has its own virtues and vices. Eg, the British arrangements are much more equitable than the American, and far less extravagant. On the other hand, there is much more innovation and (for most people) more choice in the USA.

In the past twenty years, there has been a growing tendency for governments to reorganise healthcare systems as a way of reacting to the undoubted difficulty of containing costs, while maintaining quality, and professional and public confidence. Among the best known examples of ideas currently driving healthcare systems reform are "managed competition", stemming from the Health Maintenance Organization movement in the USA, and "the purchaser/provider split" featured in the latest reorganisations in the UK and New Zealand.

See also: Cost containment; purchasing.

RJM

Health economics is the application of economic theories and methods to the study of the production and distribution of health and health services. Health economics focuses attention on the choices both explicit and implicit, that have to be made because there are not enough *resources* in any society to do everything that people *want/need* for their health, or that health professionals are able, technically, to provide.

At the macro (national economy) level, health economics attempts to describe and explain changes in the health of the population resulting from changes in a country's economic structure, eg: economic growth and recession; absolute and relative contribution of expenditure on health services; different ways of paying for, and allocating, health services.

At the micro (provider/purchaser) level, health economics is concerned with both the "technically efficient" process of allocating resources to provide a service, and the "socially efficient" provision and distribution of different health services in order to maximise overall benefit to the population. The distribution of health services between individuals and groups of people within society raises important issues of *distributive justice*.

Theoretically, health economics identifies not only the costs to the immediate provider and purchaser, but also the direct and indirect costs that fall on other people or organisations. It also involves the identification of health *outcomes* (benefits to health) and the relationship between costs and benefits (*cost–benefit analysis*). However, there are considerable technical and philosophical issues associated with measuring and valuing both costs, particularly when prices do not adequately reflect the value of a resource (eg, unpaid carers), and health in an agreed "currency", not least the valuing of one person's, or group of people's, health against another's.

Health economics has taught us that these kinds of valuations are made implicitly every time resources are allocated to one service and not to another. In making them explicit, economics brings us face-to-face with uncomfortable implications and sometimes conflicting ethical principles associated with decision-making. Furthermore, by providing a range of economic analytical procedures as aids to decision-making, there is a danger that other, more democratic, processes for allocating resources are abandoned for the appeal of the technical fix.

Reference

Williams A. Economics, society and health care ethics. In: Gillon R. ed. *Principles of health care ethics*. Chichester: John Wiley, 1994.

See also: Cost containment; equity; market; National Health Service; purchasing; quality of life; QALYs; values.

MP

Health education has its roots in the 19th century public health movement which sought to prevent the spread of infectious diseases by introducing sanitary reforms and improved hygiene. Health education was seen as the means of persuading the population to adopt behaviours which would prevent illness and thereby reduce premature deaths. Although its scope broadened in subsequent decades to encompass a range of health problems, notably child and maternal health, *sexually transmitted disease* and aspects of "lifestyle" such as *smoking*, its methods and values continued to be dominated by the medical model. The primary aim was preventing disease through the provision of information to individuals who, it was expected, would then change their behaviour and thereby reduce their risk of ill health – eg, by being immunised, stopping smoking, adopting some form of *contraception*. This model assumed that people were free to choose

how they lived their lives, individual behaviour was a prime determinant of health, information alone was sufficient to enable people to change behaviours, and behaviours were deemed appropriate or otherwise according to medical criteria.

Many underlying assumptions about this "medical model" are now rejected. Modern health education practice sees health not as the absence of physical disease but as a positive concept encompassing physical, mental and social dimensions; recognises the *fallacy* of free choice and the dangers of victim blaming; acknowledges the social and political determinants of health, particularly inequalities in health; draws on a broad educational base which aims to empower people to make informed decisions about their own health; recognises that behaviours deemed "incorrect" or "irrational" on medical criteria may be appropriate in the context of people's daily lives; respects individual *rights* and fosters *autonomy*; and is an integral part of health promotion, which aims to enable people to increase control over and improve their health.

Debate continues within health education as to which of the several models and approaches that have emerged over the last few years are the most appropriate and effective. These approaches reflect or emphasise different, though often complementary, values and ethical principles. Eg, the educational approach aims to facilitate personal responsibility, free choice and *decision-making* through developing people's knowledge, understanding, skills and self-esteem. In contrast the *empowerment* model aims to help individuals, groups and communities meet their perceived health needs through *advocacy*, negotiation and networking. The political or social-change approach addresses structural factors which reduce freedom of choice and damage health.

Reference
Naidoo J, Wills J. *Health promotion foundations for practice*. London: Balliére Tindall, 1994: 62–119.

See also: Attitudes; freedom; potential; public health.

AA

Health, illness and disease, concepts of Illness is not the same as disease; it is possible to feel ill (say, as a result of simply thinking of a bumpy flight in an aeroplane) without having a disease. Diseases are from one point of view in the same category as injuries, disabilities or handicaps, in the sense that in all these cases something has, objectively and demonstratively, gone wrong with the effective functioning of an organism. This organism might be a human being, or an organ or part of a human being or other biological entity. Malfunctioning of this sort is a common cause in human beings of the subjective state we call "feeling ill". Sometimes of course we speak of "being ill" or of "ill health" and mean a state that is verifiable as distinct from being subjective. "Being ill" in this sense can be added to the list containing "disease" or "injury" and referring to what can be objectively shown to involve the malfunctioning of an organism.

It is much harder to identify the concept of health. Of course it can always be identified negatively: an organism is healthy if it is not diseased or injured. But since the time of the World Health Organization (WHO) definition of health in 1946 ("Health is a state of complete physical, mental and social *wellbeing*, and not merely the absence of disease or infirmity") some theorists, particularly in the health promotion movement, have argued that health can be positive as well as negative. Yet "positive health" is perhaps better discussed in terms of concepts such as *welfare*, wellbeing, or fitness, which may overlap with health but are essentially different. In a similar way it is reasonable to extend "ill health" to include mental ill health (which will prevent effective functioning) but positive mental health is a dangerous idea that may discourage eccentricity and encourage conformist behaviour.

Reference
Downie RS, Fyfe C, Tannahill A. *Health promotion: models and values*. Oxford: Oxford University Press, 1990: 9–26.

See also: Disability; health education; illness; mental illness; potential.

RSD

Health visitors A community based profession with a particular role in relation to the prevention of ill health and its consequences, which includes *health education* and promotion. The health visitors' remit also covers the early detection of ill health; the surveillance of high-risk groups; and mobilisation of appropriate resources to meet identified need. The United Kingdom Central Council for Nursing, Midwifery and Health Visitors (UKCC) Code of Conduct for Nurses, Midwives and Health Visitors, 1992, is their guide for practice, but very precise and rigid rules govern child protection.

See also: Accountability; autonomy; child abuse; codes; community care; home visits; primary care; risk register.

HM

Heartsink patients refers to those patients (as individuals or as a group) who make the professional's heart sink when they are seen to be about to consult, and are seen as "difficult". Each person has her own preferences or pet hates, and one person's heartsink patient is another one's pleasure. However, the literature, mostly from general practice, tends to describe people with many symptoms, few if any diseases, who attend frequently and have little insight into their illness behaviour. Patients describe what are clearly heartsink doctors, but sensibly try to avoid them rather than write about them. *"Difficult patients"* are usually the creation of "difficult professionals".

See also: Doctor–patient relationship.

RH

Hedonism In common usage, loving luxury. In ethical theory, the view that we either are, or should be, motivated by pleasure. Its practical implications depend on how pleasure is defined (eg, quantitatively or qualitatively, short- or long-term, of the body or the mind) and on whether one, many or all persons' pleasure is to count.

See also: Utilitarianism.

KMB

Hepatitis Inflammation of the liver, frequently caused by hepatitis viruses, which may cause chronic liver disease, eg, cirrhosis and hepatoma. Hepatitis viruses A and E are transmitted by the faecal–oral route, and are common in areas with poor sanitation; hepatitis A is a problem for institutions for the mentally retarded, which led to the infamous Willowbrook experiments, where children were given virus without *consent*, to study its course and to confer immunity. Hepatitis B and C are parenterally, vertically and sexually transmitted. Hepatitis B is highly infectious by blood contact with antigen positive subjects. It can be prevented by vaccination; treatment with interferon reduces disease and infectivity. *Screening* is used in donors for *blood transfusion*, for patients receiving *dialysis*, where there is significant potential for spread to patients and staff, and to exclude *infected doctors* from conducting *surgery*, which can put patients at risk. Recent suggestions that medical students should be tested and possibly excluded if infective has raised concerns about excessive limitation of entry into the medical profession. Hepatitis B is common in Asia,

but *resource* constraints limit access to vaccination. The natural history of Hepatitis C and the risk of spread is not yet fully known and problems arise from the ability to detect it without such data.

AJP

Hermeneutics (Greek Hermes, messenger of the gods) Science of interpreting scripture, history, science or existence, and theories of whether these have independent or interpreter-dependent meanings. Not to be confused with heuristic (Greek "to find out") – non-algorithmic, trial-and-error procedures for attempting to solve a problem.

KMB

Heroes and heroic action Medical and allied work has long been seen as "heroic", in the sense that it is exhausting, dangerous and demanding while the (visible) rewards may not be commensurate. In spite of evidence to the contrary, it is still assumed that people are "called" to this work rather than select it as a career path out of a series of options. The *power* in the *doctor–patient relationship* (and, in some countries, social prestige) may join with this to persuade professionals not just that they have a super-human task but that they are in some sense super-human people. For instance, they may believe they do not suffer from illnesses or diseases like ordinary mortals, that they can go without sleep, or that they have special insight that makes them key decision-makers beyond their professional boundaries. Like Achilles's encounter with his enemy's father, Priam, near the end of the Iliad, sanity is restored when such a person recognises her own *vulnerability* and the dimensions and reality of her own human *need*.

Reference
Higgs R. Doctors in crisis. In: Litchfield P, ed. *Health risks to the health care professional*. London: Royal College of Physicians, 1995.

See also: Omniscience.

RH

Heteronomy (Greek for law of others) Being under the control of another person or (Kant) one's own unreasonable desires; hence not autonomous.

See also: Autonomy.

KMB

Heterosexual Used to describe a person who finds members of the opposite sex erotically arousing. This opposite-sex erotic preference may be expressed in fantasies and/or through sexual behaviours. An individual's heterosexuality is usually thought to be accompanied by an identity or self-image as "being heterosexual". However, many individuals may also experience sexual attraction towards members of the same sex at some point(s) in their lives and may also engage occasionally or persistently in same-sex sexual behaviours. Some of these individuals may none the less identify as heterosexual, while others may self-identify as bisexual. The heterosexual identity of an individual is often assumed to be linked necessarily with a strong *gender* identity but there is no obligatory relationship between opposite-sex preference and lack of confusion about identity as a man or woman. Eg, effeminate men and masculine women may be strongly heterosexual in their desires, and transsexuals of either sex may find either men or women sexually attractive. However, the assumed association between gender identity and heterosexuality can lead to stereotypical views about the roles of each sexual partner in a heterosexual interaction. These assumptions can be shared by doctors.

Heterosexuality is the assumed norm in Judaeo-Christian-Islamic cultures, and as such is encouraged and reinforced socially, legally, theologically and medically. However, there are cultural variations worldwide in the accepted norms for patterns of sexual behaviour and in the extent to which non-heterosexual interactions are acceptable or even obligatory.

The biological basis of sexual preference is not understood. It has been claimed variously that genes, brain anatomy, hormonal environment in utero or post-natally, learning in early infancy or choice in adulthood may underlie sexual preference, but no clear single explanation is accepted. Given the strong cultural variation in the expression of different types of sexuality, a single determinant of sexuality is unlikely.

References
Bancroft J. *Human sexuality and its problems*. Edinburgh: Churchill Livingstone, 1989.
Moore G. *The body in context. Sex in catholic thought*. London: SCM Press, 1992.
Ortner SB, Whitehead H. *Sexual meanings*. Cambridge: Cambridge University Press, 1982.

See also: Homosexual.

MHJ

Hinduism is the oldest religion in the world. It originated in north India about 4000 years ago. It is the religion of the majority of Indians; its founder is not known. Beliefs, rituals and festivals vary widely from one part of India to another. There are approximately 732 million (1992) Hindus worldwide.

Although it is a polytheistic religion, it has a concept of the supreme spirit, Brahman, which has many manifestations including three gods: Brahma, the creator; Vishnu, the preserver, and Shiva, the destroyer.

The holy scriptures are: the Veda collection of hymns; the philosophical Upanishads; the epics of Mahabharata (including the Bhagwad Gita) and Ramayana. The avatars Rama and

Krishna are the main heroes of the epics. These books are full of wisdom.

Hindus strongly believe in: reincarnation; the caste system; the signs of the zodiac influencing fate, and cremation (particularly in north India) – the cremation fire to be lit by a male child. Eating beef is strictly taboo. Hindus also celebrate sister-days and husband-days annually and fast on certain days.

Significant ethical dilemmas can arise when Hindu beliefs clash with scientific medicine. Eg: (a) belief in reincarnation can be mistaken for signs of a bizarre illness or schizophrenia; (b) the unequal privileges of the caste system (the mirror image of the British social class system) will be unacceptable to health professionals from other religions, as a guide to the allocation of health service resources; (c) a Hindu family will strive for at least one son so as to be able to fulfil the cremation rituals; (d) substances containing cow meat or cow fat, such as beef insulin or certain baby milks, will be rejected – devout followers who inadvertently use such products may suffer the pain of guilt afterwards; (e) on her husband's day a Hindu woman doctor will take annual leave, will fast and pray for his long life (the husband, if westernised, may spend that day in a pub with non-Hindu friends).

Reference
Qureshi B. *Transcultural medicine.* London: Kluwer Academic Publishers, 1994.

See also: Religion and philosophy, Eastern; transcultural medicine.

BQ

Hippocratic Oath A solemn promise: (a) of solidarity with teachers and other physicians; (b) of *beneficence* and *non-maleficence* towards patients; (c) not to assist *suicide* or *abortion*; (d) to leave *surgery* to surgeons; (e) not to harm, especially not to seduce, patients; (f) to maintain *confidentiality*

and never to gossip. Traditionally associated with Hippocrates (5th century BC); but who originally wrote or took the oath is uncertain. Clauses (a), (b), (e) and (f) remain central to modern *codes* of medical ethics. Contrary to popular belief it is not sworn by doctors in most countries.

KMB

HIV Human Immunodeficiency Virus is the causative agent of *AIDS*. Tests for the presence of antibodies to HIV are widely used as a means of showing that a patient is infected with the virus.

AJP

Holistic is used to describe an approach to medicine that takes account of the whole person, rather than focusing on solely medical aspects. Arguably, this is an essential feature of good medical practice in any system. The term "holistic medicine" is often used to describe forms of *complementary* (or alternative) *medicine*, in contrast to orthodox medicine, because the latter is perceived to be disease-orientated rather than patient-orientated.

AJP

Homeopathy is based on the observation that an individual's energetic imbalance can be restored to normal by specially prepared medicines that need to be administered in small (often ultramolecular) doses. The medicines are usually prepared from dilutions of natural products such as herbs, a variety of naturally occurring minerals, and animal products. In healthy organisms the medicinal agents chosen would produce the symptoms and clinical features of the *disease* (like cures like) and are therefore given in the disease as a treatment. There is great conceptual difficulty within conventional medical circles in reconciling the effects of the infinitesimal doses used in homeo-pathy with conventional pharma-cology. In spite of these problems, many homoeopaths in the UK now work closely with their conventional medical colleagues in a variety of set-tings, although a referral to a non-medically qualified homeopath re-quires that the referring physician makes a clear diagnosis and bears responsibility for the homoeopathic treatment. This is in spite of the fact that the majority of non-medically qualified homoeopaths have appro-priate professional indemnity.

See also: Complementary medicine.

GL

Home visits Doctors and nurses working in the community, such as British general practitioners and dis-trict nurses, are presumed to be pre-pared to visit someone who is sick and unable to get out. There is much to be gained from both parties in this: the visiting professional may be offered insights and the patient is both more comfortable and more in charge in her own home. However, it unques-tionably takes more time and an over-burdened health service is likely to continue to press for patients to attend the doctor or nurse on health service premises. Whether a patient should be able to demand this service is more a political or social question than an ethical one, but should the regulations allow for it then the decision to meet at home should be a shared and nego-tiated decision, like others in health care.

RH

Homicide The term homicide covers the offences of murder, manslaughter (or culpable homicide in Scotland), *infanticide* and killing by dangerous driving.

The last condition can be disposed of fairly quickly. In essence a person is driving dangerously if it would be obvious to a competent and careful driver that driving in that way would be dangerous.

Infanticide is a specific statutory offence in England and Wales that involves the killing of a child under the age of one year by its mother while the balance of her mind is dis-turbed by the effects of giving birth or of lactation; it thus differs very considerably from the far wider inter-pretation that is commonly placed on the term. There is no such statutory offence in Scotland where the compar-able conditions would be regarded as child murder and be subject to the mitigation of diminished responsi-bility.

Murder is the killing of a human being "with malice aforethought". There need not be an intention to kill; an intention to place the victim's life in jeopardy, or to cause grievous bodily harm, is sufficient. Since murder is a crime of intent, conditions that de-prive the perpetrator of the mental capacity to form an intent will elide a charge of murder. The rule that death must occur within a year and a day from the assault has lost its relevance in the face of modern medicine's abil-ity to extend life; the usefulness of the rule, which applies also to manslaughter and suicide, is cur-rently under review.

It is clearly not homicide to withdraw intensive support from a person who is "brainstem dead" be-cause that person is, by definition, dead. Removal of life support in the absence of *brain stem death* may be justified by good medical practice; it would, however, certainly be murder for a person outside the health care team to, say, switch off a ventilator before the patient had been declared dead with the intention of ending her life.

Manslaughter is unlawful homicide not amounting to murder. Voluntary

121

manslaughter is, in effect, murder in the presence of some mitigating circumstance; these are provocation, killing as part of a suicide pact and, most importantly, diminished responsibility. Involuntary manslaughter includes all other forms of unlawful homicide committed without malice aforethought and, is, therefore, very wide in its application – the ill-definition of the offence being mainly attributable to the degree or quality of the "unlawfulness" involved. The major authorities recognise three categories of involuntary manslaughter – that resulting from an unlawful and dangerous act, that attributable to recklessness and that due to gross negligence. In the present context, it is the last of these that causes greatest concern owing to the recent spate of prosecutions of members of the medical profession. A strong argument can be adduced to the effect that, despite the demonstration of gross incompetence in a case of medical mishap, it is wrong to convict the doctor of a criminal offence in the absence of an element of subjective wrongdoing on her part – the correct test should be based on recklessness as to the outcome.

References

Mason JK, McCall Smith RA. *Law and medical ethics* (4th ed). London: Butterworth, 1994.
Smith JC, Hogan B. *Criminal law* (7th ed). London: Butterworth, 1992.

See also: Death; euthanasia; life support systems; treatment.

JKM

Homophobia A set of negative attitudes and affects towards homosexuality in yourself or others. The innate conservatism of the medical establishment has meant this is often a prevalent attitude in medical staff which has adversely affected patient care. The advent of *HIV* infection and its associated patient *advocacy* may redress some of the previous prejudices or may add to them.

See also: Bias.

CSk

Homosexual Describes someone who finds members of the same sex erotically arousing. This same-sex erotic preference may be expressed in fantasies and/or through sexual behaviours. It may be accompanied by an identity or self image as "being homosexual" ("gay" or "lesbian"), in which case it may also be expressed in a conscious and open homosexual life style ("out"). However, many individuals experience homosexual attraction and interaction at some point(s) in their lives without identifying as homosexual and without excluding heterosexual attraction and interaction. It is often assumed that a homosexual individual will experience problems with her gender identity, but there is no obligatory relationship between same-sex preference and any confusion about identity as a man or woman. Homosexual behaviour is also seen among pygmy chimpanzees; no directly comparable behaviours are seen in other species.

The extent to which the open expression of homosexual fantasy and behaviour is socially permissible is highly dependent on culture, being obligatory in some, discouraged in others, and changing through history. In Judaeo-Christian-Islamic cultures, there are strong religious constraints on the acceptability of homosexual acts and thoughts based on (contested) scriptural interpretations. These constraints are accompanied to varying extents by social taboos and stigmatisation and by specific legal regulation. In general, these negative responses to homosexuality apply more strongly to men than women. Historically, homosexuality has been construed variously as heathen, immoral, criminal and pathological.

Currently, there is an increasing legal acceptance that it is a human right to be able to express non-exploitative, consenting sexual behaviours, including homosexual behaviours.

Medical and psychiatric opinion has also moved towards a non-pathological view of homosexuality. Certain antisocial or self-destructive behavioural traits may be observed more commonly among homosexual individuals, but their presence may simply reflect individual reaction to negative social views about homosexuality. Ignorance about and prejudice towards homosexuality persists among some doctors and medical students, and generalised (mis)perceptions about homosexuality may colour approaches to homosexual patients and medical staff, regardless of their individual pattern of sexual behaviour. Attempts to "cure" homosexuality have been largely abandoned as unsuccessful. Interventions to prevent the expression of a homosexual identity in behaviours persist. Most interventions, however, concentrate on encouraging self-identifying homosexual individuals to accept their homosexuality and build their self esteem to counteract the internalised negative social image of the homosexual.

The biological basis of sexual preference is not understood. It has been claimed variously that genes, brain anatomy, hormonal environment in utero or post-natally, learning in early infancy or choice in adulthood may underlie sexual preference, but no clear single explanation is accepted. Given the strong cultural variation in the expression of different types of sexuality, a single determinant of sexuality is unlikely.

References

Bancroft J. *Human sexuality and its problems.* Edinburgh: Churchill Livingstone, 1989.

Moore G. *The body in context.* London: SCM Press, 1992.

Ortner SB, Whitehead H. *Sexual meanings.* Cambridge: Cambridge University Press, 1982.

See also: Gender; heterosexual.

MHJ

Honesty is usually taken as the *virtue* of telling the truth and not being deceitful. Health care professionals are assumed to be honest in their dealings with patients and with each other, in scientific research, and in their daily behaviour, yet there has been some dispensation allowed over their having to be open to patients about a serious diagnosis. This is increasingly questioned but remains a live ethical issue.

See also: Empowerment; therapeutic privilege; truthtelling.

RH

Honour Like "shame", important for the ethics of societies that value rank or birth. More egalitarian societies tend to prefer "*integrity*" and "self-esteem", and "human" dignity to that conferred by official status.

KMB

Hope is to have an expectation of benefit, with a reasonable chance of it being realised; yet in medicine it is often used more to describe a state of partial ignorance when an ill person's confidence in her own health has not been sabotaged by being told that something is seriously wrong.

Reference

Yates P. Towards a conceptualisation of hope for patients with a diagnosis of cancer. *J Adv Nur* 1993; **18**: 701–6.

RH

Hospice movement In the second half of the 20th century health care professionals committed to the relief of suffering in terminal illness, especially but not exclusively *cancer*, developed inpatient and domiciliary services based in specialist units called hospices. These services, many of which were wholly or partly funded from charitable sources, specialised in

123

symptom control, and in giving practical and emotional support to the patient and family. The skills developed in hospices became widely appreciated, and are now recognised as a health care speciality, known as *palliative care*. Associated knowledge and philosophy of care was widely disseminated and became known as the palliative care approach.

See also: Care; commitment; terminal care.

FR

Hospital chaplains Appointed jointly by religious and hospital authorities to meet the spiritual and religious needs of *patients*, carers and staff, hospital chaplains offer pastoral care, *counselling*, worship and *advocacy*, provide a theological and ethical resource, liaison with visiting clergymen, and teach. While representing the *values* of their faith group, chaplains are available, never imposed on patients and respect *individual* belief. By attending to spiritual needs, chaplains or other religious representatives may become a valuable extension to the clinical multidisciplinary team.

See also: Buddhism; Christianity; conscience; God; Hinduism; Islam; Judaism; need; religion and philosophy, Eastern; respect; spirituality; theology; truth.

TSM

Hospital medicine is that part of medical care conducted in hospitals, including outpatients, day cases and inpatients. It contrasts with and complements *primary care* and *community care*, and is often divided into secondary care, providing generic services in the main specialties, and tertiary care, providing highly specialist investigation and treatment for rare or complex disorders. This latter division is somewhat arbitrary, as the work is conducted by many of the same hospital staff, though tertiary referrals are made to specialist teams

at the same or another centre. In the UK, most hospital medicine is practised formally following referral by the patient's *general practitioner* (GP) for a consultant opinion. In practice, with the increasing complexity of medicine, the result is usually a form of shared care, with the hospital staff taking on the specialised aspects of investigation and treatment, the GP retaining oversight of the patient and specific responsibility for the ongoing management in the community. Patients can self-refer to hospital accident and emergency departments and to *sexually transmitted disease* clinics.

Hospitals provide a site where specialised facilities for imaging and *laboratory tests* are available and GPs can refer directly to these. However, since their use and interpretation may require specialist clinical expertise, GPs may ask hospital consultants to initiate and follow up such investigations. *Surgery* and complex medical therapies may require the patient to be in a suitably equipped and multidisciplinary environment. Furthermore, the severity of illness may necessitate the more intensive nursing and medical care available to inpatients. Increasingly, scarce and expensive hospital *resources* are focused on those with the most extreme needs, with a greater proportion of home or community-based care for less severe illness or stages of recovery. Continuing shared care follow-up of patients with complex chronic conditions is used where specialist oversight is still required.

Teaching hospitals provide the base for *medical education* and *nurse education* for undergraduates, postgraduates, and allied professions. They also provide substantial basic and *clinical research* facilities that can not only underpin high quality specialist care but also investigate improved understanding, investigation and therapy for many diseases. Community hospitals may be clinically run, wholly or in part, by GPs, providing a range of residential and day-care facilities requiring less complex interventions or care.

The management of hospital medicine in the UK *National Health Service* (NHS) is increasingly in NHS *trusts* which negotiate with *purchasers* or commissioners of health care to provide a defined range of services at agreed contractual costs. Their activities are regulated according to rules and procedures derived from government departments and agencies. Within hospitals, the management of resources and the planning and delivery of care is conducted in clinical and non-clinical directorates, with varying degrees of devolved *responsibility*. Hospital staff are employed by trusts or health authorities, or in the case of clinical academic staff by universities, as opposed to the independent contractor status of general medical and dental practitioners. The relatively high cost of hospital medicine has led to pressure to centralise facilities, close smaller units, and transfer more care to primary and community care. It is unclear whether this is in practice more cost-effective or provides more appropriate or better quality care.

AJP

Human Fertilisation and Embryology Authority This is a statutory UK government body established to oversee the activities of centres involved in assisted reproductive techniques. The Authority has a statutory obligation to ensure that centres consider the welfare of the *unborn child* and is responsible for regulating the storage and use of donated gametes.

ALo

Human nature Most people's ordinary thinking about morality makes an assumption about the ways in which human beings are likely to or are drawn to behave: "It's only human nature". This usually implies some form of forgiveness for falling below the best standards, and expresses graphically our perplexity about the supposed dual nature of man – the mixture of good and bad impulses and actions and the mingling of attributes of devil and angel which has long perplexed sincere religious people and given copy to preachers. We may not like the sin but we often secretly admire the sinner. Modern health care risks recreating a new puritanism now the costs to the service of everyday pleasures (smoking, drinking, driving fast, having sex with more than one partner) have begun to emerge, and weighs not souls in purgatory but health outcomes via statistics and stigmatic campaigning. Whether the newly prescribed life styles will fit better with human nature than righteousness has yet to emerge.

Ethics notes the different components of will, thought, and action in our choices and allegedly free behaviours. Yet as more is known about genetic and environmental influences on behaviours, the extent of our free choice and the interaction between the psychology of what we do and the ethics of what we should do may become blurred. When someone fails (by, for instance, becoming addicted to alcohol or desperately fatigued in the long term) we are unsure whether to give her latitude and excuse by calling it an *illness* or attempt to motivate her and revitalise her *autonomy* by saying that it is a behaviour for which she has *responsibility*. The law complicates: someone who falls may claim she was pushed. In ethics, autonomy is thus both a description of an ideal and a prescription for an aim, with the hope that autonomous choosers will choose the best and for the best. Theories about human nature have in the past tended to close down on options: some modern thinkers (such as pragmatists) would see the task of ethics rather as opening up new ones.

See also: Order of preferences; psychology/morality boundary.

RH

Human rights The modern human rights movement can be seen as a consequence of the Second World War and the genocide and other state-sponsored violence which preceded and accompanied it. Promoting human rights became one of the four principal purposes of the United Nations when it was founded in 1945; on 10 December 1948 (celebrated since as human rights day) the Universal Declaration of Human Rights (UDHR) a list of basic human rights, was adopted by the UN General Assembly as a "common standard of achievement". Many subsequent international treaties and declarations have further elaborated on this list and a complex series of intergovernmental, governmental and non-governmental agencies and organisations have emerged to promote and protect human rights around the world.

Human rights focus on individuals and involve their relationship to the larger society, and most especially the state. Rights, inseparable from human dignity, are considered to inhere in people simply because they are human; rights are inalienable (governments may violate them but cannot actually grant or take them away). Rights are universal, applying to all, regardless of time or place; therefore, violations of rights anywhere are a legitimate concern of all. Rights also represent claims, or entitlement by individuals on the society. In this regard, the UDHR includes civil and political rights, which protect individuals from abuses of state power (ie, rights of non-discrimination, not to be tortured or imprisoned under inhumane conditions; right to privacy and freedom of information and assembly) and economic and social rights, in which the state is required to make resource and other commitments to help bring about realisation of rights (that is, rights to health, education, social security, work). Respect for human rights and dignity therefore defines an essential minimum for all people.

Health workers have at least four reasons for learning about human rights. First, as citizens of the modern world, they should know about this most dynamic, complex and challenging modern movement; after all, their rights and dignity as well as those of their patients, are at issue. Second, health policies, programmes and practices and clinical research may inadvertently violate human rights; such burdening of rights should be avoided, or at least strictly limited. Third, violations of each of the rights (and of dignity) have important adverse health effects on individuals and groups. Finally, promoting human rights is now understood as an essential part of efforts to promote and protect public health (the modern health and human rights movement).

Reading the UDHR is an essential first step in becoming literate about human rights.

See also: Codes; justice.

JMa

Humanae vitae An encyclical letter of Pope Paul VI, best known for the assertion that deliberately contraceptive sexual intercourse is intrinsically wrong, although use of the infertile period provided by nature is permitted. The encyclical permits therapeutic procedures that are needed to cure disease but have a contraceptive effect, provided that effect is not directly intended.

Reference
Pope Paul VI. *Humanae vitae*. [encyclical letter] London: Catholic Truth Society, 1968.

See also: Double effect; natural law; papal encyclicals.

BHo

Humanism European turn (16th century onwards) from theology to the classics (humanities), from other-worldly to this-worldly interests and from communalism to individualism. Sometimes a secular religion, replacing God with humanity; but more often a movement, within or outside religions, against *authoritarianism* or collectivism.

KMB

Humanity is broadly that state of being proper to human beings, but is usually used to describe feelings of tenderness or kindness evoked by recognising in someone else an answering state to one's own, and acting accordingly.

RH

Humour Laughter and jokes are universal human responses to perplexing or paradoxical problems. There's not much of it about in ethics textbooks, but although laughing at distress would be unacceptable, finding a way together with someone else of getting to the lighter side of an issue may make a situation bearable until resolution appears.

See also: Jester.

RH

Hydration is ensuring sufficient provision of water (and electrolytes) for severely ill patients who are unable to take fluids independently. It is of particular import in relation to the late stages of the care of terminally ill patients, where there is dispute as to whether it constitutes *treatment* and whether, however defined, it is permissible to withdraw artificial hydration. The provision of water has been considered as essential to human dignity and to have symbolic significance beyond its literal function. It had been thought that dehydration was itself distressing and so should be avoided, but this is now disputed, as the patient will slip into coma due to renal failure. Since artificial hydration will prolong the process of dying, some think it kinder to withhold or withdraw it if active treatment has ceased. In relation to the debate on *euthanasia*, it is a question of boundaries, where hydration lies between withholding or withdrawal of artificial ventilation, and feeding or antibiotics. However, failure to hydrate could be construed as implicitly showing intent that the patient should die as a result.

AJP

Hypnosis is a technique of suggestion that can produce a state of deep relaxation, the electro-encephalograph consistent with an alert but relaxed state. A person can be hypnotised or taught to hypnotise herself. The ability to be hypnotised depends more on the subject than the teacher, it being impossible to hypnotise someone against her will. Hypnosis is a successful treatment of anxiety disorders, such as a dental phobia, or psychosomatic disorders, such as irritable bowel disorder. However, there are equally successful alternative treatments. Hypnotherapy is psychotherapy during hypnosis. The memories thus recalled are less reliable than those recalled in ordinary psychotherapy, being produced when the subject is most suggestible. Hypnotherapy can also cause an overwhelming emotional reaction, if a suppressed traumatic memory is suddenly released. The use of hypnosis for entertainment can be harmful and should be regulated.

PDW

I

I-Thou The modern Jewish existentialist Martin Buber contrasts the "I-it" knowledge of scientific analysis and inference, with the "I-Thou" knowledge of mutually transforming interpersonal dialogue. Without the latter, God cannot be known, and what matters most about other persons (including persons as patients) will be overlooked.

See also: Existentialism.

KMB

Iatrogenic disease is disease that results from the actions of doctors. It ranges from side-effects of *drug* therapy, of *immunisation* or of *blood tranfusion*, through complications of *surgery* or investigation, to psychological distress resulting from medical interventions. It reflects adverse outcomes of the balance of *risk*. In an effective *doctor–patient* relationship, with informed *consent* and patient *empowerment*, a patient can determine, after discussion of risks, the acceptability of potential iatrogenic disease as opposed to the consequences of there being no intervention. *Litigation* may result if the patient considers that she was not aware of such risks or if she considers that iatrogenic disease resulted from *negligence* by the doctor.

AJP

Idealism Philosophically, the view that knowledge is of thoughts not things, or that reality is mental not material. Without ideas to organise it, knowledge is not possible: but disembodied thoughts are not known. Popularly, the pursuit of ideals that cannot be (fully) realised in practice. This can lead to disillusionment, but also can bring practice closer to the ideal.

A form of idealism informs the vocational aspects of medicine. Idealism can enable physicians and other patient advocates to identify ideal goals in patient care, medical ethics, public policy, or health service organisation; such aspirations must then be adapted to what is achievable in the "real world". The concept of ideal roles (eg the ideal father) is sometimes used in psychiatric practice.

KMB/AJP

Identity A sense of the continuity of the self through time despite physical and psychosocial changes. At certain life stages, eg, *adolescence* and midlife, *conflict* may be felt between self-perception and social expectations. Reactions to identity crises can be extreme and appropriate care treads a fine line between encouraging *autonomy* and mediating the needs of others.

References
Erikson EH. *Identity, youth and crisis.* London: Faber, 1968.
Goffman E. *The presentation of the self in everyday life.* London: Allen Lane, 1969.

AVC

Ignorance The duty to respect a patient's *autonomy* demands that she not be kept in ignorance of what's wrong with her, the *treatment* options and the prognosis. However, a paternalist would argue that some patients might benefit from ignorance and that others might be harmed by being given certain information. The conflict is between autonomy on the one hand and *beneficence* and *non-maleficence* on the other. Many *cultures*, for instance, favour a patient not being told a diagnosis of *cancer*.

See also: Empowerment; paternalism.

ALI

Illness is loosely used to mean a state of sickness or disease, but is best seen, in contrast to disease, as a subjective state: that is, to describe the situation in which a person has mind or body feeling that is no longer considered as normal, or explicable, and over which she has no control. Some have tried to restrict the domain of medicine to conditions in which physical changes can be demonstrated, but that is to misunderstand the origins and nature of ill health.

See also: Health, illness and disease, concepts of.

RH

Illness behaviour Given that most health problems are not presented for medical advice, the term "illness behaviour" was coined to describe the process by which individuals make a decision whether or not to take their symptoms to the doctor. More recently, medical anthropologists have stressed that all individuals seem to have complex explanatory models interpreting symptoms and illness, and it is in the wider context of these lay theories that patients choose to seek medical advice. This context of patients' decision-making means that medicine cannot rely on patients acting in accordance with medical rationality when it comes to responding to their illnesses.

DA

Immunisation Most immunisation programmes involve children, so *competence* is important as well as *consent*. Overall, there is a balance between the individual's and the public interest. Community immunisation programmes require the acceptance of a small risk of complications in a few in order to benefit the *public health* by reducing the incidence of an infection, which would cause a greater overall burden of disease. This raises the issue of individual *compensation*. People may show *compliance* with professional advice, eg, on measles in the UK recently although a small number

of complications have followed (perhaps been caused by) the programme. With rubella, public opposition in the UK on *inter alia* religious grounds prevented the programme being implemented as planned. Could society accept a legal requirement for eg, commercial sex workers to have a new vaccine against the *AIDS* virus? A sanction of imprisonment could promote the spread of infection (within the prison) rather than control it, and thus not on balance be in the public interest, so could immunisation be enforced?

See also: Compulsory testing and treatment; health education; public health, ethics of.

SPBD/AJP

Immunity (i) In the legal sense, exemption from specified liabilities, and in a more general sense, from *harms*.

(ii) In medical usage, it refers to innate, acquired or induced (*immunisation*) protection against infection or disease, derived from non-specific (inherent or genetically determined) or specific defence against potential pathogens. Immune responses, at an individual or at a population level, represent some of the most complex biological adaptive responses; their failure in immunodeficiency (eg, *AIDS*) or their evasion by virulent organisms, represent significant challenges to personal and *public health*.

See also: Infection control; quarantine.

AJP

Impartiality In principle, not taking sides before examining the claims of different parties to an argument. In practice, this may conflict with respecting the prior claims of existing obligations, eg, to one's own patients or family.

KMB

Imprisonment As a form of punishment, imprisonment involves depriving citizens who have been convicted

129

of crime of their right to freedom. Remand prisoners are, however, despite the presumption of innocence before trial, also detained if they are felt to be a potential risk for release pending trial. Imprisonment is not intended to deprive a citizen of her right to health. Yet the very act of imprisoning people in often crowded and less than sanitary conditions may put them at risk and behavioural patterns in prison may increase risk of injury, *drug misuse,* and *sexually transmitted disease;* the latter two may increase the risk of HIV and *AIDS,* particularly since access to the means of safer injection and safer sex may be limited as prison authorities or politicians may regard provision of needles and syringes or of *condoms* to be condoning illegal behaviour (drug misuse or homosexual acts "in public"). Once released, some conditions acquired in prison will carry penalties, not only to the individual but also her partners and others, posing significant *public health* dilemmas. In some jurisdictions, measures have been taken to deal with this more humanely, but significant impediments remain. *Mental illness* and drug dependency are more prevalent in the prison population and may require particular medical attention.

Health care for prisoners presents challenges for health care staff. In the UK, the prison medical service is run separately from the *National Health Service.* The bulk of care is provided by prison medical officers and prison warders, though in some cases NHS clinicians may have a visiting role and prisoners may be referred to hospitals for treatment. Separation of the care role from the custody role may present difficulties, as do issues of *confidentiality.* It has been suggested that there should be a more explicit separation of roles.

Patients with mental health disorders who present a hazard to the public or themselves may need to be detained in secure units, and this can be ordered through the courts. Under various sections of the Mental Health Act in the UK, patients with acute psychiatric problems may be admitted to hospital involuntarily ("sectioned"), pending treatment, and this may be construed as a form of imprisonment.

Metaphorically, patients may feel imprisoned by their disease or by the necessity of treatment and this may affect their relationship with clinical staff.

See also: Forensic psychiatry; prisoners, care of; psychiatry, use and abuse; psychopathy.

AJP

Incest Sexual relations between relatives. A part of the social order of several cultures, but prohibited in most; in the latter it may serve as a defence to maintain a dysfunctional family unit. Sophocles in *Oedipus Rex* referred to the risks of unmasking lethal or detrimental recessive genes: "monsters – husband by her husband, children by her child".

References
Isaacs A. *Sex and sexuality. A thematic dictionary of quotations.* London: Cassell, 1995.
Kaplan HI, Sadock BJ. *Synopsis of psychiatry. Behavioural sciences* (5th ed). Baltimore, MA: Williams and Wilkins, 1994.

VC

Incompetence A relative term (from Latin for unable to compete) applied to malfunctioning valves or sphincters, doctors who are not up to the job, and patients who lack *decision-making capacity.* In patients and doctors, the condition may be temporary, fluctuating, partial, permanent, or in the eye of the beholder – in any case the law presumes *competence,* and requires acknowledged expert judgment to disprove it.

KMB

Incompetent professionals One of the characteristics of a profession is that it is self regulating with defined standards of competence and performance required of its practitioners. Standards of clinical practice for doctors are proposed and monitored by the *General Medical Council* (GMC) and the medical Royal Colleges, and incompetent practice is characterised by a consistent failure to achieve these.[1] Clinical competence includes both the ability and the will to carry out the tasks required of a doctor. The lack of will to practise competently is the most serious form of incompetence and sometimes the boundary with negligent practice is hard to define.[2] When incompetence is revealed the doctor has a duty to retrain or refrain from practice. If she lacks insight then other doctors should bring the situation to the attention of the employer or the GMC so that action can be taken. The duty to protect patients from harm takes priority over a natural desire to avoid distress for a *colleague*.

References
1 Good medical practice. Guidance from the GMC. London: General Medical Council, 1995.
2 Newble D, Jolly B, Wakeford R. *The certification and recertification of doctors. Issues in the assessment of clinical competence.* Cambridge: Cambridge University Press, 1994.

See also: Negligence; self regulation.

LJS

Independence 1. A relative state, since "no man is an island", but in so far as it is achievable, important for individual wellbeing and *autonomy*; hence a goal of both *parenting* and health care. 2. Independent advice is often sought when planning or arbitrating on issues of health care and *public policy* to avoid *conflicts of interest*; few parties are truly disinterested so seeking a balance of individual views may be more appropriate.

KMB/AJP

Individual This term conveys the uniqueness and functional wholeness (indivisibility) of each member of the human species. Each is perceived as having distinct characteristics (even if an identical twin) and as having a value in her own right. In Western thought the value of the individual has often been given priority over membership of family, social group, or nation. In *medical ethics* the principle of respect for *autonomy* may appear to favour *individualism*, but in *medicine* and in *ethics* the isolated individual is a misleading abstraction. We deserve respect as individuals, but our health and our moral choices require communal support and *responsibility*.

Reference
Campbell AV. *Health as liberation.* Cleveland, Ohio: Pilgrim Press, 1995: ch 4.

See also: Identity; self.

AVC

Individualism An emphasis on the *individual* over the social group. Society is perceived as an aggregate of individuals, each of whose interests are served by negotiation and compromise. In health care, a *market* approach is favoured and there is no communal responsibility for health.

Reference
Engelhardt JT. *The foundations of bioethics.* Oxford: OUP, 1986.

See also: Communitarianism; contract; egoism; healthcare systems; individual; National Health Service.

AVC

Induction Arguing from what is known to be true in an accumulation of particular cases to conclusions about similar cases generally. In this process, something new is inferred or added (or brought to birth, as in induction of labour). Induction (literally "leading to" or "drawing out") is less certain but can be more fruitful than deduction (literally "drawing from" or "subtracting") which argues from known general principles to particular cases.

See also: Logic and logical reasoning.

KMB

Industrial medicine is now largely subsumed within *occupational medicine*. Its origins were in the defining of particular diseases associated with work in particular industries (eg, mining, deep-sea fishing) and the provision of advice to management and staff on health and safety issues at work. It includes *epidemiological research*, to demonstrate and quantify the health risks of particular occupations, and identifying and implementing means of reducing them.

AJP

Inequality That people are not born equal or with equal opportunities is all too clear, but illness or disease may exacerbate differences between people, or create a gradient where there was none. Clinical medicine struggles to return patients to their previous status quo. *Public health* policy is usually seen as trying to help people to reach their full potential. The vulnerability of a patient creates inequalities of *power* in the *doctor–patient relationship*.

See also: Equity; human rights; justice.

RH

Infallibility Within Roman Catholicism it is held that the Church as a whole is protected from error by the Holy Spirit. It is also held that the Pope is protected from error when exercising the fullness of authority in proclaiming absolutely binding teachings concerning faith or morals, either alone or together with his fellow bishops.

Reference
Chirico. *Infallibility: the crossroads of doctrine*. London: Sheed and Ward, 1977.

See also: Papal encyclicals.

BHo

Infanticide Killing an infant – a recognised practice in some early societies. Today, if done by the mother, a crime distinguished from murder in English law, and in other jurisdictions often judged more leniently. Medical involvement in allowing or assisting perinatal death is both complex and unresolved in law and ethics.

See also: Homicide.

KMB

Infected doctors and other healthcare staff pose particular ethical problems if they present a risk to patients under their care. The issue arises particularly where they are potentially infectious through the close forms of contact involved in medical care at a time when they themselves are well, as in *carrier* states. While the issue is a general one, including conditions such as tuberculosis or chickenpox, to which some patients may be especially vulnerable, it has taken on special significance in relation to blood-borne infections, such as *HIV* and *hepatitis* B virus. The settings in which theoretical or actual risk can be envisaged for such infections are "exposure-prone invasive procedures", in practice during *surgery, dentistry* or obstetrics, where it is possible that the operator could cut herself and bleed into the wound before withdrawing the hand. In the case of hepatitis B, and probably C, there is a demonstrable risk for antigen positive operators; *screening* has been implemented, with reassignment to other duties until infectivity is lost, spontaneously or after treatment. In the case of HIV, the risk is largely theoretical and much smaller. *Guidelines* have been produced, including a statutory duty for those who consider they may be HIV-infected to seek investigation and advice. There is a key role for practitioners in *occupational medicine* in providing advice to staff, clinicians involved in the patient's care and employers. Particular ethical tensions may arise where the clinician has acquired infection from a patient, for which the risk is substantially greater than the reverse. In the case of HIV, infection of the health care worker may itself lead to susceptibility to infections that could be acquired from patients; occupational medical advice will be essential, as is the case with other illnesses in clinical staff.

Where a clinician has, knowingly or not, performed exposure-prone invasive procedures while infected with HIV or hepatitis viruses, *public health* doctors must determine the necessity for *look-back procedures* for patients who are deemed to have been put at risk. Such procedures may jeopardise the *confidentiality* of the infected health care worker. Balancing the rights of all parties and conducting the process in a way that protects these rights may pose serious ethical dilemmas.

See also: AIDS; sick doctors.

AJP

Infection control describes measures used in hospital or community to contain and control the spread of contagious disease. The term is particularly applied to the former, where infection acquired from other patients or from staff may pose additional problems for patients who may already be vulnerable. Hygienic measures, especially hand washing, must be rigorously enforced as a matter of routine for all staff. Patients with certain infections will need to be isolated to avoid cross-infection – notably those infections that spread readily by touch, skin fomites, or aerosol, such as methicillin resistant Staphylococcus aureus (MRSA), chickenpox, or pulmonary tuberculosis. Community infection

control measures include *health education* and promotion, *immunisation*, enviromental control (eg water, foodstuffs), *quarantine*, and procedures for *notifiable diseases*. Ethical tensions arise where infection control measures may mean some restriction of freedom or human rights, or where they may impact on the short term efficiency of hospital practice. Sometimes infection control measures may be proposed or instituted that go beyond what can be justified on scientific grounds, whether to reassure the public (but thus condoning unjustified fears about modes of transmission) or as a covert means of restricting certain individuals or groups.

AJP

Infertility is generally defined as the inability to conceive after one year of unprotected intercourse. However, it is important to realise that only 75% of normal couples will conceive in this time and that 96% will have conceived after two years of trying. Infertility treatments are generally very poorly funded by the NHS as in the past they have been hailed to be expensive and ineffective and, since the condition is generally not life threatening, infertility is often given a low priority by purchasing agencies. However, infertility can lead to significant psychological morbidity and marital disharmony, and those affected often suffer severe feelings of *guilt*, frustration, and *anger*.

With thorough and exhaustive investigations designed to achieve an accurate diagnosis and appropriately targeted treatment, the effectiveness of fertility treatments has improved significantly in recent years. The success rates of *in vitro fertilisation* in most clinics now approach the chance of natural conception of the fertile population in any given cycle, that is 30%.

Some clinics are achieving significantly higher success rates than this in certain groups of patients.

ALo

Informed consent Medical ethics often speaks of a doctor's obligation to obtain a patient's "informed consent" to medical treatment. In doing so, it seeks to encapsulate a doctor's moral duty to provide sufficient information for a patient to make an informed and rational choice whether or not to consent to a medical procedure. In a number of countries, eg, Canada, Australia, and some American states, this obligation is reflected in the doctor's legal duty: a duty to provide the information which a prudent or reasonable patient in the particular patient's circumstances would wish to know in deciding whether to agree to the proposed medical procedure, subject to the defence of *"therapeutic privilege"*.[1] English *law* has rejected this legal duty and hence the phrase, "informed consent", is misleading in England. Nevertheless, English law does cast upon a doctor a duty to volunteer information to her patient. A patient who suffers injury as a result of a breach of this duty and can show she probably would not have agreed to the *treatment* had she been given the information, will be able to sue the doctor in the tort of *negligence*. While this duty may not impose as onerous a burden as would the "prudent patient" test, it is one that goes beyond the doctor's duty to provide information to avoid a battery action. The doctor must volunteer to the patient that information (including the inherent *risks* and alternatives) that a reasonable doctor would provide having regard to the particular circumstances of the patient (contrast the "prudent patient" test above). In general, a doctor will satisfy this requirement if she responsibly exercises her *clinical judgment* in determining what information should be provided and her view is supported by a competent and responsible body of medical opinion.[2] The court, however, remains the ultimate arbiter of the doctor's legal duty to provide information.[3] Thus, exceptionally the court may determine that particular information is so necessary for the patient to make an informed decision whether or not to consent to the treatment that a doctor who fails to provide it would be in breach of her legal duty to the patient even if she acted in accordance with a practice accepted in the medical profession.[4] Additionally, a doctor will be in breach of her duty if she does not truthfully answer any questions her patient may put to her unless the doctor forms the view reasonably that to provide the information requested would be demonstrably harmful to the patient's physical or mental health.[5]

References

1 *Reibl* v *Hughes* (1980) 114 DLR (3d) 1 (Can.); *Rogers* v *Whitaker* (1992) 67 ALJR 47 (Aust); *Canterbury* v *Spence* (1972) 464 F 2d 772 (US).
2 *Bolam* v *Friern HMC* [1957] 1 WLR 582 (McNair J).
3 *Sidaway* v *Governors of Bethlem Royal Hospital* [1985] AC 871 (HL).
4 *Sidaway ibid*, per Lord Bridge and *Smith* v *Tunbridge Wells HA* [1994] 5 Med LR 334 (failure to disclose risk of impotence was negligent even though accepted practice).
5 *Blyth* v *Bloomsbury HA* [1993] 4 Med LR 151 (CA).

See also: Consent; decision-making capacity; disclosure; truthtelling.

AG

Injury *See* Assault; emergency.

Institutionalisation The term "institutionalisation" recognises that living in an institution can have a profound effect on a person's behaviour and attitudes. The term is particularly associated with people with *mental illness*. The key insight is that it is not the mental illness alone which determines people's long term outcome; the social setting in which they live is also important. Living in an institution can cause: passivity; social withdrawal; loss of interest; loss of initiative; submissiveness; apathy, and lack of ability to make plans for the future. Wing and Brown compared long-stay patients with schizophrenia in three different hospitals which had markedly different environments.[1] The least stimulating environment led to the most withdrawn patients. The recognition of "institutionalisation" has been an important factor in the move towards caring for mentally ill patients in the community, and in improving the environment of institutions themselves.

Reference
1 Wing IK, Brown GW. *Institutionalism and schizophrenia. A comparative study of three mental hospitals, 1960–1968.* Cambridge: Cambridge University Press, 1970.

See also: Community care.

TH

Institutions involved in health care include a series of interlocking organisations with defined roles and responsibilities, such as *trusts*, *health authorities*, professional associations, educational agencies. They will have their own hierarchies and corporate value systems. It is in the nature of institutions that they may become inward looking, attending to their own structural needs and financial viability and the welfare of their members, potentially at the expense of those to whom they owe duties, such as patients and the public.

See also: Business ethics.

AJP

Institutions, medical ethics Non-university institutions have played an important part in the development of medical ethics. Perhaps this is because medical ethics has not been a traditional university subject. Some examples of important secular institutions are: the Hastings Center (near New York city); The Kennedy Institute, in Washington DC (containing the world's largest medical ethics library); The UK Institute of Medical Ethics and the Akademie für Ethik in der Medizin in Göttingen. Each of these institutions has sponsored its own journal. In some countries religious institutions, too, have played an important part in the development of the subject.

TH

Insurance industry Insurance is any system whereby the (usually financial) losses of the few are paid for by the many. Life insurance provides benefits in the event of too early death (life assurance) or of living too long (annuities, especially pension annuities). Besides proprietary companies, many life offices are mutual assurances societies, owned by the policyholders: if there are more death claims than expected other policyholders will pay, either through lower bonuses, or higher future premiums. Commercial insurance requires the premium charged to be related to the expected risk to be covered. Thus when people apply for life insurance medical evidence, or a medical examination, is often required.

Traditionally insurance has been a contract "of utmost good faith" ("uberrima fides"), so any relevant information to the policy should be disclosed. This may cause difficulties for the private medical attendant (PMA) of an applicant for life assurance, if the insurer requests information known to the PMA but not to the applicant, or if a doctor in examining the applicant discovers something previously unknown to the applicant. Failure by the applicant to disclose information that may be relevant to

135

the contract may justify the insurer in repudiating a claim.

The appropriate premium for a substandard life is usually calculated by examining the mortality rates of policyholders or other relevant medical statistics.[1] Insurers tend to decline applicants until good statistics become available as they did initially with those who were tested further even if they were HIV negative.[2] Recent advances in *genetics*, which enable the identification of asymptomatic, at-risk individuals, who may but are not certain to develop a serious or fatal illness create major ethical problems for insurers, the medical profession, and the public.[3]

Sickness, permanent health or disability insurance provides a weekly or monthly payment to those who are sick or permanently disabled. A similar underwriting process applies as for life insurance, but medical evidence (whether the claimant is genuinely fit, or what degree of disability she suffers) may also be required when a claim is made. Medical expenses insurance is how health services are financed in many countries. If there is no other provision for payment of medical costs the disabled may find it difficult to obtain cover, and those with insufficient income may not be able to pay the premiums. Everywhere there are difficulties in controlling the costs, since the patient would like the best possible treatment, which may be the most expensive, and the insurer may be reluctant to pay for this.

In many countries governments have instituted national health insurance schemes, sometimes paid for by contributions from those in work and their employers, and in other cases paid for out of general taxation. Likewise, many countries have instituted social insurance or social security schemes, which provide retirement pensions and possibly benefits in the case of unemployment or sickness to the whole population, or to those who have paid contributions while working.

References

1 Brackenridge RDC. *Medical selection of life risks.* London: The Unsershaft Press, 1992.
2 Wilkie P. Life assurance, HIV seropositivity and haemophilia. *Scot Med J* 1987; **32**: 119–21.
3 Harper PS. Genetic testing and insurance. Paper presented at *Evolution or Revolution*, The Mercantile and General Reinsurance Co plc Seminar 6–8 November, 1991, London.

See also: Insurance, medical.

PW

Insurance, medical This is insurance taken out by individuals against costs of medical care and other consequences of illness. It may, eg, cover private medical care or reimbursable costs of health service care. Policies are taken out based on varying levels of assessment of *risk*, depending on the type and scale of cover. Premiums are calculated on actuarial *probability* of risk and are loaded for those with adverse factors, such as *smoking* or greater risk of disease, in order not to confer disadvantage on those at low risk. Policies are contracts based in verity and are denied if a person knowingly concealed a risk in response to a specific inquiry. Medical assessments are conducted by doctors who are contracted, often on a pro rata basis, by the insurance company. *Conflict of interest* may arise if the company seeks information from the person's own doctor, particularly if asked to speculate about life-style in risk assessment (eg for *AIDS*). Companies may request *screening* tests for some conditions. *Genetics* and *genetic disorders* are generating increasing tensions about what may legitimately be used in assessing risk for medical insurance. Specific exclusions may apply to certain disorders or types of treatment. Potential refusal of medical insurance may inhibit individuals from seeking medical attention or advice regarding their own care or risk to others (eg, HIV testing). If this is widespread, there may be hazards to public and personal health that may be hard to remedy without statutory controls on the *insurance industry.*

When the insured seeks payment, the company's chief medical officer can request medical information from attending doctors, which again must be truthful for the policy to be valid. If the insured refuses the release of medical information, the company may refuse payment. The ethical tensions are substantially heightened if medical care is funded only by insurance, as opposed to a *national health service* with voluntary insurance cover for extras, and may necessitate statutory controls.

AJP

Integrity is wholeness, psychologically or physically. The former suggests *honesty,* and usually also maturity.

RH

Intensive care Intensive care units, or intensive therapy units (ITU), as they are also known, provide treatment for patients who are suffering from actual or impending organ failure. In addition to the ethical problems which are common to all patients, the care of the patient in the ITU may give rise to specific dilemmas.

The indications for admission include such terms as "need" and "realistic prospect for useful recovery". Since neither of these can yet be accurately quantified, selection is of necessity arbitrary. This may create ethical and professional conflicts. Since discontinuation of *treatment* may result in *death,* decisions on ending treatment may be equally challenging.

Some patients are admitted as *emergencies,* without their prior agreement, on the assumption that they would wish to have all life-sustaining methods of treatment applied. The

increasing use of *advance directives* calls this into question.

Less than 5 per cent of patients who die in an ITU are suitable organ donors, but the application of the *brain stem death* criteria is an important aspect of care.

"Elective ventilation" has been suggested as a means of improving the availability of organs for *transplantation.* Although opinion has suggested such a practice may be unlawful, this has not yet been tested and may yet give rise to ethical and legal difficulties.

JCS

Intention and motive a central feature of philosophical and legal discourse for holding an individual responsible for her wrongful actions is the attribution to her of *fault.* Other features might be that she acted *voluntarily* and, perhaps, caused some (defined) *harm.* Fault may take a number of forms: intention (most serious); recklessness (middle order seriousness) and *negligence* (least serious).[1] Usually, the criminal *law* seeks to prohibit conduct only where the fault element involves intentional or reckless conduct on the part of the individual (but notice the crime of "gross negligence" manslaughter). By contrast, in order to compensate an injured person, the civil law usually requires only proof of negligent conduct by another. For the criminal law, prohibited conduct is often defined in terms of prohibited consequences and thus the defendant's legal responsibility for that consequence may turn on whether she intended to bring it about. So, eg, murder requires the defendant to cause another's death either with the intention to kill or cause serious bodily harm. What then is "intention"?

Outside the law, an *intention* to bring about a consequence is generally taken to mean that it is an individual's purpose to bring about that

137

consequence. In other words, an intended consequence is one that the individual is seeking to achieve as her aim or object in choosing to act.[2] Certainly, the law embraces this description of intention and it is known as "direct intention".[3] However, for the law this account of intention is probably too narrow.[4] The criminal law regards some consequences as intended even though they form no part of the individual's purpose or object in acting. So, a consequence that an individual knows must occur in order to achieve her goal will, in law, also be taken to be intended. But the law may go even further and also regard as intended a consequence that an individual knows is virtually certain to follow in achieving her sought outcome, even though it is not necessarily entailed in achieving her aim or object.[5] Both of these examples of the law's broader definition of intention are described as "oblique intention".[4] However, the law stops short of regarding an individual who merely knows that there is a *risk* of producing the consequence (even if it is probable) as intending that consequence. Risk-taking of this kind is, in law, described as recklessness, which is generally considered to be a less culpable state of mind.[6]

Motive describes the underlying reason why an individual carries out a particular act or seeks to achieve a particular consequence. Motive is normally equated with an emotion underlying (and explaining) the individual's conduct, eg, jealousy, greed, spite, or love. It should be distinguished from an individual's intention, which relates to what is sought to be achieved (or is known will occur). Unlike an individual's intention, an individual's motive is irrelevant in law in determining her responsibility.[7] Hence, a good motive will not excuse an otherwise illegal act and a bad motive will not condemn a

legal act. However, an individual's motive for committing a crime may be relevant in determining the appropriate sentence.

A useful illustration of the distinction between intention and motive in the medical context arises in the situation where a doctor prescribes pain-killing drugs to a terminally ill patient when she knows that the cumulative effect of the increased dosages will almost certainly shorten the patient's life. Has she intentionally caused the patient's death and is therefore guilty of the crime of murder?[8] The doctor's good motive in relieving pain does not in itself justify this action.[9] The doctor has intentionally caused the patient's death: though not her purpose (no direct intention), it is a consequence that she knows to be virtually certain to follow (oblique intention)[10] – contrast the arguments of some philosophers, based upon the principle of *double effect*. Whether, therefore, this doctor's conduct amounts to murder has nothing to do with her lack of intent to kill or, in itself, with her good motive. It must, instead, be based upon an argument that the terminal illness alone is the cause of the patient's death[11] (though analytically difficult)[12] or that the doctor has a duty to relieve pain and thus her conduct is lawful even though the patient dies.[13]

References

1 See general discussion in Duff RA. *Intention, agency and criminal liability.* Oxford: Blackwell, 1990 and Norrie A. *Crime, reason and history.* London: Weidenfeld and Nicolson, 1993.

2 Hart HLA. *Punishment and responsibility.* Oxford: Clarendon Press, 1968: 120.

3 Smith JC, Hogan B. *Criminal law* (7th edn). London: Butterworths, 1992: 53–9.

4 Williams G. [1987] CLJ 417.

5 *R v Moloney* [1985] AC 905 (H.L.); *R v Hancock and Shankland* [1986] AC 455 (HL).

6 See reference 1: Norrie A: ch 4.

7 See reference 1: Norrie A: ch 3.

8 Skegg PDG. *Law, ethics and medicine.* Oxford: Clarendon Press, 1984: ch 6.

9 *R v Arthur* (1981) 12 BMLR 1 (Crown Ct) and *R v Cox* (1992) 12 BMLR 38 (Crown Ct).

10 *Airedale NHS Trust* v *Bland* (1993) 12 BMLR 64 (HL). Contrast, *R* v *(Bodkin) Adams* [1957] Crim LR 365 per Devlin J.
11 *R* v *(Bodkin) Adams* [1957] Crim LR 365 per Devlin J.
12 Kennedy I, Grubb A. *Medical law* (2nd edn). London: Butterworths, 1994; 1206–7.
13 *Airedale NHS Trust* v *Bland* (1993) 12 BMLR 64 (HL). per Lord Goff at 114 (also arguing lack of causal link; on which contrast Lord Mustill at 139–40).

See also: Euthanasia; homicide.

AG

Interest (Latin: it concerns) (i) A sense of curiosity or attention vital for health professionals. (ii) Financial or other advantage that may accrue from a particular relationship, action, or situation. This is of importance where it is hidden, such as when an academic is asked to review the giving of a grant to someone she works closely with: this interest should therefore be declared.

See also: Conflicts of interest.

RH

Interests A person with *decision-making capacity*, relevantly informed, is normally in a better position than anyone else to judge what is in her own best interests, since these are relative to her own world view. The professional's *responsibility* is to inform and empower the patient's decision-making, and decide on the patient's behalf only as requested or consented to by the patient. When a patient's decision-making capacity is impaired or absent, determining her best interests requires careful clinical evaluation, skilled communication with the patient and/or family, and taking the least drastic action compatible with avoiding *harm* to the patient.

See also: Empowerment.

KMB

Internalising The process whereby a set of externally imposed rules, principles, or values are "taken in" to someone's thinking, and becomes part of their moral *framework*.

RH

Internationalisation of standards An attempt to achieve common agreement on an issue, often by achieving an international consensus. Such agreements are limited by the narrow band of representatives who agree the *codes*, and an inability to enforce adherence to them. Almost all such attempts are based upon Judaeo-Christian traditions and thus fail to engage much of the world's population. Examples of codes are the World Medical Association (WMA) Declarations of Geneva (the general code of medical ethics) and of Lisbon (the code on medicine and *human rights*).

VHN

Intersex *See* Sex, determination of.

Intervention *See* Non-intervention.

Intimacy A close personal relationship (in physical or psychological terms) may be required by or be the result of medical or nursing care, but may place the patient in a vulnerable position and so confers particular *responsibility* on the professional to behave with sensitivity and propriety. Interpreting the term intimacy as sexual intimacy is the basis for considering sexual relationships between professional and patient as unacceptable.

RH

Intolerance *See* Tolerance.

Intravenous feeding is also known as parenteral nutrition, total parenteral nutrition (TPN), and hyperalimentation. The delivery of nutrients in their most elemental form into the patient's vein is used when the gastrointestinal tract is not functioning.

Long-term intravenous feeding requires infusion into a central vein with increased associated risks. The potential metabolic complications and need for intensive monitoring mean that this is usually considered an extraordinary means of sustaining life and therefore more likely to be withheld in situations where recovery is not expected.

See also: Burdensomeness of treatment; extraordinary and ordinary means; nutrition.

SA

Intuition An immediate (ie, not mediated by inference or analysis) grasp of what is at issue. Ethical "intuitions" or "gut feelings" may be unexamined prejudices. But if ethical (or clinical) intuition is the fruit of careful and critical attention to detail, sustained over years, it may sense what is salient without the aid of an algorithm.

See also: Clinical judgment; prejudice.

KMB

Invasive A term used in a general sense to refer to any invasion of a person's privacy or space and in a specific sense to refer to medical procedures that involve entering a person's body. This may include examination, eg, of female genitalia or the rectum, or procedures that breach the skin, from venepuncture to major *surgery*. Invasion may be used as the basis for an allegation of *assault*. "Exposure-prone invasive procedures" is a phrase used to describe procedures that may put a patient at risk of blood-borne infection in an *infected doctor*.

AJP

In vitro fertilisation is an assisted reproductive technique in which eggs collected from the female are incubated with a suspension of spermatozoa. Fertilisation occurs in a laboratory in carefully controlled environmental conditions and the initial cleavage and embryonic development is observed until the two to four cell stage of development, when the embryo is replaced in the uterine cavity using a transcervical embryo transfer catheter. Centres offering *in vitro fertilisation* are closely controlled by the *Human Fertilisation and Embryology Authority* to ensure the highest standards of professional practice.

ALo

Islam With the present rate of population growth it is expected that Muslims will increase from 1.25 billion in 1992 to to 2.5 billion in the year 2020. The teaching of Islam covers all the fields of human activity: spiritual and material, individual and social, educational and cultural, economic and political, national and international. Instruction which regulates everyday activity of life to be adhered to by good Muslims is called Sharia. The primary sources of Sharia in chronological order are: The Holy Qur'an, the very word of God; the Sunna and Hadith, which are the authentic traditions and sayings of the Prophet Mohamed (Peace be upon Him) as collected by specialists in Hadith; Igmaah, which is the unanimous opinion of Islamic scholars, and Aimma and Analogy (Kias), which constitute intelligent reasoning used to rule on events not mentioned by the Qur'an and Sunna through comparison with similar events that have been ruled on.

The Sharia is not rigid but is flexible enough to adapt to emerging situations in different times and places. It can accommodate different honest opinions as long as they do not conflict with the spirit of its primary sources and are directed to the benefit of humanity. Even if the action is forbidden, it may be undertaken if the alternative would cause *harm*.

The primary sources of Sharia have stressed the four widely accepted principles of ethics, namely *autonomy, justice, beneficence,* and *non-maleficence.* The Sharia has also given attention to the principle of protection of the human subject against commercial exploitation.

The ethics of contemporary Islamic medical practice are based on the instructions of the Sharia, the ethical guidelines developed throughout history by earlier doctors and scholars, and on the additions of religious leaders, leading doctors and legal regulations, which became necessary as a result of the accelerated progress of technology and science and the marked development of medical bioengineering.

The rapid expansion of scientific knowledge has made medical research a top priority for the practising doctor. Though scientific excellence may be one of the objectives of medical research, in Islam the value of "scientific knowledge" and the pursuit of high-technology medicine should not be placed above the welfare of the research subjects.

References
Serour GI. Islam and the Four Principles. In: Gillon R, Lloyd A, eds. *Principles of health care ethics.* Chichester: John Wiley, 1994.

GS

Is-ought gap The missing link in reasoning from a factual and descriptive premise (eg, "there is a cure for this disease") to an evaluative and prescriptive conclusion (eg, "we ought to cure it"). Not minding the gap is committing the "naturalistic fallacy" of deriving an "ought" from an "is" (eg, "everybody does it, so it must be right"). But the gap may be narrowed by noting that "describing facts" is itself a selective and evaluative procedure (eg, "there is a cure for this disease" reflects the perceptions and values of the doctor, but not perhaps the patient's avaricious heir).

KMB

J

Jehovah's Witnesses Religious movement (USA 19th century) whose interpretation of the Bible forbids *blood transfusion* even to save life. While a competent adult's *refusal of treatment* must be respected, Jehovah's Witnesses accept alternatives to blood transfusion that are sometimes effective (eg, use of erythropoetin). A moral dilemma may be avoided by exploring this, and also the true wishes of the Jehovah's Witnesses concerned.

KMB

Jester A role that embodies the concept that *humour* may be an effective way of communicating important or uncomfortable information. The mediaeval court jester was protected so that he was able to say the unsayable without fear for his life and so could ensure that the king had his views and authority challenged. At its best, it may have served to reduce the dangers of autocracy. As the clinical milieu, with its professional heirarchies, becomes increasingly subjected to management theories and control, and a series of orthodoxies of policy, process, and practice, there seems to be a greater need than ever for the jester. Every senior clinician or manager and every committee should have one.

AJP

Journey A common *metaphor* in educational and psychotherapeutic thinking, which also has its place in ethics, best understood when actions and ideas are examined in retrospect. *Change* is not only necessary but inevitable in individuals and systems, but modern and post-modern perspectives have questioned whether it is possible to consider this as "progress", given that almost every gain can be balanced by a loss. Thus while improvement can and should always be aimed at, and *good enough* may not be good enough for long, the analogy of the journey may partly illustrate the dynamic, interactive, reflective and multi-dimensional nature of the best in modern medical ethics. This dictionary attempts to clarify and question rather than define; more a map than a prescription, a point of departure rather than a destination.

RH

Judaism is the religion that grew out of the faith of the patriarchs and matriarchs of the Hebrew Bible. It is the earliest monotheistic faith, and has a strong ethical base in its legal system. It has much to say in the field of medical ethics because it is so committed to the preservation of human life. "*L'chayyim*", "To life", is the toast to which Jews raise their glasses. Integral to their value system is the rabbinic teaching that one may, indeed must, break all but three of the commandments and prohibitions of the legal system in order to save a single human life. (The exceptions are the prohibitions on *murder*, *incest*, and idolatry.) Within the Mishnah, the end of the second century AD legal code, we read:

"One single man was created in the world, to teach that, if any man has caused a single soul to perish, it is as if he has caused a whole world to perish. If any man saves alive a single person, it is as if he has saved a whole world." (Mishnah. Sanhedrin 4.5)

Hence doctors, physicians, are held in the highest regard (which is not always the case in modern US or British societies) because they are thought to have been given the power to heal by God. In the Jewish tradition, people do everything in order to save life. But they do not necessarily help the dying. In the commentary to the Shulchan Aruch (16th century), we read: "It is forbidden to cause the dying to pass away quickly; for instance, if a person is dying over a long time and cannot depart, it is forbidden to remove the pillow or cushion from underneath him."

The Jewish tradition's strong life-affirming tendency has made it negative on the whole about assisted *suicide*, *euthanasia*, and any form of life-shortening *treatment*. There are less orthodox authorities who take a more lenient view, but the majority is for life preservation at all costs.

References
Jakobovits I. *Jewish medical ethics*. New York: Bloch, 1975.
Feldman M. *Birth control in Jewish law*. New York and London: New York University Press, 1968.

JN

Judgment, clinical and moral *See* Clinical judgment; moral judgment.

Jurisprudence The philosophy of law: it embraces the study of the role of *law* in society; the nature of legal concepts, such as *rights*; the obligation to obey the law (and when ethics require disobedience of unjust laws); the role of the judiciary, and the relationship between law and justice. One school of jurisprudence, whose members are known as positivists, believes that law is a self-sufficient closed system that can be understood without reference to other disciplines. From this view, the questions: "what is the law?" and "What should the law be?" should be answered in entirely different ways. Other thinkers argue that legal rules must always be interpreted so as to make them as consistent as possible with ethical principles.

References
Davies H, Holdcroft D. *Jurisprudence: texts and commentary*. London: Butterworths, 1991.
Montgomery J. Patients first: the role of rights. In: Fulford A, Erser S, Hope T, eds. *Patient centred health care*. Oxford: Blackwell Scientific, 1995.

JMo

Justice A *prima facie* moral obligation to be just or fair is a common feature of many moral theories, and Aristotle's formal analysis of the obligation of justice is common to many different substantive accounts of justice. According to Aristotle justice requires equals to be treated equally and unequals to be treated unequally in relation to the morally relevant inequalities. Unfortunately, substantive analysis of what should be regarded as relevant inequalities, and indeed relevant equalities, varies widely, both with *context* and across a wide variety of substantive philosophical, political and theological accounts of justice. In the context of health care ethics justice is important in the areas of distribution of scarce *resources*, respect for *rights*, and respect for (morally acceptable) laws. Important amongst the competing moral concerns for fair distribution of scarce health care resources are: distribution in proportion to people's health care *needs*; distribution that maximises beneficial outcomes; distribution that avoids waste of scarce resources; distribution that provides equality of access to health care; distribution that provides people with maximal choices in selection of their health care; distribution that acknowledges health care workers' special obligations to their particular patients, and distribution that respects the *autonomy* of those who provide the funds and resources for health care, whether as taxpayers or as subscribers to health insurance schemes. All these criteria for just allocation of health care resources have moral justifications (and there are also other candidates) and not all can be simultaneously met. In the realms of rights-based justice and of legal justice, while again competing theories and systems share the underlying Aristotelian formal principle of justice, a similarly wide variety of competing

morally relevant criteria is offered upon which to ground rights and laws. In addition to disagreements about the substantive content of theories of justice, obligations of justice may conflict with other moral obligations. Large questions also arise concerning the *scope* of application of the various types of justice – to whom (or even to what) do we owe fair distribution of scarce resources? Who (or even what) has and should have rights? What is the proper scope of application of different systems of legal justice?

See also: Cost containment; developing world; healthcare systems; human rights; insurance industry; parsimony; veil of ignorance.

RG

Justification Even if something should be done or is right, it will usually be important to show that it is or to show why it is. This is particularly so if the action is disputed by others.

RH

K

Kantian ethics Kant (1724–1804) believed that we can and should work out for ourselves what is right, and act accordingly. Freedom is following "the moral law within"; virtue is persisting in the struggle against contrary desires. The key is rational, universalising deliberation – to act according to ground rules that all rational people could consistently adopt (eg, never to tell lies, since if everyone did, no one would believe anyone). Critics object that Kant's deontological ethics is too uncompromisingly rationalistic (sometimes lying can be justified on consequentialist grounds; sometimes emotions are a surer guide than arguments). But Kant's insistence on the *autonomy*, dignity and rights of persons, and on respect for reason rather than blind *obedience* to authority, have deeply influenced most modern ethical debate.

See also: Deontology.

KMB

Karma Literally "action", or "work". In Indian religion, right action, like contemplation, can liberate one from illusions and suffering. But wrong or foolish actions accumulate, determining one's future life or lives, and delaying liberation of one's spirit.

See also: Religion and philosophy, Eastern.

KMB

Killing vs letting die This distinction is important psychologically to many healthcare professionals and philosophically to those who see intention rather than motive as crucial in end-of-life decisions. But the moral evaluation of "letting die" in particular cases depends on how far there is an obligation to keep alive; and some acts of killing (in *self defence*, or if it is requested by the person concerned and known to be the only way to end intolerable suffering) may be morally justifiable.

See also: Euthanasia; intention and motives; treatment.

KMB

Kin designates a category of persons related through procreation and marriage. The groups they form ("family", "lineage") will be narrower than the category (kin = relations). *Cultures* differ over how closeness and distance between kin are reckoned and what is allowed as sexual or marital practice (boundaries for *incest*, consanguineous marriage). The Western emphasis on the biology of procreation distinguishes "biological" from "social" kin. Major ethical dimensions: (1) Knowledge and ignorance: (a) reconstructing biological ancestry

may uncover unknown genetic connections; (b) over-evaluation of biology leads to pressures, welcome or otherwise, to "find out". (2) Diversity: social kinship encompasses (a) a wide emotional spectrum, from the intense to the indifferent; (b) varied conventions concerning *rights*, *duties* and *obligations*; (c) different moral endorsements of substitute practices, eg, *adoption*, same sex parenting, donor or surrogate reproduction).

See also: Families.

MS

Kindness is an attribute expected in, but often missing from, the response of a health care professional to a patient. Kindness and consideration are everyday human *virtues* which seem most vulnerable to overwork, lack of sleep or professional *arrogance*, but which seem particularly to increase the positive effects of *communication* and *care* and reduce the chances of negative outcomes such as a formal complaint by a disgruntled patient. The word is related to "kin", and this suggests that a key ability is for a person to have *empathy* with another and recognise the importance and impact of her suffering even if its causes are hard to elucidate or understand.

See also: Empathy.

RH

L

Labelling may be important before a patient is anaesthetised for the operating theatre, but is probably of equal importance as a concept in health behaviour, where a "label" for a symptom or illness may be explicitly or tacitly requested by a patient. If so, it may be hard to reassure or satisfy that person without: but the inherent danger exists in the "stickiness" of such labels, that once given they are hard to remove and may have major effects. For instance, many people with a benign heart murmur have led restricted lives since being wrongly told they had valve disease of the heart. Being labelled as "insane" may be an important step on the pathway to becoming "mentally ill".

See also: Stigma.

RH

Laboratory tests in the clinical sense are studies on patient-derived samples, usually conducted remote from the patient in a specialised laboratory, eg, haematology, microbiology, histopathology. These services are run by clinical pathologists, who advise clinicians on the most appropriate tests and on how to interpret the results. The form accompanying the sample is formally a request for a *consultation* by the clinical pathologist, who has a duty to perform the test or a suitable alternative, by agreement, or to arrange that it is done elsewhere if not available locally. Laboratory staff owe the same duties to the patient as clinicians, eg, regarding *confidentiality*; they may need to confirm that *consent* was obtained for particularly sensitive tests. Since patient samples, eg, *blood* and tissue, may be hazardous, the clinician has a duty to ensure the safety of portering or laboratory staff by appropriate labelling and packaging. The laboratory must be a safe environment in which to handle material of a biohazardous nature (eg, infection or *radiation safety*). Laboratory tests are a significant part of *clinical research and trials* as markers for disease, and for the *safety* and efficacy of therapies. The use of "near-patient testing", often performed by clinicians with simple automated machines, raises concerns not only because of the lack of interpretation from a clinical pathologist but also because of the need for awareness of biosafety issues on the part of the clinician.

AJP

Language is central to ethics because it is the way in which an ethical issue is described and analysed. While the initial understanding that something is wrong may be a feeling, and not truly expressed in language, the ability to go beyond this depends crucially on expression in words. But language is seldom neutral: the way in which thoughts are expressed, or even that they are expressed at all, may contain an ethical issue in itself; so that, for instance, some expressions contain their own evaluation ("is abortion murder?") or some words are, on reflection, simply *boo words*. Thus breaking the *silence* of a previously unexpressed moral domain may entail new words or a new way of expression in order to allow objective evaluation. That some words (such as "murder" above) seem to cross the *is-ought gap*, has complicated the neat division of *fact versus value*. In everyday ethics, it is good advice for the speaker to be re-evaluating her practice regularly by assessing not only what she is trying to say but how she is actually saying it, and/or how it is being heard.

See also: Communication

RH

Law The state of *jurisprudence* is such that no answer to the question "what is law?" may be viewed as impartial between the schools of thought offering an answer. For the purposes of exposition, it is possible to distinguish between controversy as to the **status** of propositions which seek to distinguish law from similar phenomena (a methodological debate) and the **content** of such propositions (a substantive debate, involving positions on, eg, the relationship of legal rules to moral rules). The methodological debate has resolved itself into a debate symmetrical with that now being conducted in many other disciplines, and questions the possibility of description (as opposed to evaluation) of social phenomena such as law. The impulse towards such questioning has its origins partly in the increasing lack of confidence that the social sciences have placed in the possibility of a non-evaluative, external perspective on *culture* and partly in the general climate in *philosophy* (both analytic and continental) favourable to theories of *truth*, *meaning* and language which issue in an ontological or conceptual *relativism* of a fairly thoroughgoing kind. In fact, one position in that debate would question the very distinction between "method" and "substance" of the sort here used for exposition.

On the substantive issue, one of the most enduring and important questions has concerned the relationship between law and morals. Positivist writers (Austin, Kelsen, Hart) have insisted that they are conceptually distinct so that even the most *evil* law may still be called "law". Such writers see, as central to law, some strongly "factual", non-evaluative element such as *coercion* or rule-following. Others, such as Fuller, Finnis and Dworkin, have argued that law and morals cannot be analytically distinct and that legal argument is, in some cases at least, indistinguishable from moral or political argument. Such writers see evaluation as central to legal reasoning. Dworkin, eg, argues that even in straightforward cases there is an irreducible degree of interpretation (and, therefore, evaluation) occurring. Whatever is to be made of such a position, there is a clear sense in which a debate concerning the relationship between law and morals cannot be purely descriptive: whatever their conceptual relationship, it is a question for moral and political philosophy how the undeniably coercive machinery of law is properly to be used. The establishment of the limits of the law (ie, asking whether there are some spheres of human activity which are "not the law's business") involves a judgment, not a description. Indeed, critical theories of law such as the feminist and marxian, forcefully assert the politically committed nature of law, howsoever conceived. Whether lawyers, as lawyers, may be understood to have any role in establishing the limits of law, if any, depends very much on the answer to, and highlights the importance of, the conceptual question "what is law?"

RD

Law, comparative systems Most contemporary legal systems have been required to address ethically sensitive issues of medical law. In some jurisdictions, eg, in certain Australian states, the legislature has been active in promoting statutory changes to the *law* in crucial areas such as *surrogacy* and *advance directives*. In other countries, the courts have dealt with these issues on the basis of general legal principles. There is a marked difference between the approach of courts in the UK and the USA; the British courts have taken a more cautious view of the *rights* of patients and have generally acknowledged professional discretion to a greater extent than is the case in the USA. In the USA there has been a vigorous assertion of individual rights in areas such as *consent* and cessation or withholding of *treatment*.

AMS

Law and morality Law differs from morality principally in its power of *closure* – a verdict is reached and enforced. Nor do all legal principles, precedents, procedures, and judgments satisfy ethical criteria for *justice*. Some laws are morally wrong or bad, and morally appropriate conduct involves more than keeping on the right side of the law. The *law* is usually interested in *intention*, ethics often in motive. But law is influenced (albeit not always determined) by morality, and legal *reasoning* is often closer to practice than is *moral theory*. Familiarity with relevant legal principles and cases can be helpful in the study of *medical ethics*.

KMB

Learning   difficulties/disabilities
Both terms are used to describe the condition of individuals in whom varying amounts of developmental, intellectual and social disability occur before the age of eighteen.

There are three main areas of ethical contention: prevention, prevention of secondary handicaps, and general medical intervention.

(i) Prevention: the idea that the birth of a child with learning disabilities is a tragedy is predominantly a cultural norm in Western society; there are some societies where such a birth is celebrated. Despite opposition by religious groups and those campaigning for the rights of people with learning disabilities, early termination of pregnancy is widely accepted. A physician can be faced with the moral decision whether or not to treat a potentially fatal condition, a decision which may be better faced by the whole clinical team and the child's parents.

(ii) Prevention of secondary handicaps: people with learning disabilities have a moral and legal right to optimal care, including medical intervention to prevent secondary handicaps. The doctor has to balance the often conflicting interests of the patient with those of her carers. Families may want the removal of stigmatising characteristics, such as facial plastic surgery for children with Down's syndrome. It is important in these situations that the physician assess the psychological benefits to the child as carefully as she would for a child of normal intelligence in similar circumstances. Psychotropic drugs can be appropriately used to contain socially unacceptable behaviour, but might best be seen as a temporary intervention, to enable skills training and the application of behaviour change techniques.

(iii) General medical interventions: research in day services for people with learning disabilities indicates that getting general basic health care is difficult for this group.[1] Hearing, vision and cervical *screening* are often overlooked in this section of the population, despite the greater prevalence of visual and hearing problems. The difficulty of explaining procedures is often cited as the reason for individuals with learning disabilities not being encouraged to attend well woman/man clinics. These problems can be overcome with specialist training and support for the professionals.

People with learning disabilities have similar aspirations to their able peers, including marriage and raising children. The provision of family planning and pregnancy advisory services, *abortion* and male/female *sterilisation* presents considerable moral, emotional, practical and financial dilemmas for the physician, health care team, social services, the judicial system and, most importantly, for people with learning difficulties wishing, or not wishing, to use these services. The difficulties people with learning disabilities face in successfully parenting their children are revealed by UK and US research studies (eg, Whitman et al, 1989).[2] Prospective parents should receive a careful assessment of their skills and help to enable them to care for their child while this is in the child's best interests.

Reference
1 Lawrie K. Better health care for people with learning disabilities. *Nursing Times* 1995; **91**, 19: 32–4.
2 Whitman BY, Accordo JP. *When a parent is mentally retarded*. Baltimore: Paul H Brookes, 1990.

See also: Advocacy/activism; child, status of; behaviour therapy; life prolongation;

non intervention; psychiatry, use and abuse; psychopharmacology; stigma.

MC

Lesbianism An affectional and erotic attraction between women, usually within the context of a specific identity, lifestyle and sub-culture. Disclosure within medical settings is often difficult because of perceived or existing *homophobia* or assumptions that an individual is heterosexual. The lack of legal recognition of lesbian relationships in the UK has led to difficulties for lesbians/assessing fertility and *adoption* services.

CSK

Leucotomy This is a technique of dividing the white matter fibre tracts that connect the medial and anterior parts of the frontal lobe to the rest of the brain. It has also been called prefrontal lobotomy, though less often recently. Leucotomy was first publicised by Egas Moniz in 1935 and used for a wide range of psychiatric conditions in the two decades following its description. Eventually it became clear that the complications and side-effects could be quite severe and its use has been very restricted in recent psychiatric practice.

References

Moniz E. Prefrontal leucotomy in the treatment of mental disorders. Am J of Psychiatr. 1937; **XCIII**: 1379–85.

Dax EC. The history of prefrontal leucotomy. In: Smith JS, Kiloh LG, eds. *Psychosurgery and society*. Oxford: Pergamon, 1977: 19–24.

See also: Psychiatry, use and abuse; psychosurgery.

GG

Liability Health professionals are liable to censure by their *statutory bodies*, eg, the *General Medical Council*. They may also be held liable for their actions under the criminal and civil *law*. Conviction for a criminal offence leads to punishment. A finding of civil liability leads to compensation for the damage suffered by the "victim". Health provider organisations may be directly liable for defective services even if individual members of staff have not been negligent.

The general rule is that people will be held liable only for their own actions, not those of others. However, employers may be "vicariously liable" for the civil wrongs of their employees and can be sued for damages. Strictly, this is an alternative to suing the professional individually. However, it has been agreed that National Health Service *trusts* will indemnify clinical staff for money they are required to pay in damages as a result of *negligence* in the course of their duties.

References

Department of Health. *Claims of medical negligence against hospital and community doctors and dentists*. London: Department of Health, 1989: HC(89)34.

Montgomery J. *Health care law*. Oxford: Oxford University Press, 1996: chs 7 and 8.

JMo

Liberty *See* Freedom.

Life events Current interest in life events centres on the role they may play in the aetiology of life-threatening and less serious morbid conditions.[1] In Victorian times people had no hesitation in attributing illness to the stress of such dramatic life events as *bereavement*, broken engagements, loss of income, or employment.[2] Non-western societies frequently ascribe illness or injury to the violation of traditional codes of social conduct.[3]

The discovery of the part played by bacteria and viruses in disease causation, and the separation of psyche from soma, which characterised medical thought and practice in the late 19th and early 20th centuries, meant that the possible influence of social structures and psychological processes on health was largely ignored or ridiculed.[4]

In the past fifty years, however, the inability of simple causal models to account satisfactorily for vulnerability to illness or its differential course in individuals began the search for more sophisticated multifactorial paradigms and led to the revival of scientific interest in life events as precursors of disease. Social epidemiologists seek to establish objective measures of events and ways of assessing their subjective meaning for individuals.[5] Psycho-pharmacologists study possible pathways through which emotional responses to adverse life events translate themselves into physiological responses severe enough to hasten death. At present there is a growing consensus that childhood loss of a parent, eg, is a risk factor for subsequent ill-health in adult life.[6] Bereavement also appears to hasten the death of widowers.[7]

Ethical interest in life events lies in the extent to which they diminish or increase the sense of personal *guilt* for their condition felt by the sick.[8] Professionals as well as informal carers may also attach *blame* to those in their care, however morally reprehensible and therapeutically ineffective it may be.

References
1 Rahe RH. Subjects' recent life events and their near-future illness report. *Ann Clin Res.* 1972; **4**: 250–65.
2 Tolstoy LN (Trans R. Edmonds). *War and Peace*. Harmondsworth: Penguin Books, 1978, 776–9.
3 Young A. The anthropologies of illness and sickness. *Annu Rev Anthropology* 1982; **11**: 257–85.
4 Lawrence C. *Medicine in the making of modern Britain, 1700–1920*. London: Routledge, 1994.
5 Brown GW, Harris TO. Life events measurement. In: *Life Events and Illness*. London: Unwin and Hyman, 1989.
6 Bowlby J. *Attachment and Loss* (2nd edn). London: Pimlico, 1997.
7 Parkes CM, Benjamin B. Broken heart. A statistical study of increased mortality among widowers. *BMJ* 1969; **1**: 740–3.
8 Blaxter M. Why do the victims blame themselves? In: Radley A (ed) *Worlds of illness: biographical and cultural perspectives on health and disease*. London: Routledge, 1993.

MJ

Life insurance *See* Insurance industry.

Life plan indicates the idea that most people have a general aim or series of aims for their life even if vague, incoherent, or conflicting. Ethical dilemmas arise when an apparently good treatment is at odds with this, – for instance, when an elderly sportsman refused an apparently necessary amputation because of his concerns for his bodily integrity.[1]

Reference
1 Higgs R et al. Earning his heroin but seeking release while the surgeon advises amputation. *J Med Ethics* 1987; **13**: 43–8.

RH

Life prolongation Medical technology now prevents death from many previously fatal conditions.

After cardiopulmonary *resuscitation* patients who have stopped breathing with non-beating hearts may be "restored to life".

Organ transplantation can prevent untimely deaths from end-stage kidney, liver or heart disease. More controversially, "brain dead" or persistent vegetative state victims may be kept "alive" by sophisticated life-support systems.

For the great majority of patients the outcome is highly satisfactory, but when used inappropriately, patients may be condemned to a "living death". Thus, discussion is now correctly aimed at ensuring the appropriate use of these therapies. In this context patients' wishes must always be paramount; where communication is impossible patients' previous views and those of proxies must be fully respected.

See also: Advance directives (living wills); autonomy; brain stem death; dialysis; DNR orders; intensive care; persistent vegetative state; proxy; quality of life; resuscitation; transplants; treatment.

JW

Life saving This would be claimed to be the prime duty of medical personnel, particularly when faced with a choice between two or more patients. It is a less easy guiding principle in the individual, as most people would feel there was a limit to the extremes to be taken to save a life which was naturally coming to its end.

See also: Euthanasia; triage.

RH

Life support systems Apparatus for supporting the function of body systems, without which the patient will die or suffer serious harm – frequently a ventilator, but kidneys and heart may also be supported. The need for support may be temporary or lifelong.

Without the use of life support systems those who need them will usually die, so the arguments for their deployment seem compelling. However, such systems may not, for resource reasons, be available to everyone, and their use is often unpleasant or painful for the patient, who may not wish to depend on machinery.

If someone is able to express a view about life support, either when it is needed or by an *advance directive*, respect for their *autonomy* would generally dictate the appropriate action. But often, patients are too ill, or the need is too urgent, for any useful discussion. With limited resources, who should be treated? Explicit rationing systems are difficult to construct and often decisions are made on the basis of futility of treatment, or previous *quality of life*.

If *resources* are unlimited it is still possible to argue that not all interventions that can be made should be made.

It is much easier to introduce life support than to withdraw it. Morally there may be no difference between killing and letting die. But that is not how it feels in practice.

See also: Dialysis; intensive care; killing vs letting die; treatment.

PG

Limits are important to place on the application of principles in ethics (we can't do good for everyone) and to activities (everyone needs time off) or to expenditure.

See also: Boundaries; scope.

RH

Listening is now considered to be an important therapeutic activity in itself, and implies attention rather than just hearing something out. Why "telling one's story" is so helpful is not clear. It may reflect the transfer of *responsibility* for diagnosis and treatment from patient to doctor, but being listened to also conveys an important sense of being believed. It is important that the clinician hears the explicit and implicit questions that are being asked in the account and answers them. The effects of poor listening skills are evident in patient dissatisfaction, *complaints*, *litigation*, and poorly directed referrals.

RH/AJP

Litigation is the process of taking a grievance to court. This recognises the rights of the individual and the responsibilities of the person or institution challenged. Litigation is often expensive, protracted and uncertain. It can arise where one individual, group or organisation should have foreseen they might *harm* (personally or financially) another by their act or omission (the "neighbour" principle). Successful litigation is generally followed by the award of financial compensation, which is designed to restore the person harmed to the position she would have been in but for the consequences which resulted from the failure of care of the person being sued.

See also: Apology; duty of care; law; negligence.

SAMM

Living wills *See* Advance directives.

Locum is a person who acts in the "place" (Latin: *locus*) of another, having the professional skills and licence to do so. Someone "in loco parentis" acts as if he were the parent. The moral requirements may, if anything, be more stringent for such a person than for the person replaced.

RH

Logic and logical reasoning To reason or to argue logically is to use a related series of statements, one of which is called the conclusion and the others the premises. We argue from premises to a conclusion, or we support the conclusion with the premises. Logic is the study of the steps from premises to a conclusion, so that to appraise an argument from the logical point of view is to consider whether or not the conclusion does or does not follow from the premises, whether the inference is valid or invalid, or whether the premises entail or imply the conclusion.

Note that logic is not concerned with truth or falsity, which are matters of evidence or facts and dealt with by science. Sometimes this point is put by saying that logic is concerned with the form of arguments whereas science is concerned with the content. Thus a conclusion may still be true even though it does not validly follow from its premises, and equally a conclusion may validly follow from its premises but still be false, if one or both premises are false.

There is an important distinction in logic between deductive and inductive argument. Deductive arguments proceed from general or universal premises to particular or singular conclusions, or to a general conclusion (from "all to some" or from "all to all"), whereas inductive arguments proceed from the particular or singular to the general or universal, or they deal with frequencies or probabilities. Inductive arguments are common in the biological and social sciences where the accumulation of evidence makes conclusions increasingly probable, but not certain.

Mistakes in reasoning are called "fallacies", and there are many typical fallacies. eg, an argument "begs the question" if it assumes what is at stake. ("Abortion must be wrong for it involves murder".) Or an argument involves the "genetic fallacy" if it confuses the historical or psychological origin of something with its rational justification. Eg, it may be true that a patient is caused to complain because of fear or loneliness, but that is irrelevant to the question of whether the *complaint* is rationally justified.

Reference
Shaw P. *Logic and its limits*. London: Pan Books, 1981.

See also: Consistency.

RSD

Long term care Long term care or continuing care implies tending until *death*, in a residential or nursing home, or a hospital. Practical issues involve the quality of the environment, payment by family, insurance or state, training of staff, the standards of tending, personalisation, and activity programmes. The boundaries between health and social care are difficult to define. The financial and organisational consequences of changes in these boundaries, and the level of responsibility that should fall on the individuals and their informal carers, are currently much debated as tensions arise between supply and demand. Ethical considerations involve the decision to place an individual in long term care, the choices offered regarding type and location of institution, the level of *autonomy* allowed within such care and treatment at the end of life. The quality of tending reflects the value that society puts upon its disadvantaged multiply handicapped members.

Reference

Denham M, ed. *Care of the long stay elderly patient.* London: Chapman and Hall, 1995.

See also: Care; chronic disease; geriatric medicine; hospice movement; institutionalisation; palliative care; politics; quality of life; resources.

PHM

Look-back procedures are used to identify, advise and, where appropriate, screen and treat patients who may have acquired infection during treatment by *infected doctors* or other health care workers. It has been used for tuberculosis, *hepatitis* B virus and *HIV* infection. The notification of patients may cause significant anxiety and may hazard the *confidentiality* of the doctor; these need to be balanced against the risk of infection and its consequences, in both the decision to conduct a look-back and in the detail of the process used. Data from such procedures can be used for *epidemiological research* into the actual risks pertaining, and thus to help in deciding whether it is necessary to follow up subsequent incidents.

AJP

Loss and grief Responses to the loss of a much valued aspect of life, such as a job, health, a pet or a close personal relationship, often follow a similar pattern.

Grief, a feeling of deep and intense sadness, is usually the dominant emotion, but other responses may occur. Shock, emotional numbness and disbelief are usually followed by intense sadness as awareness of permanent separation grows. Despair, anger, guilt and anxiety, with physical and behavioural changes, may occur.

Ultimately the loss is usually accepted, and the person adjusts to the change in circumstances, investing emotional and physical energy in other aspects of life.

See also: Anger; bereavement; denial; guilt; life events.

FR

Love, moderated The personal and emotional components of love may make it unsuitable for professional relationships. Codes of ethics stress the exploitative dangers of sexual or emotional closeness with patients and training stresses avoidance of over-involvement. But, in the crisis of illness, more is required than technical efficiency. Moderated love entails respect for and *empathy* with the patient, a granting of value to the other through the risks involved in genuine *care*. The ethical dilemma resides in the tension between involvement and detachment. If the professional boundary is crossed in the name of care, *harm* can result to both parties, but health care is in essence personal.

Reference

Campbell AV. *Moderated love.* London: SPCK, 1984.

See also: Boundaries/limits; care; detachment; doctor–patient relationship; paternalism.

AVC

Loyalty is a faithful, firm allegiance, sometimes perhaps taken beyond the rational (such as to a royal family, or to someone who has let one down). The implication is that were the other person to be different, one's own views would be different: although this would need to be challenged, it could be justified because particular people (a mother, a lover) could never be really replaced and so are unique and are perhaps owed a special *duty*.

RH

Luck A great deal of post-Enlightenment *moral* philosophy has conceived of moral goodness as immune from luck. The moral quality of actions (and persons) should be independent of factors that lie outside the control of the responsible agent. It seems, however, that there are various kinds of situation in which the allocation of moral praise and blame is affected by factors outside the agent's control. The moral assessment of a careless action may, eg, be affected by the seriousness of its consequences in such a way that the *boundaries* of moral *responsibility* appear not to coincide with the boundaries of personal agency.

Reference
Williams B. *Moral luck and other essays.* Cambridge: Cambridge University Press, 1979.

KH

Lying is to make a false statement with the intention of deceiving someone. But can there be a good lie? "White lies" are supposedly unimportant deceptions. Medical workers are sometimes considered to be justified in deceiving patients. Some would go further to insist that we all need to lie occasionally; but perhaps that's not what they really think? It may be necessary to lie to others (eg, family, the media) to protect a patient's *confidentiality*. Lying to patients, or the perception that clinicians do so, undermines *trust* and the *doctor–patient relationship* and may impair the doctor's therapeutic efficacy.

References
Bok S. *Lying.* Hassocks: Harvester, 1978.
Kerr P (ed). *The Penguin book of lies.* London: Viking, 1990.
Nyberg D. *The varnished truth: truth telling and deceiving in ordinary life.* Chicago: University of Chicago Press, 1992.

See also: Truthtelling.

RH/AJP

M

Malingering is to pretend to be ill, usually with some ulterior motive, such as being excused from playing compulsory games or working on dictionary entries. It carries a serious accusation and should be used with caution and precision, since most people develop symptoms or become ill if pushed beyond their limits.

The perception that a patient is malingering may result from a failure of *listening* or understanding. This perception may be an expression of professional exasperation at a seemingly insoluble clinical or social problem.

RH/AJP

Malpractice *See* Negligence.

Mammography is the radiological interpretation of high quality x-ray images of the breasts and is the most sensitive method available for the detection of small breast *cancers*. It is used in *screening* programmes to decrease mortality from breast cancer by detecting small cancers that can be treated before they have spread. The disadvantages of mammography are that it is not 100 per cent sensitive for detecting cancers and it may detect suspicious-appearing x-ray abnormalities that are found to be entirely benign.

MJM

Management is not easy to define. One of the best attempts (by Mary Parker Follett) is "the art of getting things done through people", emphasising that it is about mobilising groups of individuals who are working together within some organisational structure, to achieve defined goals. It is primarily an empirical field, where there is much experience but few rules. The good manager is not defined by what he knows, but by the performance of the organisation over time, and management in a collective sense is always more than the doings of one individual. The reactions of physicians to management are interesting. They tend to start from a position of distrust, condescension, and some slight apprehension, and move on to growing amazement that there is no massive body of factual knowledge to impart, as there is in medicine. Some physicians, however, pass through that phase and in time find themselves intrigued to reflect on their own growing managerial experience within a department or service, a clinical directorate, or (it may be) a whole institution. Giving up such a role, once one has become used to it, can be surprisingly difficult for someone who still thinks of himself primarily as a clinician. For a while at least, life seems dull when you leave the business of governing.

In the *National Health Service*, the 1974 reorganisation emphasised a shift from old-style administration – defined as keeping the paperwork moving, the support services running, and resolving conflicts – to something more demanding and ambitious. But the "Grey Book", as the 1974 blueprint for reorganisation came to be called, now seems very dated in its emphasis on structures, professional hierarchies, and consensus.[1] Far more impact was made in practice by the Griffiths Report of 1983, with its insistence on one individual being managerially accountable at each level and a general management line connecting every such individual to the top of the NHS.[2]

Since the mid 1980s, not only in the UK but in other countries too, there has been a marked increase in the relative standing of managers and management in health systems. Whether the competence of managers has grown as much as their influence is more debatable, though failings are often systemic as much as they are individual – the obverse of the earlier statement about management in a collective sense transcending the doings of one person.

Management as an activity obviously goes far beyond health services, affecting most sectors of the economy and of government. There have been marked shifts in management theory over the years from an early emphasis on industrial processes and assembly lines (human work organised to achieve mass production), to much increased awareness of organisations as dependent on the combined efforts of all the people working in them. Some of the most interesting current thinking emphasises the fact that successful organisations may have substantial similarity to living organisms in their ability to react instantly to fast changing external circumstances.[3]

Finally, there are important ethical dilemmas and dimensions peculiar to management as there are to medicine.[4] Much more will be heard and written about these in the years ahead.

References
1 *Management arrangements for the reorganised National Health Service*. London: HMSO, 1972.
2 DHSS. *The NHS management inquiry (Griffiths Report)* London: HMSO, 1983.
3 Wheatley M. *Leadership and the new science*. San Francisco: Barrett-Kochler Publishers, 1992.
4 Maxwell R. Health care management: are ethics relevant? In: Gillon R (ed): *Principles of health care ethics*. Chichester: John Wiley, 1993.

See also: Accountability; business ethics; change; institutions.

RJM

Manipulation (1) Healing by using the hands to correct the arrangement of a disordered musculoskeletal system.

(2) Trying to influence the situation or change the views of others by behaving insincerely or "playing games", usually leading to one's own advantage.

RH

Market Many *health care systems* including the UK *National Health Service* have recently adopted systems based on the concept of a market in health care, including the separation of *purchasing* from provision of care. This has introduced the concept of competition to professions and organisations that are used to a more collegial ethos and where there are many de facto monopoly providers, on the grounds of geography or expertise. While it has resolved some of the inbuilt inefficiencies in previous systems, it has created instability in some instances by shifting provision over short time frames; this may prevent more strategic planning and may create maldistribution of *resources*. The contracting process requires much information on the volume and type of demand, and consistent pricing models that adequately cover all costs. What has emerged is a "managed market", in some ways contrary to the idea of allowing market forces to determine patterns of health care. Managing the market involves some return to strategic planning and collaboration; few systems have yet reached a sustainable and cost effective balance.

In addition, the commercial concept of market involves active participation from consumers and is responsive to their needs. It is probably in no one's overall interest to turn health service users into consumers in the usual sense, but it is hard to see how users of the health service can currently have proper influence over the discussions between *institutions* managing the market, as would be an appropriate consequence of respecting user influence and patient *autonomy*.

See also: Colleagues/collegiality.

AJP/RH

Marxism The humanistic and materialist philosophy of Karl Marx (1818–83), in the 20th century developed or distorted to justify both radical revolutions and totalitarian regimes, is now widely discredited by association with former Soviet communism. But many questions raised by Marx, about the economic roots of social disharmony and the contradictions of capitalism, remain unanswered – not least in Eastern Europe, where medical ethics, formerly reduced to "Marxist *deontology*" is being painfully reconstructed.

KMB

Materialism as a way of life indicates undue attention to physical needs, and as a doctrine signifies any thinking that totally discounts the *spiritual* and sees only one substance to be of importance (matter), or in history economic forces to be the dominant issues. Dialectical materialism was one of Karl Marx's theories about class struggle.

See also: Dialectic; Marxism.

RH

ME (myalgic encephalomyelitis) *See* Fatigue syndromes.

Meaning is the sense intended or contained in a statement. The clarity of *communication* is of great importance in medical ethics, so that concepts and arguments are coherent. But human interactions being what they are, actions (such as bursting into tears in a consultation) or symptoms (such as getting a headache in a particular situation) can be seen as communications beyond language to which patients and health care professionals should pay attention. Indeed, the question "what does all this mean?" from a patient holds more than just a request for an accurate diagnosis. Observations always involve some measure of interpretation, and thus some judgment about significance or meaning.

RH

Means The best means to a morally desirable end are not always evident, especially when the end (as is often the case) can be envisaged only in general terms. Determining what are good motives and right procedures and acting accordingly may be the best means of both clarifying and achieving the moral goal (eg, good will and fair mindedness may help show what is the most beneficent outcome).

See also: Beneficence; ends and means.

KMB

Medical education is the process by which entrants to medical school are changed into doctors, and by which postgraduates develop and augment their professional abilities.

Historically in the UK, the training of doctors evolved from three independent sources, the ancient royal colleges, the teaching hospitals, and the universities. At the beginning of the 19th century each awarded medical qualifications of a kind. Subsequently, the teaching hospitals linked with the universities to produce a course that allowed students to learn by apprenticeship from physicians and surgeons after undertaking a course in basic medical sciences.

Undergraduate training has been criticised at various times as being the process of accruing quantities of facts unrelated to an ability to make use of them,[1] failing to give students a scientific (and therefore a university) education, failing to train students in the professional skills they will require as graduates, and failing to allow students to address the human and emotional aspects of their patients and indeed their own problems. Medical schools have been been accused of being slow to take cognisance of the move of care into the community, continuing to educate their students largely in highly specialised teaching hospitals.

The *General Medical Council* (GMC), responsible in statute for the quality of medical education, has recently addressed these criticisms vigorously.[2] If their recommendations are fully implemented they will significantly change the nature of undergraduate medical education in the UK.

The royal colleges now have the major responsibility for specialist training, which they moderate through examination of individuals and accreditation of training posts.

Professional development after the appointment to a senior position is the responsibility of the individual concerned, although increasingly the new *National Health Service trusts* have been concerned, if only by fears of litigation, for their staff's continued development. This remains the weak area: once a position of seniority is reached a doctor can practise moderately incompetently for the remainder of his career without challenge. The GMC consider cases of "gross professional misconduct" but have no remit for more modest failures. The profession has tended to protect its weaker brethren, often at a cost to their patients. Recently the GMC has initiated a humane policy to help doctors who are failing through illness, in particular *mental illness* and *alcoholism*.

References

1 Evered DC, Williams HD. "The medical schools accept only the most gifted students and then expose them to an educational process so rigid in its structure and limited in its horizons that at graduation the medical student is the best informed but most poorly educated of all graduates." Postgraduate education and the doctor. *BMJ* 1980; **280**: 626–8.
2 *Tomorrow's doctors: recommendations on undergraduate medical education*. London: General Medical Council, 1993.

See also: Attitudes; clinical teaching; incompetent professionals; role modelling; students; support staff; training, vocational; videos.

PBo

Medical ethics Historical changes in what this term refers to can be illustrated by the fact that whereas the first important English text entitled Medical Ethics, by Thomas Percival in 1803,[1] was largely concerned with prescribing etiquette for physicians, the 1994 House of Lords Report on Medical Ethics[2] was largely concerned with discussing problematic questions related to euthanasia – itself a term which was not used in the modern sense of actively assisting death until the end of the 19th century.[3] Until the mid-20th century, "medical ethics" was generally understood to refer either to matters confined to the self-regulation of the medical profession ("discussed by clinicians with clinicians and in camera") or to treatment of medical questions in Catholic moral theology. But medicine's growing ability to prolong life, if not always its quality, combined with moral concern related to "euthanasia" and medical research in Nazi Germany, led in the 1960s to greater professional, and then academic and public attention, being paid to the moral problems or "dilemmas" raised by modern medical practice. Medical ethics today comprises (a) systematic study of and popular debate on these subjects, but also (b) the standards of professional competence and conduct which the medical profession expects of its members. In both respects it has served as a model for similar treatment of the ethics of other health care professions (nursing ethics and health care ethics, eg, overlap with it) and also of ethics related to the life sciences (bioethics), the sciences generally (science, technology and engineering ethics), and many other practical activities in society (eg, business and management ethics). In an academic context, many of these activities are studied under the rubric of applied philosophy, or practical ethics, while in public life the terminology of ethics is increasingly being used to provide a common language and agreed standards for a multicultural and pluralist society. Here too standards of medical ethics agreed by professional bodies from different countries and enshrined in international declarations have led the way. Alongside these professionally led or philosophically informed versions of medical ethics, however, others based on the specific assumptions of particular cultures or religions continue to flourish; and while philosophy plays an important role in academic medical ethics and bioethics, these are essentially multidisciplinary fields, relying no less on the expertise of students and practitioners of the relevant sciences and arts, with important contributions being made by law, theology, and the social sciences.

References
1 Leake CD. Percival's medical ethics. Huntington, New York: RE Kreiger, 1975.
2 House of Lords. Report of the Select Committee on Medical Ethics. London: HMSO, 1994.
3 Jalland P. Death in the Victorian family. Oxford: Oxford University Press, 1996.

See also: Bioethics, history of.

KMB

Medical journalism Coverage of health in the mass media has increased dramatically in the past 50 years. Most newspapers now have specialist correspondents on health. Television programmes that showed operations began in Britain to a storm of protest as recently as the 1950s, but documentaries on health are now routine – and one recent series of live transmissions from a London hospital was watched by half of the British population.

This growth in coverage coincides with a growing ethical conviction that patients have the right to know about what is happening in medicine. The journalists who produce the material hope that it will help individual patients make informed choices on their own health care and help the general public take part in important debates on, for instance, rationing of health care, genetic manipulation, and *euthanasia*. In a sense the only way to have a national debate is through the mass media, but the hope that increased media coverage leads to a more informed population is not supported by strong evidence. Indeed, some commentators have argued that the deluge of information – much of it partial, biased, and contradictory – has served to confuse people rather than educate them. Particularly when so many people, including doctors, are trying to manipulate the media to their own ends. More coverage on health in the mass media is far from being an obvious benefit. Less coverage of higher quality would be better for everybody.

Much of the medical material in the mass media originates in medical journals, and intense debates have raged over the tension between the slowness of the *peer review* system and the need to report rapidly scientific results with important implications for the public. Editors of medical journals argue that publication first in a peer reviewed journal gives some guarantee of validity and allows everybody to see all the data and make up their own minds on their worth. Journalists argue that editors are protecting their own interests and that the public has the right to know as soon as results become available. Unsurprisingly, some journal editors subscribe to the view that everybody, including the public, is best served by material appearing first in scientific journals.

RSm

Medical records One form of medical record follows a patient through life, and is held by his general practitioner; another form of record relates to a specific episode of illness, and is generally held in hospital or by a specialist. The "ownership" of either type of record is uncertain, and probably immaterial. What matters is their usefulness to those who "need to know", in order to participate in the clinical care of the patient; their protection from those who do not "need to know", and who might even make improper use of the information in the record; and their availability to patients themselves, who have a right to "subject access". This latter justified exercise of autonomy is not unlimited, there being no obligation to disclose data potentially damaging either to the patient or to third parties mentioned in the record.

See also: Data protection; next of kin.

DB

Medical students See Students.

Medication *See* Drugs.

Medicine The term "medicine" is used in different ways. In popular usage, it denotes a therapeutic substance usually taken in liquid form ("Have you taken your medicine today?"). In a very general sense, it covers the totality of medical care – doctors, nurses, hospitals, community care, research institutions – in phrases such as "what medicine has to offer" or "the rising cost of medicine". In a more focused sense, it is used to convey what those who wish to become doctors have to study – they are students of medicine, and the term covers all components of the medical course that leads to the degree MBChB or its equivalent (MD in the USA). The most confusing application of the term is to that specialty known in the USA and Continental Europe as internal medicine, the practitioners of which are internists. In the UK and much of the Commonwealth this specialty is known simply as medicine, sometimes general medicine, and those who practise it are physicians or consultant physicians (another source of confusion since "physician" is used generically in the USA to denote all doctors, specialised or not). As a rather loose generalisation those who specialise in this way become expert in diagnostic skills and in the treatment of conditions that do not require surgery. They do not deal with childbirth or disorders of the female reproductive tract (obstetrics and gynaecology) or with mental disease (psychiatry), although in practice many of the specialties tend to overlap.

Because of the expansion of medical knowledge the broad specialties of general medicine and surgery have tended to subdivide, usually on the basis of one of the systems or organs of the body, such as the heart, lungs, kidneys, gut, endocrine or nervous systems. Divisions have also occurred in relation to age: those who deal with children become paediatricians or paediatric surgeons; those who deal with the elderly, geriatricians.

The primary education and training of a doctor takes place in a university which awards the degree of MBChB (or equivalent) on successful completion of the course. The postgraduate specialist phase is regulated in the UK by one of the specialised colleges. In the case of medicine these are the four Royal Colleges of Physicians (London, Edinburgh, Glasgow and Ireland); admission to membership (MRCP) is by examination, to Fellowship (FRCP) by subsequent election.

See also: General practice; hospital medicine; medical education; National Health Service; specialism.

RHf

Mental handicap *See* Learning difficulties.

Mental illness The term is used both as a synonym for the generic 'mental disorder' and, in a more restricted sense, for those particular kinds of mental disorder that are most like physical (or bodily) illnesses.

Mental illness differs from physical illness in being more overtly value-laden both in treatment and diagnosis. Thus even the most routine treatments in psychiatry are often ethically problematic.

But diagnosis, too, raises questions of value far more often in psychiatry than in the rest of medicine. These may be general (ie, as to whether someone's mental condition is bad as such) or specific (ie, as to whether the badness of someone's condition is, genuinely, medical or, say, moral or aesthetic). Both kinds of question are involved in the judgments of *rationality* which underpin both medicolegal issues of *responsibility* and particular diagnostic distinctions, eg, between psychotic disorder and religious experience, *psychopathy* and delinquency, *depression* and sadness, *alcoholism* and drunkness, paraphilias and normal variations in sexual behaviour, and hunger-striking and anorexia.

The relatively value-laden nature of mental illness has provoked contrary responses from psychiatrists and anti-psychiatrists. Psychiatrists have sought to eliminate the evaluative element from mental illness by assimilating it to a supposedly value-free "medical model" of physical illness. Anti-psychiatrists have argued that the evaluative element in mental illness shows it to be a moral rather than a medical concept.

Philosophical moral theory, notably *prescriptivism*, reconciles these two extreme positions. It shows, contra anti-psychiatry, that mental and physical illness are equally valid species of illness; but also, contra psychiatry, that mental illness is irreducibly more value-laden than physical illness. This is because the criteria for the value judgments involved in diagnoses of mental illness are relatively (and legitimately) contentious compared with those for diagnoses of physical illness.

This has important practical consequences. It also: (a) shows psychiatry and other aspects of primary care to be the clinically more demanding end of medicine rather than (as in the "medical model") its scientifically soft end; (b) gives bioethics a new role in helping to explicate issues of diagnosis as well as treatment, and (c) links bioethics in this respect directly with some of the deepest metaphysical questions in moral philosophy and the philosophy of action.

Reference
Fulford KWM. *Moral theory and medical practice.* Cambridge: Cambridge University Press, 1989, reprinted 1995.

See also: Addiction; decision-making capacity; drug misuse; eating disorders; electroconvulsive therapy; forensic psychiatry; health, illness and disease, concepts of; leucotomy; psychiatry; psychopharmacology, use and abuse; psychosurgery; psychotherapy; sexual practices.

KWMF

Mercy may involve *forgiveness*, but in health care suggests particular compassion for those who are unfortunate or suffering. This is a quality that can be eroded by exposure and needs to be cared for in its own right (viz by reflection). Mercy killing suggests (presumably voluntary) active *euthanasia*, but is not in any sense a precise term.

RH

Merit A person deserves health care because he is ill or in need, rather than because he has earned the attention in other ways. Yet in decisions that involve putting one person in front of another (such as in *triage*, or waiting lists, or organ *transplantation*) it may be hard not to respond to the perception that one person merits attention more than another, for instance, because of his personal attention to his health care, or his contribution to

society. Only a lottery would completely eliminate these considerations, but even if they are to be discounted they are best acknowledged.

Systems of *reward* for merit among staff are problematic, presenting a tension between promotion of a meritocracy and preservation of equity. Bonuses or discretionary increments in salary are widely used and accepted; however, merit awards for doctors, which provide substantial salary increases to some, based on criteria that are not always apparent and that may preferentially reward some categories, remain contentious.

See also: Desert.

RH/AJP

Metaethics Philosophical inquiry into the concepts, theories, language and intellectual foundations of ethics – as opposed to practical ethical questions, but not unrelated to them, since the nature, content and context of moral understanding are endlessly puzzling.

KMB

Metaphor (Greek for "to carry over or beyond") – an unusual (or unusually used) word or phrase, combining a familiar with an unfamiliar idea, which can advance our understanding, especially when no current word catches the exact sense of what we want to say. Sometimes opposed to "literal". But literal (including scientific) terms are often "dead" metaphors, whose origin has been forgotten (eg, "immunity", "epidemic", "renal").

KMB

Metaphysics (Greek for "beyond physics") – the attempt to understand not things (as in the sciences) but the whole of things in terms either of religion or of philosophical inquiry into the structure of human thinking.

Sometimes dismissed as illusory: but the dismissal itself is a metaphysical judgment.

KMB

Micro/macro allocation Micro allocation refers to the provision and consumption of health services between individuals, patient groups or social groups within a country or local population. Macro allocation refers to expenditure on health services relative to a country's wealth (as measured by Gross National Product), or other services such as education.

See also: Cost containment; health economics; priorities; public policy; purchasing; resources.

MP

Midwives A group of autonomous health care workers who take personal *responsibility* for the care of women having babies. Midwifery practice is governed by statute. Secondary legislation is laid down in a set of rules issued by the United Kingdom Central Council for Nursing, Midwifery and Health Visiting (UKCC) relating to competencies, boundaries for practice, record-keeping and the administration of medicines.

References
International Confederation of Midwives. *International code of ethics for midwives.* London: ICM, 1993.
UKCC. *The midwife's code of practice.* London: UKCC, 1994.

See also: Autonomy; accountability; codes; competence; duty of care; primary care; professionalism.

HM

Military metaphors are commonly used in medicine to describe both the action of professionals and the reaction of chemicals or cells within the body. The problem comes when the *metaphor* contaminates the thinking or

action: when aggressive treatment seems to justify aggressive or unfeeling professional behaviour, for instance.

RH

Minorities Millionaires are a minority group but that is not how the term is used. It denotes members of groups who by virtue of being different in ways not valued by the powerful majority are seen as lesser; typically they lack power. Examples include black people, homosexuals, and women. Health care workers should be aware of the force of unconscious assumptions based on, for instance, class, *gender*, and age.

See also: Autonomy; doctor–patient relationship; ethnicity; feminism; homosexual; prejudice; silence; women's rights.

ALI

Minors are individuals who are considered to be insufficiently mature to be competent to make important decisions. This applies to those under the legal age of *consent*, who rely on those with parental responsibility to make decisions on their behalf and in their best interests. With increasing maturity, children are given more *autonomy* depending on the importance and complexity of the issues. Recently, minors have been recognised as having the right to make decisions about *contraception* when it is judged by their doctors that they are sufficiently mature to understand the implications of their actions. The other edge of this sword is the recent swing towards a more punitive response to increasingly young children involved in criminal activity. This is another example of the link between developing rights and responsibilities with age. To be classed as a minor limits the individual's freedom but at the same time increases the obligation which society has to care and protect that individual.

161

See also: Adolescence; child, status of; decision-making capacity.

GC

Misconduct may be professional (exercise of clinical skills) or personal. Either form may provoke disciplinary action by an employer or regulatory body, such as the *General Medical Council* (GMC), the General Dental Council (GDC), or the United Kingdom Central Council for Nursing, Midwifery and Health Visiting (UKCC), to protect the public interest. About half the cases of serious professional misconduct considered by the GMC relate to "disregard of professional responsibilities to patients": significant failures of care. The remainder involve *fraud*, improper (usually sexual) relationships with patients, *advertising, confidentiality*, alcohol or drug problems. In future the GMC will consider chronically poor performance, through a new assessment mechanism.

Reference

General Medical Council. *Duties of a doctor*. London: GMC, 1995.

See also: Accountability; negligence.

PH

Mistakes Twenty per cent of all hospital-based *negligence* claims settled out of court are for *harm* caused to patients by mistakes or other practical problems rather than by errors of clinical *judgment* – wrong operations or operations on the wrong patient or site; direct injury to patients (burns, pressure sores following long operations); retained swabs or instruments; failure of equipment. When such a problem has been identified, the doctor has an ethical obligation to notify the patient at the earliest opportunity, and to redress the damage as quickly and as far as possible.

Reference

Hoyte PJ. Unsound practice: the epidemiology of medical negligence. *Med Law Rev* 1995; **3**: 53–73.

PH

Modality in *logic* refers to the classification of propositions, as to whether they are true or false, possible or impossible, or necessary.

RH

Moderation has been seen as a key virtue in places and times as diverse as ancient Greece and Edwardian England. The notion of avoiding extremes and acting reasonably is important in health care because it enables patients and professionals to develop a consistent approach within a *trusted* and trusting relationship, and in medical ethics provides a way of avoiding excesses (say, of medical intervention) and reduce inflexibility (for instance, of adherence to rules or contracts). Its links with *tradition* may slow apparent progress, but confers stability in an environment of *change*.

RH

Moral (from Latin mores: customs, manners) – in common usage the opposite of "immoral"; in philosophy referring to questions about what is right or wrong, good or bad, in arguable matters of human conduct. Often but not always interchangeable with the more high-sounding *"ethical"*.

KMB

Moral agency Moral agents judge for themselves and act (Latin agere: to act), while moral patients bear or suffer being acted upon. Telling the two apart can be difficult. Apparent agents may be reacting to events and/or inner impressions (eg, unconscious memories) acting upon them, while apparent patients, choosing to accept their life's limitations, may enjoy greater *autonomy* of thought and *will*.

See also: Patient, moral.

KMB

Moral argument has the following structure: a major premise consisting of some general rule or principle ("Patients ought to be informed about the diagnosis"), and a minor premise consisting of a matter of fact ("This patient was not informed"), which together yield the conclusion ("This patient was wronged"). Criticism of the argument can be directed at the alleged facts of the minor premise, ("The patient *was* told") or at the major premise ("It is not the case that *incompetent* patients ought to be told").

Reference

Downie RS, Calman KC. *Healthy respect: ethics in health care* (2nd ed). Oxford: Oxford University Press, 1994: 118–134.

See also: Double effect; rhetoric; slippery slope.

RSD

Moral development, theories of The pioneering work of J Piaget, which included exploring children's understanding of the rules of games, has been followed by that of Lawrence Kohlberg, who focused on the reasons people gave for their solutions to fictional dilemmas. Kohlberg suggested that individuals moved from a morality based on power and punishment towards one based on a universal equity. The predominance of male subjects in Kohlberg's study prompted Carol Gilligan and others to explore women's moral development, which has been characterised as being based on care rather than on equity – ie, equality of attention to individual needs rather than on equality of treatment.

References

Gilligan C *et al*. *Mapping the moral domain: a contribution of women's thinking to psychological theory and education*. Cambridge, Mass: Centre for the Study of Gender, Education, and Human Development, Harvard University Graduate School of Education, 1988.

Kohlberg L. *The psychology of moral development: the nature and validity of moral stages*. San Francisco: Harper and Row, 1984.

BC

Moral distinction/difference A moral distinction (from Latin: marking apart) may or may not make a moral difference (from Latin: carrying apart). Distinctions between killing and letting die, or between *intention and motive*, eg, may be more persuasive in theory than in clinical practice.

KMB

Moral imperative A command to do (or not to do) something without further argument, because a judgment has been made that it is right or obligatory. To be moral, an imperative must arise from the agent's reflection on, recognition of, and decision to comply with, its necessity.

See also: Categorical imperative.

KMB

Moral judgment Judgment is "difficult" (Hippocrates), "mysterious" and irreducible (Kant). Moral like *clinical judgment* involves discerning what evidence is relevant, reviewing it and coming to a conclusion whose rightness may be evident, if ever, only in retrospect. Judgmentalism (a readiness to make moral judgments about other people), is easier, but neither medically nor morally appropriate in clinical practice.

See also: Bias.

KMB

Moral psychology has two different connotations: first, describing the branch of psychology that studies the development and structure of moral cognition and behaviour as psychological phenomena. Some psychologists deny an independent role for ethics and claim that moral psychology gives an exhaustive account of all moral phenomena.

Second, in moral philosophy it describes the set of background assumptions about the mental capacities of moral agents (eg, degree of rationality) in a particular moral theory.

Many philosophers deny that "psychological" moral psychology can play any role in *normative ethics* because reasoning from how people think to how they ought to think would contravene the *is-ought gap*.

See also: Moral development, theories of; psychology/morality boundary.

SH

Moral sentiments In 18th century philosophy, "higher" feelings (eg, respect, sympathy or a special "moral sense") that dispose towards, accompany and confirm rational moral judgments. Now often regarded as (if they exist) relative and fallible.

See also: Conscience; intuition.

KMB

Moral theory or ethical theory, is the body of knowledge derived from attempts to give a coherent or consistent account of ethics or morality. It includes both (a) *metaethics'* interest in what words like "right" and "wrong" mean, and whether they reflect the way things are or just the way we see things, and (b) particular *ethical systems*, such as *utilitarianism*, *Kantian ethics*, or *social contract* theories, whose advocates' interests are more prescriptive. Although conducted at a remove from practical ethics, moral theorising uncovers genuine complexities and the distinctions it draws can be helpful in organising practitioners' thinking, at least initially. Its main practical disadvantages are (a) that moral theorising can degenerate into a decontextualised or one-dimensional fight to the death between rival systems, and (b) that final victory in such battles is rarely if ever won, because uncovering the genuine complexities of ethical thinking is almost always an interminable process (rather like psychoanalysis – indeed some philosophers regard theorising as a form of therapy). Moral theory's

most appropriate contribution to *medical ethics*, therefore, may be rather like that of the life sciences to clinical practice – as Aristotle remarked of ethics generally, it is "adequate if it achieves the amount of precision which belongs to its subject matter". This may be why the *principles* of bioethics approach, criticised by many theorists, is valued by many practitioners. In this context it is also worth remembering Cardinal Newman's observation that people who cannot give a reason, nevertheless may have a reason, and that in the original Greek, theory means not just intellectual speculation but also reflective contemplation.

KMB

MRSA Methicillin-resistant Staphylococcus aureus *See* Infection control.

Multidisciplinary teams are groups of health and related professionals who act together in delivery of integrated care across a range of disciplines. The complexity of health care requires that such teams are increasingly needed. Their effectiveness in working together as *colleagues* requires a common ethos, information base and therapeutic approach to the patient. It must be underpinned by a recognition of each other's professional skills and negotiated boundaries of *responsibility*. Key workers may be identified for some functions. Acknowledgment of who has ultimate clinical responsibility is essential. It may be necessary to agree if a leadership role is required and who should have this, in particular whether it should be a doctor. Ideally, in an *empowerment* or *mutual participation model* of care, the patient should be explicitly included in the multidisciplinary team. Duties owed by the physician to the patient must extend to the whole team, who are part of the confidential network. The composition will be determined by the context, but could involve, eg, physician(s), possibly including several specialists, nurse, psychologist, dietitian, *pharmacist*, physiotherapist, occupational therapist, and social worker. Increasingly, clinically orientated managers should be part of the team.

See also: Ancillary staff; confidentiality; paramedical professions, teamwork.

AJP

Münchausen syndrome The term, dedicated to the memory of Baron von Münchausen who travelled widely and told false stories, is applied to persons who invent false illness stories, causing themselves to be treated needlessly in different hospitals for the fictitious complaints. Their stories are dramatic, untruthful, but usually convincing.

Such persons are not thought to relish the pain and inconvenience of operations and investigations, but they do like the care and concern that is associated with these. The dilemma for doctors is that the correct way to work is to believe and empathise with the patient: patients do not want a doctor who questions or disagrees with their symptoms. Similarly, the care and concern that these people appreciate when in hospital are needed for genuine patients.

Reference
Asher R. Münchausen's syndrome. *Lancet* 1951; I: 339–341.

RM

Münchausen syndrome by proxy Used mainly to describe a form of child abuse in which a parent (nearly always the mother) invents or causes illness for his or her child. Similar abuse of adults, incapacitated by age or other disability, by their relatives also occurs.

Doctors dealing with children rely on the parent's story. If that story is false, massive and dangerous over-investigation and treatment follows. On the one hand, doctors are blamed for not recognising that a mother's story is false, while on the other, they are accused of being callous and too prepared to doubt a mother's story, and of accusing her of Münchausen syndrome by proxy *child abuse*. The methods used to uncover the mother's deception occasionally include unusual strategies such as covert video surveillance of the mother with her child, and are the source of considerable ethical debate.

Reference
Meadow R. Münchausen syndrome by proxy. *BMJ* 1989; **299**: 248–50.
Southall DP *et al.* Symposium on covert video surveillance. *J Med Ethics* 1996; **22**: 16–32.

RM

Murder *See* Homicide.

Mutilation To maim, or permanently spoil the positive features of a person has no part in good medical practice. No doctor should take part in operations which are not for the benefit of the patient, (and properly consented to by him), unless circumstances are exceptional. Thus to assist in *torture* or punishment is clearly wrong: yet one person's mutilation may be another's *cosmetic surgery*. The law and ethics both, for instance, forbid a surgeon, without prior permission deciding while the patient is asleep that "he would be better off without this mole". The *castration* of persistent sex offenders, recently proposed by some legislatures, may be the beginning of an unpleasant *slippery slope*. A man who has been circumcised as a child may also claim that a piece of his body which would have contributed to his sexual pleasure has been removed at a time when, infant and sexually inactive, he was doubly unable to give *consent*.

See also: Complicity.

RH

Mutuality suggests interchange (Latin mutare: change), or reciprocal exchange of something between people (such as support or attention) and *reciprocity* in that relationship. As usually conceived the best life cannot be lived in isolation, and the best moral solutions and human *welfare* take into account the *dependency* of one upon the other as well as respecting the *autonomy* of each. Early modern medical ethics has been weakened (remediably), and Thatcherite politics flawed (fatally), by a poor understanding of this.

RH

Mutual participation model A system of care in which patient and clinician participate in *decision making* as partners. The phrase also describes the outcome of an effective *doctor–patient relationship*. It is in many ways the result of successfully empowering patients to work in partnership.

See also: Empowerment.

AJP

Myth (Greek for story) – tall tales about the gods or the origin and destiny of the universe. Discredited by popular rationalism, but surviving in popular culture (eg, urban myths). Many enduring religious myths share common features and have been rediscovered as archetypes of human experience, embodying perennial insights.

KMB

N

Narrative ethics A new name for the oldest way of exploring and expounding ethical issues (*myth*, history, parable, fable (auto-) biography). Retelling a case by recounting the patient's life story, lived *values* and experiences of illness (and the stories told by different professionals and relatives) complements and contextualises moral principles and clinical *perspectives*, often clarifying the ethical crux in the particular case.

See also: Context.

KMB

National Health Service A state-run *health care system*, funded through taxation and in particular the UK system (NHS). It works on the principle of providing universal and comprehensive health care that is free at the point of delivery. It is a very large and complex organisation, comprising many elements of clinical provision, *purchasing* and planning. It has been subject to many organisational changes and reforms as a result of changing political imperatives and attempts to enhance cost effectiveness of *resource* utilisation and *accountability*. The most significant change has been the concept of separating purchasing and planning, ie defining health needs, from provision of care, ie the delivery of services to meet the needs. Purchasers or commissioners (health authorities) contract for a level of service and are informed by *public health* professionals. Providers (some of whom have been organised into *trusts*) include *general practitioners*, *community care* agencies, *hospital medicine*, health promotion, and ambulances. The boundaries of responsibility for some aspects of provision between the NHS and other statutory, private, or voluntary agencies are not always clear, with some functions increasingly being contracted out. Yet there is very strong support for the concept of the NHS in the public mind, which serves as a check (regulative ideal or maybe sacred cow) for some proposed changes.

The NHS is staffed by a wide variety of professions and trades, each with its own values and overseen by its own professional body and/or trade union, some of which have explicit *self-regulation* and some of which are involved in negotiating terms and conditions of service. GPs are independent contractors. Historically, *management* and the professions have mutually agreed their areas of responsibility and authority. However, each reorganisation modifies the dynamic and may jeopardise the delicate balance, as eg in discussions over local pay bargaining or constraints on what staff may say publicly about organisational matters that have a professional impact (*whistleblowing*).

The principles on which the NHS is based accord with the vocational approach to health care and offer the best prospect of *equity* in its delivery. Compared to insurance based and private health care systems, which tend to be least available to those with the greatest need (eg those affected by *poverty* or alienation), it is generally less costly in overall terms. However because these costs fall on the public purse, they are subject to other competing pressures on the national economy and to perceptions about need.

It is a widely held view (or canard) that the demand for health care now exceeds the capacity of a national economy to support it, as a result of increased expectations, improved technology, and increasing age and morbidity of the population. This means that a NHS is necessarily subject to resource constraints. While the issue is now more widely debated, there is little structured or explicit rationing (eg, *cosmetic surgery* and treatment of *infertility* are excluded by some purchasers). Restriction of access or treatment may indirectly and inequitably result from funding limitations resulting from resource allocation and problems in implementing the contracting process. While decisions are ostensibly in the hands of planners and purchasers,

they are often de facto made by providers. Clinicians and managers attempt to balance medical needs and financial prudence, posing major ethical dilemmas. Yet it may only be from knowledge of the individual, their circumstances and their needs that rational decisions can be made, provided there are broad principles to guide and there is a system of regulation and accountability for the decisions. These issues are rarely articulated or rehearsed publicly yet they go to the very heart of the nature of the *responsibilities* of the clinician to the individual and to the public health.

There are many conditions that fall as costs to any health service whose origins are beyond the scope of that service (eg poor housing) and whose effective treatment is also not in health service hands. There are cases where a smaller amount of money spent elsewhere (such as in effective preventive measures) would also reduce larger health service expenditure. International comparisons appear to show that health statistics deteriorate when the gap widens between rich and poor. These sorts of consideration have moved many to try to take health service planning and policy issues beyond the narrow confines of the particular national health service structure.

See also: Cost containment; gatekeeping; poverty.

AJP/RH

Natural family planning (NFP) Modern scientific natural methods (originally known as the rhythm method) are used by women to identify the fertile days when pregnancy can occur; to avoid a pregnancy, abstinence is practised. Ethically acceptable to all creeds and cultures, the Double-check-method (mucus, cervix, temperature) is highly efficient (Pearl 2.2%)

whereas the Billings-method (mucus) is less efficient (Pearl 22.3%).

See also: Contraception.

AMF

Natural law theory asserts that moral norms can be derived from reflection on human nature. A static approach to it has produced claims of unchangeable norms regarding the uses of certain human faculties and organs. More dynamic approaches admit development in our knowledge of human nature and a need to revise norms accordingly.

Reference
Curran E, McCormick A, eds. *Readings in moral theology no 7: Natural law and theology.* New York: Paulist Press, 1991.

BHo

Necessity (from Latin: what will not yield or "cede") (i) what cannot but be; (ii) the opposite of free will; (iii) principle whereby a wrongful act may be justified as the only way to avoid a greater evil – eg, *surgery* would be *assault* without not only *consent* (if the patient has *decision-making capacity*) but also the necessity to save life or preserve health.

KMB

Need A need is what is necessary for a person to exist (eg, sustenance) or to flourish (eg, health). Basic needs include common biological needs, and, arguably, culturally specific goods, such as education. Needs are often set in opposition to wants. Since the mediaeval era, in which it was argued that those with superfluous goods had a duty to help the needy, the concept of need has been closely tied to *justice*. Health care could be said to be a human right, that is, a need of all persons which when unmet demands immediate attention. The difficult question is: "Attention by whom?".

Reference
Wiggins D (ed). Claims of need. In: *Needs, values, truth* (2nd ed). Oxford: Blackwell, 1991.

See also: flourishing; human rights; interest.

RCr

Needs assessment for the local population is critical to planning and *purchasing* of health service provision and in the UK *National Health Service* is formally one role of *public health* departments in health authorities. As full needs assessments are complex and labour intensive, they are in practice focused on major areas of health need, whether determined by prevalence of disease, local factors such as poverty, sizable elderly or ethnic minority communities, or costly aspects of health care. Community or patient involvement is variable.

AJP

Negligence A patient who wishes to succeed in a medical negligence action must prove three things: the existence of a *duty of care*; breach of that duty, and that damage resulted.

Negligence (breach of the duty of care) may be defined as a failure to come up to the standard to be expected from colleagues with similar training, skills and experience. Or, more simplistically, "being negligent is getting wrong that which another practitioner more often than not would get right"[1].

In legal terms, the judge's comments in Bolam[2] have become a standard for assessing a practitioner's performance: ". . . a doctor is not negligent . . . if he acts in accordance with a practice accepted as proper by a responsible body of medical men . . . merely because there is a body of opinion who would take a contrary view".

The payment of proper and prompt *compensation* for established negligence is a basic principle of the civil *law*.

168

References
1 Hay S. *Are you negligent?* London: Economist Publications Ltd, 1987.
2 *Bolam* v *Friern Hospital Management Committee* [1957] 2 AER 118.

See also: Informed consent.

PH

Neighbours may be interested parties in health care decisions in a number of ways. They may be informal or even formal carers for the elderly or vulnerable living alone. They may provide company, advice, or security to the lonely or anxious. They may be the unwilling recipients of attention from the paranoid, or actually at risk when living near the confused or disturbed. The quality of relationships between neighbours is often used to judge the moral health of a society, and may be the limiting step in establishing or maintaining health care in the community. To religious thinkers like Jesus Christ they symbolise people we come across, and are thrown together with, rather than connected to by friendship or blood: in such eyes our *care* for them should be measured against our care for ourselves.

RH

Neural tube defects are the range of *congenital malformations* affecting the development of the nervous system, including anencephaly and spina bifida. These occur spontaneously or may be induced by teratogenic agents. They can be identified during pregnancy by *screening* methods including alphafetoprotein estimation in blood, *amniocentesis* and/or ultrasound imaging. Parents may need *counselling* to help reach decisions about whether or not to screen, about inducing *abortion* if a defect is identified, or in preparation for a child's disability. Spina bifida presents a range of disorders from a fully correctable skin defect without disability through to significant limb paralysis. There is much debate about whether spina bifida constitutes sufficient reason for abortion, as intellect is unimpaired, with strong views being expressed by, among others, those affected. Anencephalic babies may survive for some time after birth and pose similar dilemmas regarding supportive therapy as patients with *persistent vegetative states*. The use of their organs and tissues in *transplantation* presents particular concerns.

AJP

New age movement A loose yet complex network of sometimes divergent ideas, insights and practices including those connected with *complementary medicine*, *spiritual healing*, and *personal growth*. Common to all is the affirmation of a *spiritual* dimension to life, and challenge to a scientifically reductionist world view as we approach the new millennium.

Intuitive inner wisdom tends to be valued above systems of external authority. Personal and planetary transformation are held to be closely connected. While some esoteric and apparently trivial practices may be criticised as naive, even dangerously exploitative, serious practitioners, particularly in the fields of health and *healing*, would maintain that their work is disciplined, rigorous and respectful of people.

References
Bloom W, ed. *The new age – an anthology of essential writings*. London: Rider, 1991.

See also: Ecology; holistic; intuition; paganism; reductionist thinking; religion; spirituality; wisdom.

HA

Next of kin is the closest family member to a person/patient who, in legal terms, is entitled to a share in the estate in the case of intestacy. Medically the term is often used for the person who, by blood or marriage ties, or by the patient's request, is designated as the closest relative for the purposes of information giving or as a *proxy* for *decision making*. In the case of an *incompetent* patient or after death, there may be dispute about who is the next of kin, especially if the patient had not instructed previously. Specific problems may arise between *homosexual* couples and parents/siblings. Disputes or uncertainties over next of kin may present difficulties regarding *confidentiality*, information giving and involvement in clinical decisions, and clinicians may be obliged to arbitrate.

See also: Power of attorney.

AJP

Night visits *See* Out of hours work

Nihilism (from Latin: nothing) (i) Extreme scepticism or relativism about all metaphysical claims and moral values. Difficult to maintain consistently or coherently if "all" includes nihilism itself. Often a term of abuse used by defenders of the status quo in society or philosophy against radical critics or even moderate reformers. (ii) Therapeutic nihilism is grave medical doubt about the value of any medical treatment.

KMB

Non-intervention may be a preferable line of action in situations where intervention may be harmful or carries too high risks. Since there is often pressure (internally and externally) on professionals to intervene, it is important to see non-intervention as an action in its own right, appropriate or not as the case may be and, if so, entirely justifiable.

RH

Non-invasive treatments are preferable to invasive ones, other things being equal, on the basis of *risk* of *harm* and the principle of *parsimony*.

RH

Non-maleficence Not doing *harm*. The *prima facie* moral obligation to avoid doing harm is common to a wide variety of moral theories. In the context of health care (and whenever we are trying to benefit others) it requires us to minimise the harmful effects of our interventions and achieve net benefit.

RG

Non-voluntary Term applied to *euthanasia* when it is not voluntarily requested by the patient: preferable to "involuntary" (which can also mean "unintentional") and to "compulsory" (which could mean "required by law"). Non-voluntary euthanasia is not necessarily contrary to the patient's wishes: but because these are not known or expressed, the crucial element of any possible moral justification is absent.

KMB

Normal An adjective which can be applied with more or less precision, from its statistical use (normal distribution) to its subjective or conventional – "she felt back to normal" (health); "the normal way to behave".

KMB

Normative ethics is concerned with establishing basic ethical principles or standards ("norms" – from Greek for builder's rule or square). Examples include normative theories (eg, *deontological* or *teleological*), normative principles (eg, the *principles* of *bioethics*), and *declarations* or statements either on the core values of medicine or on specific duties of doctors and nurses in particular circumstances.

KMB

Notifiable diseases are those conditions that clinicians have a statutory requirement to report. They are infectious diseases that may necessitate *public health* control measures, such as *contact tracing*. Notification also provides a means of epidemiological surveillance, though its reliability depends on the reliability of clinician reporting. Examples in the UK include tuberculosis, measles, acute meningitis, rabies, yellow fever, malaria, leprosy, cholera, and food poisoning. Notification also places certain formal restrictions on the use of public facilities by patients while they are deemed a public health hazard. Clinicians may be concerned about *confidentiality* in the reporting of individuals, but there are some safeguards as to the use of this information by public health doctors and their staff.

AJP

Nuclear war Whether or not there can be an ethical or just *war*, nuclear war is different.

Nuclear weapons are so powerful that their effects are inevitably indiscriminate; so-called "collateral" damage is a euphemism for the destruction of civilian and non-military targets. The use of such weapons amounts to genocide; death will occur in several forms, including: vaporisation; direct blast damage to the human frame (eg, being hurled at 50 feet per second into a brick wall at three miles from a one-megaton bomb); severe crush injuries from falling masonry, and slow death from radiation sickness. Large-scale nuclear war would have serious ecological effects on the planet, possibly precipitating a nuclear winter. Any medical response would be only of a peripheral significance; so the *responsibility* of the medical profession must be to warn populations of the catastrophic consequences of nuclear war.

Some argue that the destruction of Hiroshima and Nagasaki shortened the Second World War and thus saved lives. In 1945, however, only one country (USA) possessed nuclear weapons and so their use then reflected a unique historical period (ie, there could be no threat of nuclear war when only one side had these weapons).

Nuclear deterrence is rational to the extent that neither side starts a (nuclear) war, which would result in Mutual Assured Destruction (MAD). It therefore relies for its effectiveness on leaders being rational and war not being started by accident. It is unsafe to assume that leaders of nuclear weapon states will always be rational.

As there is no absolute guarantee that once created, a nuclear weapon will not be used, some argue that the mere possession of nuclear weapons is unethical (cf gas warfare).

Knowledge of good and evil has been with mankind since the dawn of consciousness. The evil that the human race could do to our planet was limited before 1945. The mastery of nuclear fission and fusion brought with it potentially unlimited power for destruction; it created God-like power for some humans. This knowledge will remain with us – it cannot be unlearned short of a total catastrophe to our planet. In the long term, we must master our shadow side or perish.

References

British Medical Association Board of Education and Science report. *The medical effects of nuclear war.* Chichester: Wiley, 1983.

Gladstone S, Dolan P. *The effects of nuclear war.* United States Department of Defense and Energy Research and Development Administration, 1977.

IR

Nurse education in the UK is responsible for meeting the needs of health care providers who require a well qualified highly competent nursing and midwifery workforce. This is achieved by:

- preparing registered midwives and nurses in one of four specialties, ie, children's nurses, adult

171

nurses, mental health nurses and learning disability nurses

- preparing specialist practitioners, eg, district nurse; intensive care nurses
- providing continuing education programmes to enable staff to maintain/advance their knowledge and skills. This should include short courses, bachelor's, master's and research degree courses.

These activities enable the individual practitioner to meet the requirements of the United Kingdom Central Council for Nursing, Midwifery and Health Visiting for professional updating and preparation for specialist practice. From 1996 nurse education has been based in universities and research is a central activity alongside teaching.

Until recently nurses and *midwives* were trained "on the job". Limited theoretical input was provided by the School of Nursing and Midwifery, whilst clinical skills and the application of theory were learned through practical work experience.

Much of this learning was through unsupervised trial and error. Students were exploited and used as "pairs of hands", often being substituted for qualified staff. This led to concerns about the ethics of exposing two equally vulnerable groups, students and patients, to potential risks. Furthermore, nursing students, unlike all other health care professionals did not receive an academic award on completion of training.

The high student wastage rate, the increased dependency of patients and the complexity of new technologies led to a major reform of nursing education. Diploma programmes with equally weighted theoretical and clinical components were introduced. Students are now supervised for 80% of the course and trained clinical

supervisors work with students during placements. Increasingly, simulated clinical environments are being used to improve the preparation of students for clinical work, thus improving patient care as well as enhancing learning.

With the rapid changes in health care the scope of professional practice is extending and new roles are evolving, placing more demands on the qualified nurse and midwife. It is critical that education equips future practitioners for such realities and initial preparation at degree level is increasingly necessary and likely.

Nurse education is funded by the *National Health Service* (NHS) and a return on the investment is required which is monitored through performance indicators, eg, pass rates and recruitment targets. Under-performance results in reduced funding. This raises potential ethical dilemmas for teachers when recruiting and assessing students. Ethical issues can arise when selecting course content and clinical experience.

Ethics and ethical decision-making is a central component of the undergraduate diploma and degree courses, supported by a growing literature and research base. These course components are likely in the future to be shared with students from other health care disciplines, eg, medicine.

SJS

Nursing Since its early history nursing has carried with it an idea of nurturing. The exact nature of nursing is difficult to pinpoint since activities vary with culture, context, demand, role, and relative position of the practitioner. However, it aims to assist people to live with the effects of *illness* or *disability* and to obtain, retain or regain their optimal state of *health* or independence within the limits of any existing constraints.[1] Awareness has grown of the necessity to care holistically for patients, considering their social and psychological *welfare* alongside their physical *wellbeing*, and respecting their uniqueness, integrity, and right to dignity.

Debate has continued over many years about whether nursing is a profession and the development of a discrete body of research knowledge has been a recent response to this challenge. It is difficult to separate the effect of nursing intervention from medical, but increasing emphasis has been placed on determining outcomes and measuring standards specifically of nursing care. Efforts have been made to ground nursing practice in health rather than in illness.

Nurses are accountable to society (criminal liability), to the patient (civil liability), to their profession (through the United Kingdom Central Council (UKCC) for Nursing, Midwifery and Health Visiting), and to their employer (assumed by the courts to exist in any *contract*) as well as to themselves (a *moral* dimension with no recognised means of enforcement).

Since 1953 the International Council of Nurses has issued an international code of ethics for nurses which outlines four fundamental responsibilities of the nurse: to promote health, to prevent illness, to restore health, and to alleviate *suffering*. Although largely non-specific this code does emphasise the *confidentiality* of the nurse–patient relationship.

Since 1976 the Royal College of Nursing (RCN) in the UK has published its own Code of Professional Conduct. Coverage is essentially the same but the UK version additionally deals with matters such as handling potentially violent patients; strike action (which until 1995 could "never be justified"); and patients' right to information about their own case.

In recent years both the UKCC and the RCN have issued a range of statements to guide their practitioners in such matters as record keeping, *resuscitation*, administration of medicines, *conscientious objection*, and harvesting of organs.

References
1 Scottish Office Home and Health Department. *The role and function of the professional nurse.* Edinburgh: HMSO, 1992.
Burnard P, Chapman CM. *Professional and ethical issues in nursing. The Code of Professional Conduct* (2nd ed). Harrow: Scutari, 1993.
Dimond B. *Legal aspects of nursing.* Hemel Hempstead: Prentice Hall, 1990.

See also: Accountability; care; codes; competence to practise; duty of care; guidelines; healthcare systems; health education; holistic; incompetent professionals; misconduct; multidisciplinary teams; nurse education; professionalism; quality assurance; statutory bodies.

HM

Nutrition The ingestion of nutrients for maintenance of body structure and function is essential to sustain human life. Artificial nutrition requires delivery via enteral feeding tubes or a cannula in the vein. Debate concerns categorising artificial nutrition either as a form of medical treatment which may constitute extraordinary means of sustaining life, or as a supportive measure which cannot ethically be withheld.

This may arise: (a) When the patient is insentient and recovery is not expected. The judicial ruling in the Tony Bland case, 1993, confirmed that medical treatment including artificial nutrition can be lawfully discontinued in some cases. These must be referred individually to the courts. (b) When the patient knowingly refuses nutrition as a means of ending life.

The right to refuse nutrition in specific circumstances may be expressed as an *advance directive*.

See also: Burdensomeness of treatment; extraordinary and ordinary means; hydration; intravenous feeding; persistent vegetative state (PVS); treatment.

SA

O

Obedience (from Latin, to hear) – traditionally required in religious and military communities (hence, until recently, in nursing) with respect to superiors in the hierarchy. Religion and ethics also require obedience to *conscience*. Some medical procedures require unquestioning obedience: their objectives are most likely to be achieved if the reasons are understood and agreed to by all involved.

KMB

Objectivity (i) Seeing objects "as they really are", or "as they are in themselves" is, arguably, an ideal, never fully realised even in science. (ii) Philosphers disagree on whether any non-tautologous moral judgment can be objectively true. (iii) Objectivity may be shorthand for the desirable state of mind of clinicians who try to exclude their own personal opinions or *prejudices* when making medico-moral judgments.

KMB

Obligation to society Health care professionals are in the relatively unusual situation of having strong obligations (to *care* for, not to *harm*, etc) to the individual at the same time as more broadly and explicitly to society, in terms of the *public health*, the public purse, future generations and so on. There may be *conflicts* between these different *roles* and obligations.

See also: Accountability.

RH

Occam's razor is a philosophical principle derived from William of Occam (Ockham), which is also used in clinical diagnostic analysis. The principle is not to multiply entities (explanations or assumptions) beyond necessity. In medicine, respect for the principle would have one to try to resolve a set of symptoms or clinical problems under one overarching diagnosis or explanation. In general it is helpful, with notable exceptions in the elderly, where multiple pathologies often coexist, and the immuno-suppressed, where multiple pathogens are commonplace. Occasionally its unthinking application leads to far-fetched connections between two events that occur coincidentally (the eight-legged horse principle: "if I see four grey and four piebald hooves under a gate, I don't think I'm seeing an eight-legged horse").

See also: Parsimony.

AJP

Occupational medicine Formerly known as *industrial medicine* occupational medicine is the clinical specialty that addresses the interface between work and health. A largely preventive discipline, its aim is to minimise work-related health problems. Ethical principles followed by members of this sector of the medical profession are second to none, with especially clear guidance emanating from the Faculty of Occupational Medicine of the Royal College of Physicians, London. The Occupational Health Service should be independent, impartial, accessible and, above all, confidential. While paid by management, the occupational physician is no lackey and has an overriding *duty of care* to ensure the health, welfare and *safety* of all employees, regardless of role or status. Similarly, he has an ethical responsibility to protect the employer from the potentially inappropriate sequelae of employment of an unfit worker.

Referrals to occupational health should be made with the informed consent of the employee and adherence to the Access to Medical Reports and Health Records Acts should be maintained. Occupational health records are the property of the Occupational Health Service and when not in use should be securely stored. Data kept on electronic systems come under the provisions of the Data Protection Act and should not be accessible to other systems. At no time should these records be available to any third party without the explicit *consent* of the individual employee. This generally applies even to requests from lawyers, though if the request comes from the courts, by subpoena, compliance is unavoidable.

On extremely rare occasions an occupational physician may feel it necessary to reveal information about an individual to protect others (examples would be of a seriously mentally ill employee who lacked insight or, say, of an HIV-infected surgeon who refused to stop operating). Even then, *confidentiality* should be observed and the minimum information given to management sufficient to protect others without revealing detailed information regarding the employee.

Increasing awareness of the need for better work-place health care has resulted in a burgeoning legislative framework over the past decade. No longer the province of the casual practitioner, occupational medicine has responded by increasing its numbers of trained and appropriately qualified doctors, who are aware of their ethical duties.

Reference

Guidance on ethics for occupational physicians. A report of the Faculty of Occupational Physicians of the Royal College of Physicians. London, November, 1993.

See also: AIDS; data protection; infected doctors.

AMH

Ombudsman The Ombudsman, an officer of Parliament, investigates complaints from citizens about a failure in service or maladministration by a health service authority that has caused personal hardship or injustice. The authority concerned must first have an opportunity to deal with the complaint. The Ombudsman is not a substitute for a court or tribunal.

The Ombudsman's independent investigations can cover such issues as poor communications, lack of openness, neglect and inadequate respect and care of patients. If, on investigation, the complaint is justified the Ombudsman will ask for redress from the health service authority and seek an assurance that systems and procedures have been changed to prevent a recurrence of the failure.

The Ombudsman is also empowered to investigate complaints against practitioners in primary care (family doctors, dentists, opticians, pharmacists) and complaints about the clinical judgment of doctors, nurses, and other professionals.

Reference

Bi-annual reports of the Health Service Commissioner's selected cases are published by HMSO and the *Directory of Ombudsmen* is published by the British and Irish Ombudsman Association.

See also: Complaints; openness; procedures; respect.

WR

Omniscience Because medical training involves the (partial) digestion of a vast amount of information there has been a tendency for the fantasy to arise that doctors know everything, and by extension can legitimately make judgments about anything. It is not difficult to become seduced by this fantasy but for professionals it is wise to be open and willing to say: "I don't know", both for moral and medico-legal reasons.

See also: Empowerment; heroes; openness.

RH

Oncology (from Greek for a swelling) is the study of *cancer*.

175

Ontology (from Greek for Being) is the study by *metaphysics* of being in general, or the essence of things, eg, whether it is material or mental. The ontological argument is one of the traditional, but philosophically disputed, proofs for the existence of *God*.

KMB

Openness is linked to truthfulness and *veracity* as a modern virtue in the professional relating to patients. The distinction would be that openness refers to a general style and goes beyond individual questions of whether this or that is a truthful statement. It is also limited by professional considerations and proper *boundaries* between work and personal life. For instance, some might see that a professional sharing a similar personal experience of his own with a patient might be helpful, while others would cite the risk of trivialising the complaint, upstaging the patient or taking over the consultation. Plato suggested that doctors use truthfulness like a drug (differing doses, different situations). While this might make us feel uneasy, the analogy perhaps is better with personal openness for a professional; in the consultation it is a powerful but relatively dangerous drug, to be used sparingly and with care.

See also: Truthtelling.

RH

Order of preferences This makes a distinction between immediate (first order) desires or preferences and deeper or longer term *aims* and *values* (higher or second order). The autonomous individual could be considered as one who is able to reflect on and moderate his first order preferences (for instance, to consume a whole bar of chocolate) with reference to his second order concerns (say, to be slim and fit). This can be useful in moral

debate in health care when considering autonomous choice in *dependency* states or *consent* in *research*, where a first order choice is surrendered in order to achieve second order goals.

Reference

Dworkin G. *The theory and practice of autonomy.* Cambridge: Cambridge University Press, 1988.

See also: Autonomy; human nature; responsibility.

RH

Origin of ethics Moral rules in human societies always indicate priority systems, ways of life to be aimed at, as well as sometimes serving practical purposes. Through these ethics, humans have tried to solve a problem which they share with all intelligent animals, namely, how to arbitrate conflicts of motive. They have done this in their own special way, through thought and language. Darwin reasonably suggested that any species that had reached our degree of intelligence would have had to take this step of developing morality. Unsatisfactory though our various ethical systems always are, they are probably a necessary condition of our species-life.

References

Darwin C. *The descent of man.* Princeton: Princeton University Press, 1981, reprint of the 1871 edition: ch 3: 71.

Midgley M. *The ethical primate; humans, freedom and morality.* London: Routledge, 1994.

See also: Argument, moral; conscience; ethical systems; human nature.

MM

Orphan drugs are relatively expensive *drugs* that are exclusively used for treatment of rare diseases, such as rare *genetic disorders*. Their development, manufacture and distribution may need to be subsidised, usually by the state (hence, orphan), since there would otherwise be insufficient market or motivation for their continuing production by the *pharmaceutical industry*.

AJP

Orphans *See* Adoption and fostering; child, status of.

Osteopathy A method of diagnosis, prevention and treatment of ailments, primarily by physiomedical means, based on the principle that much of the pain and disability which humanity suffers stems from abnormalities in the function of body structures as well as damage to these by degeneration, trauma, inflammation or any other structural change. Osteopathy recognises abnormal function, in the absence of pathology, as a common, or even likely, cause of symptoms. Many osteopaths now work closely with their conventional medical colleagues. In the UK, as far as the General Medical Council is concerned, if a medical practitioner refers a patient to an osteopath then he must do so with a clear diagnosis and must bear responsibility for the osteopathic treatment provided, in spite of the fact that members of the Register of Osteopaths now have statutory recognition and appropriate professional indemnity.

See also: Chiropractic; complementary medicine.

GL

Outcome is the result of an action or intervention, eg, of a treatment or in a *clinical trial*, or as a consequence of a *management* change. An outcome measure in evaluation, *research* or *audit* should be defined in advance if it is to be used as a criterion of success and should be chosen to reflect the impact of the intervention concerned. In clinical practice the desired outcome may be subjective in nature, which may cause problems in measurement or validation, though *quality of life* measures attempt to resolve this. In the *National Health Service*, there is a tendency to use what is measurable rather than what is necessarily important (for instance, league tables). Outcomes, however, are being increasingly used in *purchasing* and specifically in the application of *evidence-based medicine*. Outcome may be contrasted with process or content, where an intervention is assessed with reference to the process itself (eg, change) or the intent of a decision.

AJP

Out of hours work Night, weekend, and holiday work may be seen in a different way from routine daytime service. *Emergencies* may happen at any time, and established inpatients must be cared for around the clock, but most health service work follows the pattern of work elsewhere and tries to plan new contacts with patients during the working day. The traditional understanding of a doctor or nurse as never being completely off duty has been linked with specific contractual obligations, for instance for British general practitioners to offer 24 hour cover for their patients. A greater understanding of the need for professionals to have recreation and family contact like others, and the destructive nature of chronic caring stress, challenges this approach. A professional has a duty to care, but there are *limits* to this and these *boundaries* may need to be reviewed regularly, and renegotiated. The apparent paradox is clear: which is easier to get at 3am, a pizza or a prescription? With recent changes in urban life, the two appear to become inversely related, but is this as it should be?

RH

P

Paganism (from Latin for rural) originally a denigratory term referring

177

to countryfolk not worshipping the Judaeo-Christian God. More recently rehabilitated by advocates of *New age movements* and of pre-Christian Greek or Roman virtues such as pride and self-sufficiency.

KMB

Pain is a complex psycho-sensory phenomenon which in many ways defies definition. The World Health Organisation definition – "pain is an unpleasant sensory and emotional experience associated with actual or potential tissue damage or described in terms of such damage" – alludes to the fact that pain is inextricably linked with emotion and can exist in the absence of physical signs of injury.

In experimental models pain arises secondary to tissue damage, but in "life" the relationship between such damage and the experience of pain is variable and subject to powerful modification by the central nervous system. Two extreme examples are that in times of great stress such as war soldiers can run without pain despite severe injuries, but conversely some psychiatric conditions present as pain with apparently no cause. Some pain can serve a biological function, resulting in the removal of part of the body from a potentially damaging source such as fire. However, long term pain may result in physiological and psychological changes leading to loss of both function and quality of life.

Pain is the commonest symptom presenting for medical advice. Despite this, however, modern medicine concentrates on diagnosis-making and specific treatment, with the consequence that symptom control may be overlooked. The development of pain clinics in the 1960s attests to the high prevalence of unrelieved pain in the community.

On top of the complex physiology of pain, cultural attitudes may also hamper the progress of its management. The Latin for pain is poena, which also means penalty, thus suggesting that pain may be considered as retribution. The pain of childbirth was, and in some ideologies still is, regarded as life-enhancing. Fortunately, the use of chloroform by Queen Victoria in labour allowed the advance of obstetric analgesia during the 19th century.

Thanks to pain pioneers such as John Bonica in Seattle there has been some progress. Labour can now be a pain-free experience, and the *hospice movement* has dramatically improved pain control in those with advanced cancer. More recently a concerted effort to improve the treatment of postoperative pain has met with success. The remaining challenge of pain is chronic pain, the most significant of which is back pain. Almost half the patients referred to pain clinics have back pain and it is hugely expensive in terms of sick leave, lost output and long term disability benefit. The challenge of this pain is to promote activity and the leading of a normal life. As yet the problem remains unsolved, but the use of *multidisciplinary teams*, combining different methods of pain relief in conjunction with physical and psychological rehabilitation may offer the greatest hope of success.

See also: Palliative care.

WJG

Palliative care is defined by the WHO as the total care of someone who has an incurable and progressive illness. The primary aim of total or holistic care is not to prolong life but to improve or to maintain *quality of life* for as long as possible, and to ensure that *death* is achieved with *dignity* and in comfort.

Palliative care is ideally provided by an interdisciplinary team working in partnership with the patient, spouse/partner, and family. Medical and nursing care, while maintaining necessary active treatment for as long as is appropriate, aims to improve quality of life through good symptom control. While addressing the physical needs of the patient the team also seeks to meet social, emotional, and spiritual needs and supports the partner and family prior to and after *bereavement*.

Palliative care should be gradually and increasingly integrated with the medical care of a patient with any chronic but progressive and life-threatening condition. Such conditions include *cancer*, *AIDS*, motor neuron disease, multiple sclerosis, and life threatening cardiovascular and respiratory conditions.

In the terminal phase of such illnesses great emphasis is placed on the control of distressing symptoms and on maintaining the patient's quality of life for as long as possible. Sometimes the best way of achieving symptom control in palliation is to continue active treatment. The team seeks to adhere to the patient's wishes as far as possible (eg, by respecting a previously signed *advance directive* or living will). It seeks to ensure that the patient dies with dignity and in comfort and that the family receive appropriate support.

See also: Care; holistic; hospice movement; pain; spirituality; suffering; teamwork; terminal care.

VM

Panacea A panacea is the dream of a universal remedy for all ailments. There have been, and will be, many false panaceas for sale to the public. They are sold for conditions as diverse as *AIDS* and *cancer*, supported by unsubstantiated claims of efficacy. The damage they cause includes the false hope of a cure, financial debts, and side-effects.

PDW

Papal encyclicals are letters by popes addressed to a part, or the whole, of the Church, and occasionally to a wider readership. Statements therein concerning faith or morals are normally described as authoritative but not infallible. Some encyclicals deal with issues of medical ethics: eg, Evangelium Vitae, on the value and inviolability of human life, 1995.

See also: Humanae vitae; infallibility.

BHo

Paradigm is a particular way of looking at an issue, particularly in the sense of a conceptual framework within which scientific or other theories can be constructed or presented. There has been some claim recently of the need for, or existence of, a "paradigm shift" when people begin to look at things in a completely new way.

Reference
Kuhn T. *The structure of scientific revolutions.* Chicago: University or Chicago Press, 1970.

RH

Paramedical professions A term for health care workers other than doctors and nurses. They comprise a wide range of clinical and support staff who are essential to provision of health care and who increasingly participate in *multidisciplinary teams* in *hospital medicine* and the community. Some have direct *patient* contact, such as clinical psychologists, physiotherapists, dieticians, *pharmacists*, radiographers, ambulance staff, *health visitors*, and *receptionists*; laboratory technical staff (MLSOs) perform *laboratory tests* on patient samples. Most have their own professional standards, codes of conduct, and training schemes. In the past, they have tended to work under the direction of a doctor, but increasingly they are functioning as parallel professionals, who have agreed roles and responsibilities in delivery of health care. They have common values with doctors and *nurses* on issues such as *consent* and *confidentiality*, but may have distinctive ethical principles relating to their own area of work.

See also: Ancillary staff; receptionists.

AJP

Parasuicide is applied to suicidal acts performed without the intention to kill oneself. These gestures often serve, intentionally or otherwise, as a cry for help. They may also be a form of attention-seeking, and are relatively common in adolescents and those with personality disorders. Usually, non-lethal drugs or small amounts are used; notifying a person who will ensure prompt treatment is another means of ensuring the relative safety of the attempt, but on occasion an intended parasuicide leads to death. The behaviour patterns and aftercare required are different from those associated with *suicide*. Parasuicide may invoke negative feelings among staff, who may regard such patients as diverting attention and limited resources from other patients.

See also: Adolescence.

AJP

Parents and parenting Parenting, with its biological, psychological and social functions, begins before a child is born and continues after he leaves home. In the first phase, mother and baby are an inseparable psychobiological unit. As the child grows, parenting must adapt constantly to meet the evolving needs of the maturing person.

See also: Adolescence; child, status of; families; good and good enough; paternalism; potential.

CD

Parsimony has a bad press in the sense of meanness or niggardliness in the spending of money, but is an important principle in health care when proper economy is used in choosing the most efficient or effective means of achieving a particular end. It is the extension of *Occam's razor* into practical health care, and suggests that, other things being equal, one should always choose the simplest and most economical way of reaching a particular health goal. In place of hi-tech we should prefer low-tech or even no-tech.

RH

Partiality implies taking sides in an issue where even-handedness might be expected. It is implicit and important in *advocacy*, but destructive in *public health* or *resource* allocation. This *conflict* is why some general practitioners have not embraced *fundholding* with enthusiasm.

RH

Partner notification is a term for *contact tracing* of sexually transmitted diseases, particularly used in respect of *HIV* and *AIDS*. The identification of partner(s) by the index case enables advice and assistance to be given to ensure that partners who may have contracted infection are warned by the index case or by health professionals, directly or through contact slips, of the need to seek *screening*, treatment and *health education*. It attempts to balance *confidentiality* with the duty to warn and the protection of the *public health*.

AJP

Partnership is a part of the aspiration for professional–patient relationships which sees in them the *potential* for *reciprocity* and mutual investment, a sharing between peers with different expertise.

See also: Doctor–patient relationship; empowerment; general practice; practice; primary care; teamwork.

RH

Patent Inventions, notably new medicines and devices, may be patented to protect against unauthorised production and competition. Patents may relate to a new active substance, its use or its process of manufacture. Grant of patents may be refused through prior art and/or obviousness. The increase in development times of new medicines has led to the erosion of patent lives and to the pharmaceutical industry focusing increasingly on products with large multinational sales.

Patenting of biological systems is morally problematic. European patent law (which weighs possible harm to animals and the environment against possible benefits) has been more reluctant than law in the USA to allow it. Developments in *genetics* (transgenic animals, the human *genome*) are likely to make the ethical problems increasingly acute.

See also: Drugs; medicine; pharmaceutical industry.

DF/KMB

Paternalism is generally thought of as the control of other people's lives, exercised in the name of their own "best interests" but irrespective of their wishes. Such control clearly undermines individuals' personal *autonomy* and ignores any *right* or *responsibilities* they may have. Paternalism goes against the very grain of the Kantian imperative to treat *persons* as ends in themselves.

We should be careful to distinguish paternalism and moralism. On the former we may have a proscription "don't do that, it's bad for you", while on the latter we would have "don't do that, it's wrong".

The principle of respect for autonomy is widely recognised as a cornerstone of modern medical ethics, but there is debate concerning the tension between respecting a person's autonomy and providing for his *welfare*, or best interests. Is it necessarily the case that respect for autonomy and acting in a person's best interests irrespective of his wishes are mutually exclusive? Konrad, eg, argues that, in the context of the *doctor–patient relationship*, because illness necessarily diminishes the patient's autonomy, medical paternalism aimed at restoring the patient's health, and so his autonomy, is justifiable.[1] However, where a patient's illness has affected his cognitive capacities to the extent that he is (temporarily) incapable of fully autonomous choice, it is dubious whether (considerations of *advance directives* aside) acting in his best interests constitutes genuine paternalism.

As in so many areas of moral and political philosophy, it is instructive to think of the case of children. We sometimes act against our children's wishes, perhaps by *deception* or in their ignorance, but this is usually thought justifiable if it is done in their best interests. One of these interests is the development of the capacities requisite to their autonomous management of their own lives. Where children lack these managerial capacities, acting in their best interests irrespective of their wishes might not be considered as "paternalism" (at least not in the sense this term has been adopted in biomedical ethics) since their wishes cannot be fully autonomous. If such a view is accepted, it is no great step to the conclusion that paternalism is always wrong.

CAE

Reference
1 Konrad MS. A defence of medical paternalism: maximising patients' autonomy. *J Med Ethics* 1983; **9**: 38–44.

See also: Child, status of; decision-making capacity, empowerment.

Paternity The common law determines parentage (whether motherhood or fatherhood) by reference to a person's genetic ancestry. However, in the case of fatherhood there was one exception: the presumption of legitimacy. The need for certainty led the common law to hold that the father of a child born within a marriage was presumptively deemed to be the husband's. The presumption could be rebutted by proof that the husband was incapable of being the father, eg if it was shown that he was infertile or lacked the opportunity to have procreated the child. In modern times the presumption was more likely to be rebutted by the husband establishing through *blood* tests or *DNA fingerprinting* that he was not genetically the father.

In the context of modern assisted reproductive technology, the common law was, however, inadequate. Under the common law, subject to the presumption of legitimacy, the father of a child born following *artificial insemination* or *in vitro fertilisation* using donated sperm was the donor even though he was to play no further part in the child's life. This was unsatisfactory since it denied the social (and legal) reality of who was really the child's father, namely, the partner of the child's mother. Consequently, the UK Human Fertilisation and Embryology Act 1990 reverses the common law rule in the context of assisted reproduction. First, the donor of sperm is deemed not to be the father of the child (s. 28 (6)(a)). Second, the partner of the woman receiving the infertility treatment is, in law, the father of the child. If she is married, the presumption of legitimacy continues to apply (s. 28 (5)(a)) and even if the presumption can be rebutted by genetic testing, the husband is still the father under the Act unless it is proved that he did not consent to her undergoing the infertility treatment (s. 28(2)). Similarly, where an unmarried couple receive "treatment services" under the Act "together", then the Act deems her male partner to be the father of the child (s. 28(3)).

In one situation the "donors" of the genetic material are, unlike in the other situations of assisted reproduction, intended to be the child's social "parents" after its birth. As a consequence, the 1990 Act reflects this by continuing to recognise the genetic parents of the child as its legal parents. Where a child is born following a *surrogacy* arrangement using the genetic material of one or both of the infertile couple and all the parties (including the surrogate and her husband, if any) agree, the commissioning couple may then apply to the court for a "parental order", which will deem them to be the parents of the child (s. 30).

In two situations the Act creates, on the face of it, the rather curious situation that the child is legally (though obviously not genetically) fatherless: first, where donated sperm is used but under the Act no one else is deemed to be the father – eg, if the woman is treated alone or her husband did not consent to her insemination – and, of course, the donor is not the father either; and second, where the sperm is used after a man's death, eg, to inseminate his widow (s. 28 (6)(b)).

See also: Human Fertilisation and Embryology Authority.

AG

Patient, moral is a term sometimes used to refer to individuals who have no awareness of right and wrong and so are not regarded as moral agents who can be held responsible for the consequences of their actions, eg infants, those with severe mental disability, and most but arguably not all non-human animals.

Reference
Regan T. *The case for animal rights*. London: Routledge, 1984.

See also: Moral agency.

KMB

Patients are, or should be, the focus of all health care. Yet all too often patients report treatment and attitudes that suggest that they are a nuisance, not the reason for the health care industry existing. Patients have *rights*, differently described and differently enshrined throughout the world, often not legally enforceable. However, the fact that patients' rights can be discussed at all demonstrates a profound change in attitude in the latter part of the 20th century.

No longer can a doctor be simply autocratic. Patients no longer necessarily accept whatever they are told. Young medical and nursing students learn that one of the four generally accepted principles of medical ethics is respect for (the patient's) *autonomy*, including when the patient wishes to do something against the health care professional's advice.

Patients have a right to equal treatment, irrespective of class, social origin, ethnic origin, and so on. Treatment should be allocated on a non-discriminatory basis, and patients increasingly feel they have a right to complain if this is not so. They are also beginning to play a major role in deciding what health care should be provided. Purchasers of health care increasingly treat the public in general, and regular patients in particular, as partners in decision-making.

This would suggest that patients should be described by a different term. "Patient" suggests suffering patiently, rather than being an equal partner. Yet equality between health care professionals and patients is not yet assured. Schemes focusing on "patient centred care" are now legion throughout the USA and UK. The idea that care should ever have been anything but "patient centred" indicates that until recently patients have played a passive role in health care. Now, however, patients, including those who need advocates for their case, are asserting themselves and describing health care in not necessarily flattering terms, as seen through their eyes.

See also: Advocacy/activism, consent, doctor–patient relationship; empowerment; healthcare system; paternalism; purchasing.

JN

Patient's Charter A set of standards determined by the UK government that patients can expect from *National Health Service* staff and institutions, which are extensions of the Citizen's Charter. They focus on items such as rights of access to care and *equity*, as well as on specific targets for waiting times. While ensuring *accountability* and delivery of certain basic standards, some are seen to be promoting the importance of measurable items over more qualitative aspects of health care, potentially diverting attention or resources from quality issues.

AJP

Pause This concept refers to the pause that is required when someone has to make a reasoned moral decision which may have mortal consequences. It is fuelled by the intuitively felt moral weight we attach to life and death decisions. Such decisions reach deep into our constitution as moral agents. The ability to heed such complex intuitive responses is fundamental to the caring professions. We cannot argue that the pause, in and of itself, resolves a moral issue one way or the other, it merely alerts us to the seriousness of the decision being made and allows lingering misgivings or unresolved questions to emerge for consideration. In this way the pause can indicate that the stated or statable reasons, and a decision based on principles which result may not have done full justice to what is at stake in a particular decision. The phenomenon of the pause is therefore congenial to the kinds of reflection and discussion found within writing on *narrative ethics* and the ethic of *care*.

References
Gillett G, Euthanasia, letting die and the pause. *J Med Ethics* 1988; **14**: 61–8.
Gillett G. The pause and the principles. In: Gillon R, Lloyd A, eds. *Principles of health care ethics*. Chichester: Wiley, 1994; 743–752.

GG

Peer pressure describes the way in which the behaviour of an individual is affected, explicitly or implicitly, by the attitudes, actual or perceived, of his peer group. It is an important factor in health-related behaviours such as *smoking, drug misuse*, sexual behaviour, crowd violence and some culturally defined behaviours. In some cases, peer pressure is based on attributes of role models that are considered desirable; in others, there is pressure (the dare) to challenge authority or social norms in a way that the individual would normally reject. If *health education* and promotion is to be effective it must appreciate the way in which peer pressure operates. In some cases it has been possible to utilise the role of key individuals in social groups as agents of health behavioural change, in effect changing peer pressure to achieve a desired health promotional goal (eg, safer sex). This could, however, be regarded as a potentially hazardous tool for social control. The behaviour of health professionals is strongly affected by peer pressures.

AJP

Peer review is the process of asking peers to make (usually anonymous) judgments on the worthiness of scientific papers for publication or research proposals for funding. It may also be applied to the process of asking peers to make judgments on the performance of colleagues. Peer review of papers or grant applications has been criticised as slow, expensive, arbitrary, biased, and anti-innovatory, but the system persists for want of a better alternative. Peer review, although central to science, has itself been largely unexamined, but evidence is now appearing that blinding reviewers to the identity of the authors of a paper or grant proposal will improve the quality of the review. Peer review is, I believe, like democracy: far from perfect but the best system yet devised.

See also: Authorship; bias; fraud; plagiarism; research.

RSm

Persistent vegetative state defines the behaviour of a patient in whom brain damage has put the cerebral cortex out of action without affecting the brain stem. The patient can breathe and has brain stem reflexes (pupils, eye movements, gagging) and has long periods of wakefulness (eyes open) – thus distinguishing this state from *brain stem death* and from coma. With the cerebral cortex either destroyed or disconnected there is no evidence of psychologically meaningful response to the environment – no commands obeyed, no words uttered and no awareness of self or surroundings. The paralysed limbs are usually spastic, but may withdraw from a painful stimulus which may cause facial grimacing. A loud sound may cause reflex blinking. The patient is awake but not aware and is therefore unconscious.

Acute brain insults that produce the vegetative state are severe head injury and failure of the oxygen supply to the brain from cardiac or respiratory arrest, when resuscitation was in time to save the brain stem but too late for the more vulnerable cerebral cortex. After days or weeks in coma the patient wakes to a vegetative state. Some patients with progressive brain disease progress slowly into a vegetative state over a period of years.

Diagnosis depends on clinical observation as there are no reliable radiological or laboratory tests. Patients can regain consciousness after being vegetative for weeks or months, but the longer they have been vegetative the more likely they are to remain very severely disabled. This state can be declared permanent after one year, probably sooner after non-traumatic insults.

Many vegetative patients die within the first year, usually from respiratory or urinary infection. But those who live a year can survive for many years, even without antibiotics to treat infections. Continued survival depends on tube-feeding and several countries have declared it ethical and lawful to discontinue this treatment once the vegetative state is permanent. Such continued treatment is considered not to be beneficial and therefore not in the patient's best interests.

References

The Multi-Society Task Force on PVS. Medical aspects of the persistent vegetative state. *N Engl J Med* 1994; **330**: 1499–1508, 1572–79.

Jennett B. Vegetative survival: the medical facts and ethical dilemmas. *Neuropsychol Rehabil* 1993; **3**: 99–108.

The permanent vegetative state. Review of a working group convered by the Royal College of Physicians and endorsed by the conference of Medical Royal Colleges and their Faculties of the United Kingdom. *J R Coll Physicians*, 1996; **30**, **2**: 119–21.

See also: Death; hydration; nutrition; treatment; unconsciousness.

BJ

Personal growth Given individual poor functioning and the *potential* to do better, the concept of personal growth has arisen to cover maturing and integrative processes which may be enhanced by particular psychological work by an individual, usually under instruction or therapeutic supervision but sometimes just through experience which has been reflected on. While sceptics may question how many Californian therapists are needed to change a light bulb [A: one, but the light bulb must really want to change], or may reasonably demand evidence of efficacy from different approaches, experience from continuing care and *general practice* confirms that the process is real and the experience rewarding.

RH

Personality is the integrated aspects of any individual, particularly related to his behaviour, as it presents or appears to others. It is unique to that individual, but may be characterised by others in general terms. Where a person's behaviour brings him to the attention of the psychiatric services without there being a formal psychiatric illness he risks being classified as having a personality disorder. Personalities can be changed temporarily or permanently by external agents such as drugs or *psychosurgery*; but whether this is morally justified, either generally or in particular cases, remains a key issue.

See also: Prozac.

RH

Personality change Development of *personality* begins at birth and continues throughout the lifespan. In the general population, some degree of continuity in an individual's personality characteristics can be observed throughout but with modifications consequent upon the ageing process. Differences between individuals are strongly influenced by socialisation experiences, including early caretaking and with some degree of interaction between this factor and genetic heritability. Later socialisation experiences will modify earlier trends but major personality change is uncommon. Change may be considered beneficial and culturally sanctioned, eg, following religious conversion, and is considered to be a positive outcome of psychoanalytic treatment. Negative features of personality change may warrant investigation. Examples include change following severe, life-threatening trauma leading to post traumatic stress disorder, during the prodromal (earliest) phases of severe *mental illness* (eg, paranoid schizophrenia), and in the setting of traumatic or progressive cerebral pathology. This is especially marked in the frontal lobe syndrome.

JC

Persons and personhood Derived from the Greek word for the mask that denoted an actor's stage character, the word "person" is now widely used in medical ethics to denote someone who (or which) has full *moral* status of the sort that moral agents accord themselves. "Personhood" is the possession of such full moral status. While it is sometimes argued that there is little point in using these terms of art, their relevance to medical ethics is particularly obvious in the contexts of *abortion, embryo research* and the definition of *death*. In each of these contexts it is necessary to distinguish those human beings whom we ought to treat with full moral *respect*, including acknowledgment of and respect for their "right to life", or right not to be killed, from those human beings who do not require such full moral respect, and whom (or which) it is therefore morally justifiable to kill (or treat in ways that would kill them if they were alive), even if they are not aggressors. (It is widely, though by no means universally, agreed that even persons, ie, those who have full moral status, may, if they are aggressors threatening one's own life or the lives of others, forfeit their right to life and be justifiably killed in *self defence* or in defence of the lives of those others

whose lives they threaten.) Thus, if an embryo is a person we must not kill it except in morally justified defence of self or others, or experiment on it except for its own benefit. If a fetus is a person we must not kill it (abort it) except in morally justified self defence or defence of others. If a brain dead human being is a person we must not remove the heart and other organs for *transplantation*, but rather treat him just as we ought to treat other very sick patients. In specifying the attributes of personhood, or the criteria by which we may differentiate entities that are persons from those that are not, vigorous philosophical and theological debate continues. The capacity for *consciousness* seems to be a necessary but not sufficient condition for personhood (it is not sufficient unless all conscious entities including all non-human but conscious animals are persons, with full moral status including a right to life). The capacity for *self consciousness* is regarded by some as both necessary and sufficient for personhood (but this view implies that newborn infants, if they do not yet have the capacity for self consciousness, are not persons and thus do not have the right to life of persons).

RG

Perspective is important in practical ethics to give shape to the realities of a moral dilemma or *conflict*. Even were individuals to accept the same overarching rules or *principles* they would still interpret them in their own way, and each person would bring to the debate a different experience and possibly a different priority set of *values*. Discussion of a case, however graphically presented, cannot move from theoretical two dimensionality into three-dimensional realism without accepting the fact of, and examining the evidence of, the different perspectives of the actors involved.

Reference
Campbell A, Higgs R. *In that case. Medical ethics in everyday practice.* London: Darton Longman and Todd, 1982.

RH

Pharmaceutical industry The pharmaceutical industry comprises a heterogeneous group of national and international companies who discover, develop, register for sale, and market medicines and devices for use in the diagnosis, prevention, treatment and alleviation of *disease* in humans and animals. However, others representing science, shareholders, government, academic medicine, prescribers, patients, politicians, regulators and lawyers are concerned in these endeavours. They have different and potentially conflicting goals, eg, in relation to cost of medicines, access and extent of use, *advertising*, promotion and the protection of *public health*. It is not surprising that tensions, often concerning ethical issues, develop. Most important new medicines have emerged from pharmaceutical company *research* laboratories. Nevertheless, some industrial failures, including faults in drug development, unsubstantiated *claims*, improper advertising, profiteering, failure to protect employees against *safety* hazards and the occurrence of unexpected serious and sometimes persistent adverse effects in patients have resulted in increased *litigation* against companies, and in the last thirty years led to *regulation* of companies by government agencies. Some now believe the industry faces an increasingly hostile environment with greater costs and longer times required to develop new medicines and that therefore the pace of discovery and profitability will now decline.

See also: Animal experiments; biotechnology; business ethics; clinical trials and research; commercial interests; cost–benefit analysis; cost–risk analysis; drugs; health economics; market; medicine; patent; prescribing.

DF

Pharmacists are health professionals whose role is to dispense prescribed or over-the-counter *drugs* and to give detailed advice on their use. They can check the correctness of doctors' prescriptions and for potential drug interactions. Community pharmacists are independent practitioners working in retail premises and dispense prescriptions mainly from general practioners. Hospital pharmacists dispense and advise in that setting, are also involved in purchasing and audit of drug use, and participate in formulating prescribing policies. They may oversee preparation of *chemotherapy*, intravenous preparations and parenteral nutrition. Specialist pharmacists are increasingly part of *multidisciplinary teams* in specific clinical areas.

See also: General practice.

AJP

Pheresis or apheresis is the process by which *blood* is separated on-line by centrifugation from patients or donors with a part (plasma, white cells, or platelets) being removed and the remainder being returned. It may be used therapeutically or to obtain blood products for *donation*.

AJP

Philosophy Etymology might lead us to expect a philosopher to be a lover (Greek: philos) of wisdom (sophia). That definition would have made more sense in past centuries, when "philosophy" referred generally to all modes of human enquiry into the world and our place within it. At least since the seventeenth century, however, the notion of "science" has been squeezing "philosophy" out. Modern philosophy, to speak roughly,

187

engages with the questions not dealt with by natural science.

Philosophy now is best characterised by reference to both its methods and its subject matter. Its methods tend to be non-empirical. In certain areas, such as some contemporary philosophy of mind, scientific results do matter. But even here constructing philosophical theories based on these results is primarily the result of reflection and argument.

Those interested in medical ethics should not think that other areas of philosophy are irrelevant. The nature of the mind and its relation to the *body* and to *personhood* eg, will have many implications for, say, psychiatric ethics. Metaphysics is an attempt broadly to characterise the nature of the world itself. One particularly important debate here, now tied up with philosophy of language, concerns the reality of the world, or of aspects of it. Take a moral judgment such as, "It was wrong of you to insult that patient". Are there properties such as "wrongness" for us to refer to? Can moral judgments be true or false? If moral properties are mere "projections" of our sentiments, does this have any implications for our everyday lives? And can there be moral knowledge? Here, epistemology can help. Philosophy of religion, too, matters to medical ethics. If God does not exist, is everything permitted? Finally, of course, the area of ethics as a whole is of importance to medical ethics.

RCr

Phronesis *See* Practical reasoning and practical wisdom.

Placebo is an inactive preparation (or intervention) that is used in two principal ways. In *clinical trials*, placebos may be used as controls against which an active *drug* (which they are made to resemble in appearance, taste, etc) is being tested, so that the patient (single-blind trials) or the patient and doctor (double-blind trials) are unaware who has been assigned active treatment; this is to prevent *bias* in reporting. Sham *electroconvulsive therapy (ECT)* and *pheresis* procedures have also been used as placebos. Placebo treatments are used where a doctor considers that there is no need for active therapy (if there is none or where a patient will recover spontaneously), but that the patient will benefit from feeling that he is receiving something. It makes use of the "placebo effect", in which patients who believe they are receiving a treatment gain benefit from that perception, even though they are not receiving a pharmacologically active agent. Some regard this as a form of *deception* and *paternalism*, denying the patient *autonomy*, while others regard it as a justifiably beneficent approach that uses the doctor's knowledge in the interests of the patient and avoids the harm from inappropriate therapy.

See also: Beneficence; control groups; lying.

AJP

Plagiarism – an important type of *fraud* – covers about 25 per cent of complaints to the US Office of Research Integrity. The definition is difficult but its working one includes: "both the theft or misappropriation of intellectual property and the substantial unattributed textual copying of another's work. It does not include *authorship* or credit disputes."

Reference
Anonymous. ORI provides working definition of plagiarism. *ORI Newsletter* 1994; **3** (December): 3.

See also: Research.

SL

Pluralism is a philosophical approach which recognises as valid more than one principle of being, or a description of an approach in society which recognises and respects the claims of different groups (especially ethnic groups) to maintain their own customs and *values*, and to be able to live and control their own lives in accordance with them.

See also: Culture; ethnicity; race.

RH

Police are endowed with considerable power, and with expectations of its trustworthy use. They are most vulnerable to unethical practices when under pressure to produce results.

Difficulties may arise when police request information about a suspect or a victim of crime (eg, *rape*), who is currently receiving medical attention (eg, in accident and emergency departments or mental health settings); clinical staff may be uncertain of the extent to which they are obliged to assist in the pursuit of the criminal. Police surgeons are medical professionals who are contracted to act on behalf of the police in medical assessments or procedures, and may provide a valuable interface with other clinical professionals.

Checks on abuse are provided by the rule of law, disciplinary and ethical codes, threats of exposure and public opinion. Public opinion can also be fickle, inciting police to unethical behaviour, eg, excessive and unnecessary application of power and force upon unpopular *minorities*.

To withstand proclivity towards unethical practices, police require a general consciousness of *justice* and human dignity, and a well-informed moral rectitude.

References

Alderson J. *Human rights and the police*. Strasbourg: Council of Europe, 1984.

Haggard P. *Police ethics*. Lampeter: Edwin Mellen, 1994.

See also: Criminal behaviour; forensic psychiatry; imprisonment; power; prisoners, care of; role; torture:

JAI/AJP

Politics (from polis, Greek for city) is a means of governing (Greek for steering) communities, whose members have diverse and (in relation to resources) often incompatible interests, by their consent. Political consent to conflict-resolving recourse to force (of arms, or the market) is self limited, since beyond a certain point, deprivation of liberty or goods leads to revolution and/or tyranny, destroying politics. Modern politics, with coalitions of interests represented by political parties, is sometimes described as elective oligarchy (rule by the few), rather than true democracy (rule by the people). Because politics employs *rhetoric* and rumour ("the swiftest of all curses" – Virgil), and because "money talks", universal education and transparent regulation of financial interests are necessary for politics to flourish. At the least, politics demonstrates that "jaw-jaw is better than war-war" (Winston Churchill); at best, it aspires to a vision of the good "without which the people perish" (Isaiah).

In free pluralistic states, politics offers both a context and process for the resolution of dilemmas in medical ethics. On some issues, notably those related to resource allocation and organisation of health care delivery, political opinion tends to diverge along modern party political lines. On others, such as *abortion* and *euthanasia*, religious bodies may exert political influence. But on others again, related to new scientific developments, political opinions can be more unpredictable. When the science is complex, and the calculations of partisan political (dis)advantage perilous, scientists need to be politically sophisticated and the public to be scientifically sophisticated.

See also: Cost containment; healthcare systems; dirty hands debate; health economics; National Health Service; public health; public policy; resources.

KMB

Pollution (from lutum, Latin for mud) In primeval thinking, the action of dangerous quasi-material forces, which defile (make foul) or infect (stain) whoever or whatever comes into contact with them, making them in turn dangerous until cleansed or purified. The notion is related to feelings about viscous materials which resist physical or conceptual ordering, eg, sticky body fluids outside the body or oil on water. The concept of environmental pollution (chemical, smoke, noise) may be more scientific, but still draws on the primeval dread of invasion by the uncontrollable.

See also: Ecology.

KMB

Population policies began in the 1960s by setting targets for fertility decline. Over the decades policies have evolved to include emphasis on individual rights as well as societal needs. The 1994 Cairo International Conference on Population and Development also encompassed *gender* equality, the education and empowerment of women, and sexual health, including safe motherhood and freedom from *sexually transmitted diseases*. Disputes arise over the balance between an emphasis on slowing rapid population growth and a holistic approach to reproductive and sexual health that might be better dealt with more directly in the health and social sectors.

See also: Women's rights.

DMP

Positivism The view that we can know only what is posited by the senses and science. A rather dogmatic form of empiricism, associated with late 19th century evolutionary optimism, and, in the early 20th century with logical positivism, with its claim (which cannot be verified empirically) that all non-tautologous statements which cannot be verified empirically are meaningless.

KMB

Postmodernism (a cluster of ideas deriving from architectural and literary criticism and in philosophy influenced by Nietzsche) distrusts the power of ethical theorising adequately to represent or resolve real-life moral problems. It prefers a more indirect, *eclectic* and *context*-led approach, designed to draw out the many possible perspectives on an ethical issue, and to draw the reader into engagement with the moral claims of others who differ from him.

KMB

Potential suggests the high possibility of further improvement or development, and is important in medical ethics in several ways. Few definitions of health make sense without a reference not just to what a *person* is (or, in the negative as ill-health, what a person has for the moment lost) but also what that person might become. Sometimes, judgment about potential can be crucial in deciding how much effort will be put into a therapeutic programme or how long to continue it. In defining a person, particularly when discussing the *fetus*, some would feel that potential persons should be accorded the same status as actual persons, just as we may see children as potential adults with particular needs rather than in a second class of their own.

See also: Child, status of; health, illness and disease, concepts of; Personal growth.

RH

Poverty By convention, the term 'poverty', when unqualified, is used to denote a level of material or economic deprivation, variously defined from different points of view; and it is this type of poverty whose effects on health and disease have been most extensively investigated. It is important to recognise, however, that cultural and spiritual deprivation also can have baleful effects on health; and that material deprivation can predispose to these other forms of deprivation, though there is happily no iron law in this matter.

An association between poverty and ill health has been recognised for decades and is well researched.[1] There is no real dispute that a quantitative association of some magnitude exists; and not much dispute that poverty can be a "cause" of ill health. But ill health can also give rise to poverty; and this is sometimes thought to be a major factor in explaining the association. There are also uncertainties as to the relative importance of various aspects of poverty as causes of ill health – these include unhealthy and overcrowded housing, faulty nutrition, unhealthy life styles, lack of safe facilities for children, and an increased liability to unemployment.

Ill health consequent on poverty can be palliated by access to good health care; but the root of the evil lies in social conditions, and can be tackled only by social measures, directed primarily to narrowing what has recently been a widening gap in resources between rich and poor, and secondarily to encouraging general education and knowledge of health.

Reference

1 Whitehead M. The health divide. In: Townsend P, Davidson N, eds. *Inequalities in health*. London: Penguin, 1992.

See also: Equity; human rights; justice; public health.

                                                              DB

Power may refer to the ability to influence or control events in the natural world or in other persons. In the first case, we often speak of modern medicine's (impersonal) power to cure diseases and extend life span. In the second, we may refer to the *doctor–patient relationship* as one of power asymmetry, in that the physician generally is better able to influence or control the patient than vice versa.

The physician's power over the *patient* may have several aspects or origins. The physician possesses knowledge and *skills* that the patient lacks. The physician, through selection and training, may have a more domineering or persuasive personality. The physician may be of a higher social class. And the society or *culture* may have granted to the physician special authority to decide upon the truth of important matters, such as whether an individual is diseased or healthy, sane or insane, etc. In a two-party relationship, however, one party may be superior to the other in one aspect of power while remaining inferior in another.

Social scientists frequently analyse interpersonal relationships in terms of power asymmetries; and feminist scholars have paid special attention to hidden power imbalances in *gender* relationships. Medical ethics, by contrast, has until recently paid much less attention to power as an explicit feature of the doctor–patient relationship and as a specific ethical problem in medical practice. However, when a relationship grants an individual power, that person becomes ethically responsible for how that power is used or abused. And failure to study the power aspects of a relationship may lead to incorrect ethical conclusions, by suggesting either that power is not an issue, or that power can somehow be equally distributed between the parties.

Common exercises of physician power that stand in need of ethical analysis include the power to control information about the *individual* and the illness; the power to make *treatment* decisions; and the power to allocate limited medical *resources*.

References
Brody, H. *The healer's power*. New Haven, Conn.: Yale University Press, 1992.
Ladd, J. Medical ethics: who knows best? *Lancet* 1980; **2**: 1127–9.

See also: Authority; autonomy; empowerment; experts and expertise; feminism; paternalism; responsibility.

HB

Power of attorney A power of attorney is the power given to another *person* to exercise legal rights on behalf of the donor. In principle, a patient could authorise another person to consent to treatment on his behalf. However, such an authorisation could never override the patient's own choice, and under the common law it would automatically be revoked if the donor became unable to understand the nature of the grant. Thus, it is not possible for patients to appoint a *proxy* to take decisions about their care when they become incompetent to decide for themselves. The Enduring Powers of Attorney Act 1985 provides for powers in respect of dealings with property to continue to have effect after the donor becomes incompetent, but it has no application to consent to treatment. The Law Commission[1] has suggested that a similar provision might be made in relation to consent to health care.

Reference
1 Law Commission. *Mental incapacity.* Law Com No 231 (1995).

See also: Next of kin.

JMo

Practical reasoning and practical wisdom Aristotle's phronesis or prudence – deliberation which gives equal weight to what one ought to do morally and what one can do in practice, and which leads to a decision and effective action. It may use algorithms or syllogisms, but sound judgment is its key feature.

KMB

Practice (i) The actual exercise of professional care in a medical system is defined by what people in that walk of life customarily do (medical practice) or what is considered best to do (good practice) or what I usually do (my practice). Although such activity is difficult to measure or encapsulate precisely, because medical care has important *outcomes* this activity (in spite of the dangers of self-reference) takes on an identity of its own. There are some important contrasts with theory, regulation and academic instruction, and the rules of thumb developed to encourage good practice often translate poorly, and are seldom actually written down (often with good reason): "Always do a rectal examination or you'll put your foot in it".

In practical medical ethics the contrast with theory is both important and stark. Abstract thinkers have all the time in the world and are still allowed not to come to a conclusion, whereas professionals in practice have to decide what to do or not do, usually here and now. There is no sharp division between what is ethics and what is something else: a moral decision may be influenced by *communication*, sociological insights, the last meeting of the trust board or the blood urea level. The particular and the complex must constantly be examined side by side with the general and the universal.

(ii) **Practices** as organisations describe the groups of people who work in, or who are associated with, defined community buildings delivering *primary care* to a specific group of patients. The practice is usually supervised by, or employed by, a group of general practitioners in partnership. On good days the professional group will form a team and will increasingly be expected to develop their own style and standards and be explicit about their own *values. Conflicts*, moral and otherwise, may arise about issues of *power*, employment, *responsibility*, family care and so on. There are always the old quips: "I'm afraid Dr X is at a practice meeting." "Oh, doesn't he know how to do it yet?".

See also: Ancillary staff; complexity; concrete vs abstract; general practice; teamwork.

RH

Pragmatism (from Greek for businesslike) View that what is right or true is shown by whether it "works" or not. Philosophical arguments for this (USA early 20th century: CS Peirce, William James) have more sophisticated and long-term criteria for what "works" than has most popular or political usage of the word.

KMB

Pre-embryo The term embryo generally refers to the developing human prior to the second trimester (13 weeks), after which it is referred to as a fetus. During the embryonic stage of development substantial morphological and structural changes occur and the major organs take shape (organogenesis). This is why this stage of development is so susceptible to the adverse effects of *drugs* and environmental teratogens. However, with the advent of *in vitro fertilisation* (*IVF*), and an increased understanding about the early stages of development during the prefetal stages, there is now controversy about this terminology. It is clear that those stages of cleavage which develop from the fertilised egg (the zygote) up to the morula stage (16–32 cells; days three and four) have cells of equivalent totipotentiality and no one of them is identifiable definitively as destined to give rise to placenta or to the embryo proper. Thus in this context it is impossible to be precise about what is meant by the term embryo. The blastocyst stage (from day five onwards)

is the first time when two lineages of cells can be distinguished: the inner cell mass, those cells that will give rise to the primary germ layers of the embryo; and the trophectoderm – those cells that will give rise to the extraembryonic components, including membranes and placenta. The three germ layers become distinct by the primitive streak stage – at about 14 days of development. Prior to this time the developing zygote has been called the pre-embryo, and it is up to this period that *embryo research* is allowed under licence in terms of the *Human Fertilisation and Embryology Act 1990*.

See also: Fetus and embryo; safety.

PBr

Prejudice (literally: pre-judging) 1. "not being founded on reason cannot be removed by argument" (Dr Johnson). Usually someone else's opinions.

2. In spite of Dickens's comments in Nicholas Nickleby about the one-eyed Squeers – "there is a popular prejudice in favour of two" – the word usually implies a misjudgment or false assessment. People working in busy *primary care* would be in difficulty without its positive features ("this is the sort of person who might well be suffering from x") but since it precludes open-mindedness and leads to biased and unfair judgment about minority or alien groups its negative enactment is not only immoral but also in many systems illegal.

See also: Bias; boo word; discrimination; minorities.

KMB/RH

Prematurity defines babies born before 37 weeks completed gestational age (CGA). Neurodevelopmentally intact survival is rare before 22 weeks, but occurs in over half those born after 27 weeks.

Decisions concerning starting, withholding or withdrawing life-sustaining *treatment* pose ethical dilemmas for health care professionals and parents (*proxys*). Informed proxy decision-making requires accurate prognostic information and understanding of treatment/selective non-treatment options.

Treatment may be withdrawn or withheld if it is in the infant's best interests to do so, eg, if death is imminent, if treatment is futile, or if burdens of treatment far outweigh benefits. Persistent unreconcilable disagreements may require legal intervention to determine lawfulness of treatment withdrawal.

See also: Burdensomeness of treatment; viability.

VL

Premenstrual syndrome A cyclical collection of symptoms preceding the menses, which is physiological. Although sex hormones can affect behaviours, and some women have severe symptoms, there is at present no biological explanation that distinguishes women with PMS from those without. There are multiple remedies and treatments, all of which have a very large *placebo* effect. Although the distress is real, there is debate as to whether a gynaecological disease exists at all, rather than the syndrome being an expression of changing mood, underlying depression, personality disorder, or some other predisposition to physiological fluctuations.

SB

Prenatal diagnosis is the identification of diseases of the *fetus* and may be made non-invasively (eg, by scanning) or invasively (when a needle is used to obtain samples of fluid, placenta, or fetal blood). As invasive

techniques carry a risk of fetal loss or damage, and all prenatal diagnosis may lead to requests for termination of pregnancy, the ethical clash about fetal "rights" and women's domain over their bodies is obvious.

Prenatal diagnosis has more purposes than merely allowing termination of affected fetuses: it has the beneficent purpose of informing and preparing parents for the birth of an affected child, and allows some forms of in utero treatment, or referral to specialist centres for delivery to allow postnatal treatment. The specific ethical conflicts (separate from the *abortion* debate) relate to (a) the degree of disability that is considered to justify termination, particularly late termination, as diagnoses are often made late; (b) whether there is a detrimental effect on adults with *disability* when a distinction between normal and abnormal is made in utero; (c) whether it is wrong for parents to bring sick children into the world (a particularly *utilitarian* argument); and (d) the doctor's duty regarding informed choices.

Geneticists concerned about being accused of *eugenics* often place an extremely high priority on client *autonomy*. However, there is a question, particularly for those obstetricians performing invasive procedures, whether there is a limit to fulfilling the requests made by mothers for diagnosis and treatment. If there is a very remote risk of abnormality, or a very high risk to the mother (eg with fetal surgery), do doctors have to accede to informed choices for prenatal diagnosis and treatment when they are concerned about fetal or maternal harm?

See also: Abortion, ethical aspects; amniocentesis; chorionic villus sampling; congenital malformations; genetic counselling; genetic disorders; neural tube defects; risk assessment; risk–benefit analysis.

SB

Prescribing of *treatment*, usually *drugs*, is the action taken by a doctor in dealing with disease. In the widest sense it is the recommendation to the *patient*, but it usually refers to the written prescription given him to take to a *pharmacist* for drug dispensing. It specifies the active drug, may define a particular manufacturer's brand or formulation, the dose and dosing frequency and amount. Drugs may only be prescribed by registered medical practitioners (except for over the counter medications) and the clinician thus takes formal *responsibility* for their use. The doctor is expected to inform the patient why the drug is being used and how to take it and to warn of possible adverse effects (*disclosure*); this information and the degree of *empowerment* of the patient will affect his *compliance*.

Prescribing across a professional boundary may cause *resource* and *responsibility* problems. For instance when a hospital budget cannot carry a medication considered appropriate, the patient may be asked to accept a private prescription or to approach his GP, who may refuse to take responsibility because the drug is unfamiliar, or because of practice protocols. The patient is thus left in limbo. Similarly, a specialist nurse may feel it appropriate to prescribe but be unable to do so because of professional rules. New players have emerged in the regulation of prescribing. Pharmacists rightly expect a greater say in prescribing and have a role in protecting the patient when a possible *harm* is detected (such as drug interaction). Prescribing is an activity with defined expense, in nationalised systems largely falling on the government purse, and so the state may increasingly seek to control doctors' freedom to prescribe as well as regulate for public *safety*. Pharmaceutical companies will usually wish to oppose these moves and influence doctors to prescribe more and newer medication. Patients should know more about their medication but information packs, covering every eventuality, carry no sense of likelihood of *risk*. The prime responsibility to hold these issues in a good moral balance remains with the person who prescribes.

See also: Cost containment; National health Service; pharmaceutical industry.

AJP/RH

Prescriptivism is a theory of the meaning of moral and other value terms associated particularly with the Oxford moral philosopher, RM Hare. It holds (a) that an essential part of the meaning of such terms is that they are prescriptive or action-guiding, (b) that (contra descriptivism) this part of their meaning is not entailed by the descriptive criteria for the value judgments they express, and (c) that value terms differ from other prescriptions (such as orders) in being universalisable. Like Hume's theory ("no ought from is"), prescriptivism is non-naturalistic. Combined with minimal (and plausible) assumptions about human nature it is however broadly consistent with utilitarianism. It has important practical implications in particular for mental health.

Reference
Hare RM. *Moral thinking: its levels, method, and point*. Oxford: Clarendon Press, 1981.

See also: Facts vs values; is-ought gap; mental illness; moral theory; universalising; utilitarianism.

KWMF

Pressure groups are people acting in concert in advocacy for a particular cause. On health issues they often come together around a single disease, approach to therapy or access to care (eg, *AIDS*, obstetrics, and *complementary medicine*). They may comprise groups of *patients*, representatives of their peer group

195

or supporters of particular forms of therapy, and vary in the extent to which they are truly representative of those for whom they speak. They may exert pressure on clinicians, decision-makers and politicians, directly or through the media and/or may use other lobbying tactics. They can have beneficial effects by drawing attention to a clinical issue or *need*, but can distort *priorities* and create tensions between different statutory and/or voluntary agencies.

See also: Advocacy/activism.

AJP

Prima facie (Latin for at first sight) In *deontological* ethics it refers to a *duty* one always ought to obey except when it is in conflict with another equally binding duty, in which case one has to take all the circumstances (not simply the consequences as in *utilitarian* ethics) into account and come to a considered opinion about which duty is the more important.

Reference
Ross, WD. *The right and the good*. Oxford: Clarendon Press, 1930.

KMB

Primary care is the term used to cover all services related to a *patient*'s first place of seeking medical help, and the resources which relate to generalist or community health care around his home. It is contrasted with specialist (secondary) care in hospital or super-specialist (tertiary) referral. Primary care is poorly represented in most professional training programmes and probably therefore poorly understood. It is heavily dependent on people rather than technology and therefore may appear to be expensive while being (usually) under-resourced. The meaning and consequences of the recent push to a "Primary care led NHS" remain obscure to most commentators.

See also: General practice; hospital medicine; medical education; National Health Service; sexually transmitted diseases; specialism.

RH

Primum non nocere A Latin phrase usually translated as "first do no *harm*". It has been pointed out that health professionals probably always *risk* harming their patients on the way to helping them, even if the harm is small, so in the terms of timing, the harm does often come first. The sense is probably rather "as an overriding issue, or whatever else you do, don't do harm". Intervention freaks beware.

See also: Beneficence; Hippocratic Oath; non-intervention; non-maleficence.

RH

Principles *see* Autonomy; beneficence; justice; non-maleficence, parsimony; shadow.

Priorities Within tight resource constraints it would seem sensible enough to define priorities. Actually, however, this is rarely done in a rigorous sense. A brave attempt was made by the UK government and was published in Priorities for Health.[1] The document gave priority to improving health care for elderly people, people who are mentally ill or mentally handicapped, and children. It gave less priority to obstetrics, because of declining birth rates, and suggested that some money should be switched from obstetric services. This latter proposal led to a howl of protest: how dared government suggest taking *resources* away, rather than redeploying them within obstetrics to raise standards? When the government next attempted a statement of priorities,[2] it included a longer list of services to be developed and none to be cut back. That basically has remained the position since then. Government is reluctant to get into the business of rationing in the sense of formally denying any services to anybody. Nevertheless more will be heard of this topic in the years ahead because there simply is not enough money in the *National Health Service* to do everything that would bring some benefit to somebody. The debate about how to ration is long overdue.[3]

References
1 DHSS. *Priorities for health and personal social services in England*. London: HMSO, 1976.
2 DHSS *Priorities in the health and social services: the way forward*. London: HMSO, 1977.
3 Smith R. Rationing: the debate we have to have. *BMJ* 1995, **310**: 686.

See also: Cost containment; public policy.

RJM

Prisoners, care of In the UK medical care in prison is provided by the Directorate of Healthcare for Prisoners (DHCP). In smaller, lower security prisons, the doctors are usually contracted in on a part-time basis from a local *National Health Service* practice. Care in larger prisons is usually provided by full-time DHCP employees. Most prison nurses are prison officers who have undergone a short nursing course. The quality of care provided in these prisons has been much criticised.

The main ethical problems spring from the dual role of prison doctors as clinicians and prison managers. As well as treating prisoners, prison doctors are usually part of the senior management team. This can lead to conflict over issues of policy, eg on HIV. Doctors have been accused of pressurising prisoners into having HIV tests, breaching medical *confidentiality*, and sanctioning unnecessary restrictions on patients in order to allay the fears of staff and prisoners or maintain the good order of the prison.

Prison doctors also are asked to submit reports regarding a prisoner's possible release and certify that a prisoner is fit for punishment in the prison's internal disciplinary process. They are also necessarily involved in decisions about compassionate release. Doctors working in prisons are therefore necessarily part of the process of punishment and, in some cases, can have an influence on the effective length of a prisoner's sentence. The possession of knowledge about drug use or *sexual behaviour*, eg, may therefore pose particular ethical problems for doctors in the prison context.

See also: Imprisonment.

ASa

Privacy (from Latin for withdrawn from public life) allows individuals time and space to express their own thoughts and feelings to themselves or to those closest to them without (or before) having to articulate them coherently or consistently in public, at the risk of being misunderstood or prejudged by unsympathetic or even impartial third parties. Privacy is essential for sexual, religious, and imaginative impulses to flourish, and necessary to people making important life-choices, including those related to medical treatment. An important reason for medical *confidentiality* is to protect privacy.

KMB

Private medicine is the practice of medicine by independent practitioners on a fee-for-service basis, as distinct from a state-run *National Health Service* (NHS). Patients may self-refer to a specialist or go through a private general practitioner. Fees may be covered by health insurance, which may be obtained by the individual or provided as a company benefit. It may be conducted in separate premises or in private wards and clinics in NHS hospitals. Many private specialists work in NHS hospitals and do part-time private practice. Clinical academics are limited in how much they can earn for personal gain, and may prefer, or be obliged, to pay some fees earned to hospital/academic funds. Performance in the private sector is accountable to the *General Medical Council*, though there are less explicit mechanisms of professional oversight. *Patients* may use private medicine to avoid waiting and inconvenience and/or for more comfortable facilities; they may wish for the personal attention of a chosen senior clinician. Some doctors prefer private medicine because of greater direct contact with individual patients, without the interposition of trainees. Coverage of the range of medicine varies in different countries and centres, but acute problems and some *chronic diseases* are often less well catered for. It may be construed as setting double standards for those able to pay and as a potential diversion of specialist and trained staff from the NHS, or as a way of relieving the NHS of some patients who can afford it, depending on one's political and social perspective.

See also: Accountability; general practice; insurance, industry; insurance, medical; specialism.

AJP

Probability is the mathematical approach to determining whether an event or an association has occurred by *chance* or because of a linkage, causally or otherwise. Various means are used to quantify probability or statistical significance in *epidemiological research* and in *clinical research and trials* using "p-values" and confidence intervals. High degrees of probability suggest a strong, even a causal, relationship (such as between smoking and lung cancer), while low degrees may be due to chance, confounding variables, or to an indirect link (such as between riding bicycles and prostatic disease, or cholesterol levels and suicide). The more tests applied to any

data set, the greater the probability of a chance association appearing to be significant. In clinical trials, probabilities are used to determine the impact of a novel treatment against current standard or no therapy (*placebo*) and to determine the size or power of a study to identify a given impact.

AJP

Procedural ethics In *law, politics*, and *medical ethics*, parties disagreeing or in doubt about what ought to be done may yet agree on the best process or procedures by which to determine this. Examples include trial by jury, a "peace process", and "guided *consensus*" in neonatal intensive care. Sharing information, listening, time for reflection and joint decision making are key features. This can be particularly important for resolving complex ethical questions related to scientific advance in culturally diverse societies. In these contexts, increasing public and professional participation in deliberative processes (eg, consensus conferences) may be necessary to avoid the imposition of conflict-laden remedies by *experts, bureaucracy*, or uninformed media campaigns.

See also: Due process; Research Ethics Committees.

KMB

Procedures is a term often applied to medical interventions used in diagnosis or treatment that fall short of what would normally be construed as *surgery*, such as venepuncture, endoscopy, diagnostic imaging, and *pheresis*. While a useful word to avoid alarming patients, it may engender confusion about the need to seek explicit consent. Another usage is in guiding and documenting (proper) procedures or formal/informal protocols, such as in investigating or treating patients, in *research* or in *management*.

AJP

Professional courtesy *Patients* have the right to expect to be "treated" – in both the general and specific senses of that word – with "courtesy and consideration".[1] This involves more than correct etiquette. As a minimum, it requires health professionals to respect their patients' *dignity* and *privacy*; to obtain valid consent in the light of information patients might hope to understand; to protect the *confidentiality* of the confidences entrusted to them; to control personal *prejudice*; and to mobilise all the available resources from which their patients might benefit. Ideally, doctors and other health professionals should possess and practise qualities of caring, sympathy, *compassion*, and sensitivity.

Professional courtesy is also used to describe the provision of professional services to colleagues and their families, often with the implication or intent to offer more favourable services in terms of speed, convenience or special attention. It may be seen as a legitimate "perk" for insiders or could be construed as inequitable. Attempts to bypass systems may have perverse effects and inadvertently reduce the quality of care. If things go wrong, it may be difficult for the patient to seek or obtain redress, especially if the clinician is a close colleague. Some now consider it to be anomalous within the more tightly regulated health care environment and to create ethical tensions that seem to outweigh the generosity that underlies it.[2]

References
1 *The duties of a doctor.* London: General Medical Council, 1995.
2 Levy MA, Arnold RM, Fine MJ, Kapoor WN. Professional courtesy – current practices and attitudes. *N Engl J Med.* 1993; **329**: 1627–31.

See also: Attitudes; beneficence; benevolence; bias; informed consent; professionalism; respect.

SM/AJP

Professionalism Professionalism is the demonstration in practice of the aptitudes, attributes and attitudes to which practitioners lay claim and which might reasonably be demanded of them by those entrusted to their care, and by their colleagues "of good repute and competency".[1] Its hallmark is commitment: (i) to the individual patient, requiring *professional courtesy*, continuing competence, personal *integrity*, and advocacy of the patient's interests; (ii) to the *healthcare system*, ensuring continuity of relevant care of the highest possible quality for all without discrimination, and (iii) to the profession, entailing active "allegiance to the bodies providing collective professional responsibility"[2].

References
1 Lord Justice Lopes, 1894, as quoted in: *Professional conduct and discipline: fitness to practise.* London: General Medical Council, 1993:6.
2 *Core values for the medical profession in the 21st century.* Report of a conference held on 3–4 November 1994 at BMA House, London: BMA *et al.*: 15.

See also: Accountability; attitudes; advocacy/activism; competence to practise.

SM

Professional–patient relationship *See* Doctor–patient relationship.

Professional responsibility can be considered in three parts. Clinical responsibility for a patient normally rests with a hospital consultant or principal in *general practice*. It may be delegated to a less experienced doctor providing he has the necessary training to discharge it in the particular clinical situation. All doctors have a *responsibility* to maintain and adapt their professional *skills* through continuing *medical education* and to place themselves under the care of a medical colleague when suffering from illness. The medical profession has a corporate responsibility to ensure that by *audit* and *peer review* acceptable clinical and ethical standards are maintained.

199

See also: Accountability; clinical judgment; colleagues/collegiality; competence to practise; self-regulation.

JSH

Promise keeping Whether, and, in particular, why, promises ought to be kept, are age-old questions that continue to vex jurists and political and moral philosophers. Promise keeping is a *rights* issue: "Promises create rights".[1] In the act of making a promise, a person places himself under a duty to the party to whom he makes the promise and this duty is correlative to the right which his act of promising ascribes to the promisee. In as much as duties ought to be taken at least as seriously as rights, promises made ought to be kept.

Some exceptions spring to mind. First, where promise keeping conflicts with more urgent moral concerns the latter may take precedence. Eg, I promise to attend your party tomorrow night but my daughter is taken seriously ill tomorrow afternoon. Furthermore, promises made as a result of *coercion* or while the promiser is under *duress* may be distinguished from authentic promises, those made voluntarily and autonomously – think of the prospective candidate for a coronary bypass operation who promises he will give up *smoking* simply because he is led to believe this is the only way of securing his candidacy. To this extent at least, there is an analogy with the doctrine of *informed consent*. Similarly, possession of relevant information is a prerequisite for a promise fairly to be called *voluntary* and *autonomous*. With informed consent doctrine, there is invariably an obligation on the health care professional to make appropriate *disclosure*; with promise making, it can be argued that the onus always lies on the promiser, not the promisee, to ensure he is apprised of all relevant facts before making a promise. Such information should include reasonable predictions as to the ability to fulfil the duty (self-)imposed by the promise.

References
Komrad MS. A defence of medical paternalism: maximising patients' autonomy. *J Med Ethics* 1983; **9**: 38–44.
Steiner H. *An essay on rights*. Oxford: Blackwell, 1994: 76.

CAE

Prophylaxis is the use of *drugs* (or devices) to prevent the occurrence (primary prophylaxis) or recurrence (secondary prophylaxis) of a condition to which a patient is susceptible. An early use of the term was for *condoms* to prevent pregnancy, or *sexually transmitted diseases*. The most common use of prophylaxis is where antibiotics are given to people at increased risk of infection due to defects in host defences. As with *immunisation*, its use requires identification of a person or population at risk for disease and assessment of the level of that *risk* and any risk (eg, toxicity, generation of bacterial resistance) resulting from prophylaxis, as well as its efficacy. Cost-effectiveness should be considered in terms of the costs of the drug or device and any monitoring required, set against the costs of disease episodes prevented. Prophylaxis has greatly improved the outlook for many patients with immunodeficiency (including *AIDS*) and chronic lung disease and following *transplantation*.

See also: Risk assessment.

AJP

Proportion In ethics this term is used to indicate the relationship that should exist between the good and bad effects of an action. The school of proportionalism holds that, in order to ascertain the rightness or wrongness of an action, one must take into account all the non-moral goods and evils involved.

Reference
Hoose, B. *Proportionalism: the American debate and its European roots*. Washington DC: Georgetown University Press, 1987.

See also: Double effect.

BHo

Prostitution/sex workers The ethics of prostitution, which involves the exchange of sexual services for money or in kind, are fiercely contested. Within *feminism*, prostitutes are conceived both as victims of a patriarchal world order and as the most radical of feminists, who refuse to give sex away for free. The medical profession is more interested in the practical effects of prostitution. The focus is on prostitutes, who are defined in terms of their high numbers of sexual partners who, in turn, are associated with risks for *sexually transmitted disease (STD)* and associated problems of reproductive health.

While it is recognised that men as well as women work in the sex industry, male prostitutes have remained less visible. Several reports have noted high prevalences of STD in study groups of male prostitutes, who work primarily with other men, although they may also report sex with women.

Morbidity in prostitutes has caused less concern than the transmission of disease. Prostitutes, and sometimes their clients, are considered a high *risk* or core group for STD transmission and a pool of infection for the population at large. Recent studies have qualified this picture. Low prevalences of infection have been reported and explained, in part, by the use of *prophylaxis* (*condoms*) with clients. High prevalences in other study groups have been associated with *poverty* as much as partner numbers and, specifically, disadvantages of age, social class, ethnicity, and gender.

Public health efforts to control disease/prostitutes include compulsory registration, *screening* and the detention of those found infected as well as the provision of free, accessible and confidential health services.

Medical approaches are informed by legal measures and popular stereotype. Abolitionist policies, enshrined in international agreements and most national laws, deal with prostitution as a form of slavery to which criminal penalties are attached. Particular concerns are expressed about child prostitution and trafficking from poor to richer regions. In practice, laws deriving from abolitionism penalise sex workers, especially those who work visibly, more than clients or managers and they fail to distinguish between individuals who are forced to work and those who choose to work on their own behalf.

State systems of medicine and law have contributed to – indeed, some hold them responsible for creating – the *stigma* associated with prostitution. It is rarely possible for prostitutes publicly to declare their job and enjoy the same range of civil rights as other people, including access to health care. *Human rights* activists are particularly concerned about the detention of "infected prostitutes" in many states.[1]

Health workers have opposed compulsory registration and screening, through which they police prostitution on behalf of the state. They have also established services that do not deal exclusively with STD transmission but address a wide range of health issues. On occasion, prostitutes have been enrolled as health professionals themselves. These approaches are justified on the basis of practical as well as ethical considerations.

Reference
1 Delacoste F, Alexander P, eds. *Sex work: writings by women in the sex industry*. London: Virago Press, 1988 (first pub 1987).

See also: AIDS; HIV; power.

SD

Proximity Good moral *judgments* may be hard to make without a measure of *empathy* and the use of moral imagination, so being close to the main actors in a decision, physically or psychologically, appears to be of importance. There may be an optimal *distance*. It may be hard to make good judgments about our *neighbours* (Not In My Back Yard – the NIMBY effect), which gives extra force to Christ's injunction to love them, or about people who are alien or far away unless their plight is brought close to our attention. However, there is probably some rule of thumb about *beneficence* which suggests we need to set *boundaries* to our helpfulness. Charity should begin at home (though it may not end there).

RH

Proxy (from procuracy, the office of one who acts for another) A proxy may give or withhold consent to *treatment*: (a) if legally authorised by the patient (eg, if *powers of attorney* provide for this); or (b) as parents acting in, but not against, the best interests of children, too immature to understand the implications. Proxy consent from unauthorised relatives of a patient who lacks *decision-making capacity* has no legal standing. But seeking it, where possible, is courteous and circumspect – at least for treatment. Research involving such patients is, strictly, illegal.

See also: Child, status of; next of kin; substituted judgment.

KMB

Prozac is the proprietary name of the drug fluoxetine. The drug is an effective treatment of depressive illness, obsessive compulsive disorder, and bulimia nervosa. It may work by inhibiting the absorption of serotonin, a neurotransmitter, into the neurone from which it was released. This leaves more serotonin, in the synapse, to enhance neurotransmission. Some psychiatrists believe that Prozac causes patients to become violent or suicidal, but large studies have not confirmed this. Other authors believe that Prozac can change *personality*, when taken by people without *mental illness*, but there is no convincing evidence for this belief.

See also: Depression; psychopharmacology.

PDW

Prudence (from Latin for foresight) popularly regarded as caution, but in philosophy often identified with *practical reasoning and practical wisdom*. Prudence avoids both rashness and timidity, and determines the best means to the best ends. In medical ethics, *non-maleficence* is often the most prudent principle.

KMB

Psychiatry, use and abuse The abuse of psychiatry is the use of psychiatric disease labels not for legitimate medical purposes of diagnosis and treatment but as a means of repression and control.

Abuse of this kind became institutionalised in the former USSR and its satellites: political dissidents were admitted to psychiatric hospitals and treated with neuroleptics on the grounds that they were said to have "delusions of reformation" or to be suffering from "sluggish schizophrenia". Sporadic cases of abuse occur regularly in all countries.

The abuse of psychiatry can be understood as a misuse of one its most important legitimate uses, namely involuntary treatment. A suicidal patient suffering from depressive delusions of guilt eg, has lost the capacity for rational, and hence autonomous, choice. In most countries, therefore, psychiatrists have legal powers to treat such patients without their *consent*. The abuse of psychiatry is the abuse of these powers.

The factors that allow abusive practices to become widespread include poor standards of professional training, inadequate resources, over-politicisation of psychiatry and lack of appropriate legal controls.

The underlying vulnerability of psychiatry to abuse arises from the relatively value-laden nature of the concept of mental illness. This has been taken by psychiatrists to show the need for a more scientific definition of *mental illness* and by anti-psychiatrists to show that mental disorders are really moral rather than medical concepts. Both kinds of theory are important. The former underlines the need for careful clinical assessment as the basis of decisions about compulsory treatment. The latter underlines the need for shared decision making within a well balanced *multidisciplinary team* representing a range of relevant values including those of the patient.

The importance of shared decision making is reflected in the multidisciplinary checks and balances against the abusive use of the psychiatrist's powers of involuntary treatment, which are a feature of modern mental health legislation.

References

Bloch S. The political misuse of psychiatry in the Soviet Union. In: Bloch S, Chodoff P, eds. *Psychiatric ethics* (2nd ed). Oxford: Oxford University Press, 1991: ch 24.

Fulford KWM, Smirnoff AYU, Snow E. Concepts of disease and the abuse of psychiatry in the USSR. *Br J Psychiatry* 1993; **162**: 801–10.

See also: Autonomy; compulsory testing and treatment; decision-making capacity; depression; guilt; human rights; informed consent; multidisciplinary teams; patients; racism; rationality; refusal of treatment; suicide; values.

KWMF

Psychogeriatrics is a branch of psychiatry concerned with patients aged over 65 that in the UK has become a formally established specialty. A comprehensive psychogeriatric service provides domiciliary visiting by specialist doctors, nurses, and social workers, and a range of day care and outpatient facilities. A number of inpatient assessment beds are also required, as are some longer stay inpatient places, but the aim is to help an old person with *mental illness* to live in his own home if possible. This policy can raise ethical problems in striking the balance between the rights of the *patient* and those of his carers.

See also: Autonomy; dementia; geriatric medicine.

GE

Psychology/morality boundary remains a source of confusion in many ethical dilemmas. To what extent should applied ethics be setting the standards of what is objectively best, even if seldom obtained in action, and to what extent should it take into account, explore, condone, or even support less good actions because it is part of observed human behaviour or *human nature* to behave in this way or in that particular *context*? An example might be the problem of respecting *autonomy* in clinical medicine when it is apparent in practice that the most mature adult's choices are often constrained by circumstances or partly determined by *culture* or upbringing, and that a measure of dependency is not only a normal but even a desirable trait in civilised social behaviour. Failure to explore or resolve those issues does no favours to either philosophy or psychology, and allows the continuation of a dichotomy where there should be partnership and the exhibition of *practical reasoning and wisdom*.

See also: Absolutism; context; dirty hands debate; order of preferences; wisdom.

RH

Psychopathy has four contemporary meanings. Besides lay use as a term of opprobrium ("psychopath"), it has been applied in the past as a single diagnostic label and is currently retained as a legal category of mental disorder within the English Mental Health Act, 1983. It can also be used as a broad generic term to encompass a wide range of poorly delineated psychopathology exhibited by individuals with severe personality disorder, leading to antisocial or other dysfunctional social behaviour. The onset is in childhood or adolescence, there is a longstanding persistence over time without marked remission or relapses, and these abnormalities constitute a basic aspect of the individual's usual functioning. The question of whether to define psychopathy in terms of abnormal behaviour or abnormality of personality is still not resolved, although contemporary taxonomists place increasing emphasis on the latter.

See also: Mental illness; personality.

JC

Psychopharmacology is the study of *drugs* acting on the mind. These drugs can be roughly divided into three groups: medicines used to treat patients with psychological symptoms, such as *tranquillisers* for the anxious and anti-depressants for the depressed; those agents used to change feelings in normal individuals, such as caffeine and alcohol; and drugs of misuse such as amphetamines, cocaine and heroin. A major ethical consideration is the problem of ensuring there is fully *informed consent* to take the medications, in the clinical or research context, where patients' mental capabilities may be impaired owing to their illness. Nevertheless, even psychotically disturbed patients can usually understand the *risks* and benefits of medicines offered to them.

See also: Depression; drug misuse; mental illness; Prozac.

ML

Psychosurgery comprises a set of procedures designed to modify the course of psychiatric disorders through operations on the brain. The most famous of these has been prefrontal lobotomy or *leucotomy*. After its first use in 1935 the idea had fairly wide acceptance; some would claim there was widespread abuse of the technique in the 1940s and 50s. The side-effects included blunting of affect, loss of personality and motivation, and cognitive rigidity. Operations are most commonly done for disturbed affect but some are done for repeated episodes of violent behaviour. The operation has dramatic effects in some patients and is offered to a very small proportion of psychiatric patients at the current time. The most common indications are anxiety disorders, obsessional symptoms, and depression. Stereotactic techniques, which use computer directed interventions in precisely defined brain centres, have recently been used and the mortality and morbidity figures are very low.

References

Klenig J. *Ethical issues in psychosurgery*. London: Allen & Unwin, 1985.

Mersky H. Physical manipulation of the brain. In: Bloch S, Chodoff P. *Psychiatric ethics* (2nd ed). Oxford: University Press, 1991.

See also: Mental illness; personality; psychiatry, use and abuse.

GG

Psychotherapy There is no standard recognised definition of psychotherapy or agreement on boundaries with *counselling* or other talking therapies. Previously, anyone could practise as a psychotherapist and the United Kingdom Council for Psychotherapy was set up to create a register of appropriately trained practitioners abiding by a code of ethics. Psychotherapy can bring about harm as well as benefit. Individuals whose personalities are fragile, whose hold upon reality is tenuous, or who are unable to recognise and face up to their personal problems, may be harmed by psychotherapy. In addition, recipients of individual therapy may sometimes achieve personal fulfilment only at the cost of others. There are also the dangers of manipulation, and of the therapist's own *values* and *attitudes* influencing those of the client.

References

Clarkson, P, Pokorny M ed. *The handbook of psychotherapy.* London: Routledge, 1994.

Masson J. *Against therapy.* London: Harper Collins, 1993.

See also: Mental illness; stress.

RCo

Public health, ethics of A modern definition of public health is "the science and art of preventing disease, prolonging life and promoting health through the organised efforts of society". Historically, communicable diseases have been a major focus for public health and the field now includes *chronic disease* control and *health education* and promotion, as well as the promotion of effective *healthcare systems*. The focus on "the organised efforts of society" provides most of the organisational, political and ethical challenges of public health in every country. Accepting that *war* is the largest threat to public health,[1] public health workers (doctors and other professionals) see that many health problems in both developed and developing countries are determined by deprivation, *poverty* and *inequality*.

The task is to work – often from positions within the establishment – at lobbying and *advocacy* and in *politics* at promoting *equity* and *justice*, while at the same time promoting *empowerment* and *freedom* of choice for the people. Public health workers are often more aware of the problems of *paternalism* than many other health professionals, but they are no less affected by the unequal distribution of

knowledge and skills between professionals and the public. What is the public interest and how is it to be determined? This seems to be the major challenge for many public health workers throughout the world.

Focuses on "lay epidemiology" and qualitative methods are both intended to enable people to express their own values and attitudes to health and quality of life. There is a tension between the long term perspectives of public professionals and the necessarily short term views of patients and their needs, or politicians and their imperatives.

Reference

1 Rose, G. *The strategy of preventive medicine.* Oxford: Oxford University Press, 1992.

See also: Epidemiological research; human rights; immunisation; infection control; National Health Service; needs; needs assessment; notifiable diseases; purchasing; resources.

SPBD

Public policy results from government action; it may also reflect no government action. Policy in action takes many forms: in medicine alone policies range widely – from, eg, the law on *abortion* to *community care*. Ethical principles have a place, though not always explicit, in every policy; but they signify more in some policies (say, income support) than in others (say, agriculture prices). The borderline between ethical and political factors can be narrow. For some politicians unemployment benefit or hospital waiting lists, for example, may have as much an ethical as a political aspect.

The basic principles of medical ethics apply more widely. The principle of *beneficence* is reflected in policies designed to benefit us all. Governments seek to avoid policies that carry a risk of *harm* or *maleficence*, though there can be conflicts – eg between the economic "beneficence" of a motorway and the environmental "maleficence" of pollution. The rights or *autonomy* of individuals often present difficulty – for instance, if the local schools admissions policy prevents a child getting a place in the school of its choice. Governments readily acknowledge the ethical principle of *justice*, but serious problems can arise in allocating *resources*. A hospital closure can be fully justified by resource priorities, but it may be condemned as unjust by those who work in the hospital or who are its patients.

The ethical dimension to public policies should be complemented by high ethical standards in public bodies. That implies no taint of corruption or improper patronage, and government as open as possible, with strict *confidentiality* when required. There may be fears that longstanding ethical values – a vocational dedication to public service and a spirit of cooperation between public bodies – will be eroded by new, more competitive, forms of *management*. It remains, however, an ethical duty to ensure that public policies are administered to the highest possible standard.

References

Thomas R. *The British philosophy of administration*. London: Longmans, 1978. This includes a large bibiography.

McDonald O. *The future of Whitehall*. London: Weidenfeld and Nicolson, 1991.

Pratchett L, Wingfield M. *The public service ethos in local government*. Leicester: CLD; De Montfort University, 1994.

See also: Accountability; business ethics; cost containment; healthcare systems; National Health Service; politics; public health; resources.

PN

Publicity The making public, intentionally or otherwise, of information (or misinformation). Because stories about health and disease are of great interest to the public (though not always in the public interest), publicity commonly includes presentation in the media of personal health information, as well as issues regarding specific diseases and treatments, and health service provision. The former raises issues regarding *confidentiality*, if health professionals divulge patient details without *consent*, or even confirm news stories derived from other sources. The media have a great capacity to disseminate information as part of *health education*, but can distort or unbalance a debate. *Pressure groups* may use the media for *advocacy* of particular causes. Publicity about the abilities of individual doctors may be construed as *advertising* by the *General Medical Council*.

AJP

Punishment Healthcare staff may – albeit rarely – be called to be involved in official punishment schedules (such as administering a lethal injection) and will need to assure themselves of the justice of this work. There is no justification for being involved in immoral acts such as *torture* (there is no "fair play" to see). However, many treatments are so arduous and so difficult for a hospitalised patient to escape from that they become like a torture to the patient; and if the patient does not respond, there is alarming evidence that the professionals may be tempted to redouble their activity and adopt an even more punitive attitude.

Reference

Main T. *The ailment and other psychoanalytic essays*. London: Free Association Books, 1989.

See also: Blame; capital punishment; guilt; mutilation; prisoners.

RH

Purchasing One important element in Mrs Thatcher's prescriptions for the *National Health Service* published in *Working for Patients*[1] was to separate purchasing from provision. There were two main arguments for this. First, it has allowed all main provider units in the NHS to be freed from direct management by the health authorities and hence to be run by their own *trust* board in a more flexible, less anonymous way. Second, it gives the health authority the duty of concentrating on how best to commission services for its local population without being unduly swayed by loyalty to its own staff and institutions. Some of the advertised benefits – particularly that money would follow the patient – have not happened, and it has never been clear how compatible GP *fundholding* and health authority purchasing would prove in the longer term. Nevertheless, the purchaser/provider split is seen by many managers as a step forward. It has aroused substantial interest internationally and is, eg, even more clearly displayed in New Zealand than in the UK.

References
1 *Working for patients*, London: HMSO, 1989.

See also: Cost containment; healthcare systems; needs assessment; public health.

RJM

Q

QALYs The allocation of scarce *resources* between clinical interventions needs to be informed by data on what is given up by society (the opportunity cost) and what is gained: the enhancement in the length and quality of a patient's life (and that of his carer, particularly in the cases of the elderly and the mentally ill).

Disease-specific measures of relevant quality of life, combined with cost data, provide relevant information for resource allocation decisions within therapeutic categories (eg, counselling or no counselling after breast cancer surgery) but efficient resource allocation within the *healthcare system* requires outcome measures which can be used to provide indicators of benefit across all therapeutic categories

(eg, from coronary care to hip replacements).

The concept of the quality adjusted life year (QALY) was initially used by the US Office of Technology Assessment in the late 1970s and popularised in the UK by Williams and others. The approach uses a generic measure of *quality of life* and either prospectively or using "expert judgments" tracks patient progress before and after an intervention.

The generic measures used, initially the Rosser index and now the EuroQol in the UK, the Torrance measure in Canada and the Quality of Wellbeing in the USA, have been criticised in terms of their validity. They encompass, to varying degrees, processes by which descriptors have been identified, measured, and valued for physical, social, and psychological aspects of the quality of life.

When combined with survival data, they demonstrate the cost of producing one year of good-quality life (a QALY). The cost-per-QALY estimates of different interventions can then be ranked and, in principle, used to inform resource allocation across the whole range of acute therapeutic categories.

In practice the QALY approach remains contentious because of disputes about the validity of competing generic quality of life measures and because of poor cost data. Advocates of the QALY approach continue to assert the approach is crude but unavoidable. The World Bank advocates the use of a similar measure, Disability Free Life Years (DALYs), to inform the policy process in developing countries.

References
Drummond MF, Stoddart GL, Torrance GW. *Methods for the economic evaluation of health care programmes*. Oxford: Oxford University Press, 1987.
EuroQol Group. EuroQol – a new facility for the measurement of health-related quality of life. *Health Policy* 1990; **16**: 199–208.

Kaplan R. A quality of life approach to health resource allocation. In: Strosberg MA, Wiener JM, Baker R, Fein IA, eds. *Rationing America's health care: the Oregon plan and beyond*. Washington DC: Brookings Institute, 1992.

Maynard A. Developing the health care market. *Economic J* 1991; **101**: 1277

Rosser R, Kind P, Williams A. Valuation of quality of life. In: Jones-Lee MW, ed. *The value of life and safety*. Amsterdam: North Holland, 1982.

Williams A. Economics of coronary artery bypass grafting. *BMJ* 1985; **249**: 326–9.

World Bank *World development report 1993: investing in health*. Oxford: Oxford University Press, 1993.

See also: Cost-containment; developing world; quality assurance.

AMy

Quality assurance Everyone has an interest in the quality of health care and mechanisms to improve it. Good quality health care has many characteristics including good technical care, good interpersonal *communication*, *respect*, and the enabling of recipients of care to make informed *choices*. The quality of care does not solely depend on the abilities of individual health care practitioners but also reflects organisational function and support.

Quality assurance (QA) is one of several terms that describe mechanisms for quality improvement based on systematic evaluation of the quality of care. Other terms include medical (or clinical) audit, continuous quality improvement (CQI), total quality management (TQM), quality improvement, and quality assessment. There are some distinctions between these terms but the definitions are not exact. Some use QA as a general term for all systematic quality improvement schemes.

QA is often associated with external monitoring of performance against pre-set standards – a feature of health care in the USA for many years. In the UK external assessments of performance have involved only few areas, eg, the Health Advisory Service assessment of the quality of long stay services and quality assurance of clinical pathology.

Medical (clinical) audit was introduced and funded as part of the 1989 UK health reforms and is now the focus of quality improvement throughout the *National Health Service* (NHS). Audit is done by those who deliver care, and is the process of comparing an aspect of the quality of care against pre-determined standards; if indicated, making appropriate changes to solve problems and reassessing to determine if care has improved.[1] Medical audit refers to doctors assessing medical care; clinical audit encompasses the work of the whole clinical team.

CQI and TQM originated from industry and are based on the view that quality concerns everyone in an organisation: quality is about meeting the needs of customers, and that flaws are faults in systems not people.[2] Distinct from external QA, these approaches aim to improve quality through internal, unthreatening analysis of the causes of *mistakes*.

References

1 Russell IT, Wilson BJ. Audit: the third clinical science? *Quality in Health Care* 1992; **1**: 51–5.
2 Berwick DM. Continuous quality improvement as an ideal in health care. *New Engl J Med* 1989; **320**: 52–6.

FM

Quality of life Attempts to assess life's quality as opposed to its length arise in both *euthanasia* and health care rationing debates. The assumption is that death may be preferable to some states of life, or at least that, if we have to choose between allocating resources for mere survival or for improved states of health, survival need not be the trump card.

The problem is determining criteria for quality. Singer and Kuhse have argued that we have no obligation to prolong the life of severely handicapped infants, but is their quality of life to be measured by assessment of mental ability or only by reference to clearly irremediable suffering?[1] Similar problems arise in some end of life decisions. If the patient cannot tell us, who is to judge a life to be not worth living? In the rationing debate Williams and associates have proposed measuring Quality Adjusted Life Years (QALYs), thus combining survival criteria with factors such as mobility, pain, and functional independence.[2] This may help in comparing treatments for the same condition, but if QALYs are applied to different patient groups contestable values are introduced. Eg, Harris has argued that they are inherently ageist.[3]

Quality is, by its very definition, value laden, since it implies describing the nature of something in comparison with that which is inferior or superior to it. Although there is widespread agreement about some of the detriments to a happy life, the inevitable subjectivity in what we count as happiness or a worthwhile life must cast doubt on the validity of ethical judgments made on this basis. Yet judgments have to be made, especially in view of increasing demands on health care *resources*. No simple formula may ever be found, but unless questions of quality are constantly debated, the emotional appeal of survival will always win the debate over resource allocation.

References
1 Kuhse H, Singer P. *Should the baby live?* Oxford: OUP, 1985.
2 Williams A. The value of QALYs. *Health Soc Serv J*. 1985; Jul 18: 3ff.
3 Harris J. QALYfying the value of life. *J Med Ethics*, 1987; **13**: 117–9.

See also: Justice; life prolongation; moral judgment; treatment.

AVC

Quarantine Isolation, sometimes under legal compulsion, with the aim of preventing the spread of infection, has been practised for many centuries. Its very variable efficacy could be accounted for only in the post-Pasteurian era, with the understanding of such factors as subclinical infection, carrier states, insect vectors, and zoonoses.

For most diseases for which quarantine was used, like smallpox, plague, and cholera, the ethical conflict is between individual liberty of movement and the supposed or genuine public good. With *sexually transmitted diseases*, additional motives of social disapproval and ostracism are often evident under the cloak of *infection control*. Quarantine of prostitutes was employed extensively in the USA following an act in 1918, and the authorities in Cuba are attempting to control *AIDS* by quarantine of *HIV*-positive people.

Reference
Bynum WF, Porter R. *Companion encyclopaedia of the history of medicine*. London: Routledge, 1993.

See also: Carriers; compulsory testing and treatment; non-voluntary; public health.

HL

Queuing represents one form of *rationing* which Rudolf Klein calls[1] rationing by delay (as opposed, eg, to rationing by denial or by price). In the *National Health Service* it is most obviously manifested in hospital waiting lists for elective (meaning non-emergency) admissions. Less obviously it also applies to waiting for a specialist outpatient appointment. Hospital waiting lists have been a fact of life throughout the history of the NHS. In 1975 Enoch Powell noted the size of the waiting list, which was then around 500,000, as one of the enduring constants of the NHS.[2] It is not the size of the list that matters but the length of the wait. In recent years government has demanded from NHS managers a determined onslaught on the waiting list and has set charter standards of not more than eighteen months, with many purchasers setting tighter targets locally. Rightly or wrongly the custom in the NHS has always been to classify cases by urgency, so that the queue is not in fact a single list. Queues for elective surgery are also common in other large public hospital systems, such as Australia, New Zealand, and Sweden. But that certainly does not mean that they are inevitable or acceptable.[3] And they are typically not a feature of insurance-based systems where money can genuinely follow the patient.

References
1 Klein R. Rationing in the NHS: the dance of the seven veils – in reverse. *Br Med Bull.* 1995; **51, Pt IV**: 769–80.
2 Powell E. *Medicine and politics: 1975 and after.* London: Pitman Medical, 1976
3 Yates J. *Why are we waiting?* Oxford: Oxford University Press, 1987.

See also: Gatekeeping; Patients' Charter; purchasing.

RJM

Quietism refers to the doctrine and practice of passive quiet contemplation and withdrawal from the active world. It has been extended in a pejorative sense to the political or social arena, particularly when there is a practical *moral* problem to be addressed, or when circumstances seem to demand a response from right-minded people. In this sense the quietist avoids, ostrich-like, the moral challenge, and might thus be accused of acting immorally.

RH

R

Racism "Racism" encompasses both attitudes and ideologies, actions and structures. Racially biased attitudes as well as racially discriminatory policies and practices would both, thus, be instances of racism. Biological racism – the notion that "races" have distinct biological characteristics that are mirrored in achievements, intellect and behaviour – has given way to more subtle forms of racism, articulated mainly through the neutral language of *culture*, lineage, belonging, and ideas influenced by sociobiology such as "natural" fear of strangers and preference for one's own group. This contemporary form of racism is sometimes referred to as the "new" – or "cultural" – racism. The once popular psychological definition of racism as *prejudice* combined with power is inadequate for two broad reasons. First, racism is not just the preserve of the powerful; indeed many of the worst excesses are committed by the socially disadvantaged. Second, engagement in racist actions does not necessarily rest on racist attitudes; eg, the racially discriminatory policy of "virginity testing" of Asian women at British ports may well have been carried out by those who were opposed to it but saw it as a job. The latter exemplifies "institutional racism", the idea that racism has its roots in the social structures of the society and that therefore institutions need to ensure that their policies do not inadvertently discriminate against certain minority ethnic groups.

Individual and institutional racism in a health service deprives people of rights and undermines human dignity; medicine has a poor history of serving non-white people. Examples include the medical legitimation of slavery and colonisation.[1] Contemporary examples of racism in medicine include the differential modes of referral and differential treatment of black and white psychiatric patients.[1,2]

References
1 Littlewood R, Lipsedge M. *Aliens and alienists: ethnic minorities and psychiatry* (2nd ed). London: Unwin Hyman, 1989.

2 Ahmad WIU. *'Race' and health in contemporary Britain*. Buckingham: Open University Press, 1993.

See also: Bias; discrimination; ethnicity.

WA

Radiation safety Radiation, whether natural, diagnostic, therapeutic (*radiotherapy*) or from *nuclear war* presents a classic example of balancing *risk* or *harm* and benefit (*risk-benefit analysis*) and requires an assessment of risk to determine an acceptable level of *safety* for the context in which it is found or utilised. This necessitates careful quantitative analysis of the impact of radiation on biological tissues.

X-rays are flux of energy quanta that penetrate the body, yet some of the radiation is absorbed and a shadow image of the absorbing structures in the body can be produced on film or screen. The concentration of absorbed energy is called radiation dose, measured in Gy (ie, J/kg), which in diagnostic radiology range from 0.1 to 100 mGy, in cancer radiotherapy from 40 to 70 Gy. Natural background varies between 1 and >10 mGy per year.

The mechanism underlying the biological effects of radiation is its ability to break chromosomes due to double strand breaks in DNA but only 5% of double strand breaks lead to a chromosome break, 95% are repaired. Chromosome breaks may have a variety of biological consequences: large deletions or dicentric chromosomes result in loss of unlimited proliferative capacity of the cells and cell death. Small deletions or balanced translocations, compatible with cell survival, may result in mutations in somatic or germ cells.

Acute side-effects of high radiation doses are due to the loss of unlimited proliferative capacity of stem cells in tissues such as bone marrow, skin and mucosa, yet the same cellular effect is also responsible for the anti-*cancer* action of *radiotherapy*. Chronic side-effects of high radiation doses are mainly due to specific radiation effects on endothelial cells leading to loss of capillaries, atrophy, fibrosis, and necrosis. A threshold dose exists for both effects, after which the risk of damage increases steeply by up to 5% for each percentage dose increase. In curative radiotherapy, a risk of severe chronic side-effects of 1–5% has to be accepted if the patient is to have the optimal chance of uncomplicated cure.

The main risks after low doses as in diagnostic radiology (<0.1 Gy) are impairment of fetal development after in utero irradiation, increase in heritable mutations after germ cell exposure, and induction of cancer.

Radiation does not cause typical *congenital malformations* but may impair brain development, leading to microcephalus and severe mental retardation. The risk is highest between weeks 8 and 15 postconception, there is evidence for a threshold of about 0.1 Gy. After 1 Gy to the uterus during weeks 8–15, the risk of severe mental retardation is 40%.

Radiation is an inefficient mutagen. The risk of a person who received a radiation dose that is compatible with further fertility (a few Gy) producing a child that will suffer from a condition caused by a radiation-induced dominant mutation is 0.1 % or less.

Radiation may cause leukaemias and cancers in the exposed tissues. Latency is 5 and 20 years for leukaemia but may range from 10 to >40 years for cancers. The most sensitive organs for cancer induction are bone marrow, lung, stomach, colon, the breast of women under 30, and the thyroid of children under 10; the most resistant are cervix, rectum, larynx/pharynx, and lymphoid tissues. There may be no threshold; the risk may increase proportionately to accumulated dose. A total body dose of 1

Gy may lead to an additional cancer mortality risk of 5%. In diagnostic radiology, the highest exposure, eg, from abdominal or thoracic computed tomography (CT) (~0.01 Gy) may be associated with an additional cancer risk of up to 0.05%. The benefit a patient draws from medical radiation exposure has to be balanced against the estimated long term risk of radiation-induced cancer.

See also: Nuclear war; safety.

KRT

Radiotherapy High energy rays and particles damage tissues, particularly dividing cells such as cancer cells. Radiotherapy remains the most effective agent against some chemosensitive cancers, such as Hodgkin's disease, and in the early stages of a number of diseases radiotherapy can be curative. Though perceived as damaging and unpleasant, new techniques that direct radiotherapy more specifically to cancer cells minimise side-effects. The tolerance of local tissues determines the *cost–benefit* ratio of treatment and late complications, irrelevant when palliating patients with advanced cancer, are important considerations in curative treatments. Because of capital cost, expertise and technical support, radiotherapy departments are limited to regional centres, making access a problem for some patients.

See also: Autonomy; beneficence; cancer; doctor–patient relationship; empowerment; limits; palliative care; radiation safety; resources.

RTP

Randomisation is a process used in *clinical trials* to ensure that the allocation of participants to different treatment or *control groups* is random and not subject to selection *bias* by the patient or doctor derived from explicit or implicit preference for a particular

approach; it can also avoid inadvertent bias arising from differences between different centres and time of trial entry. Randomly generated numbers ensure balanced allocation. Randomisation explicitly introduces *chance* into treatment decisions in clinical trials, emphasising the need for *equipoise* in trial design and an agreed *uncertainty* about relative efficacy.

See also: Placebo.

AJP

Rape derived from the Latin, rapere, to seize, was described by Brownmiller as "nothing more or less than a conscious process of intimidation by which all men keep all women in a state of fear".[1] In England and Wales, the current legal definition of rape, based on the 1956 Sexual Offences Act, statutory modifications and case law recognises that both women and men can be sexually assaulted. A man commits rape if he has sexual intercourse with a person (whether vaginal or anal) who at the time of the intercourse does not consent to it, or is reckless as to whether that person consents to it (Criminal Justice and Public Order Act, 1994). Consent is legally defined in terms of age, mental capacity, and the jury's interpretation of the facts as presented to them.

Cases of rape are underreported, because of fear, *stigma*, or suspicion of the responsible authorities. Prevalence studies from the USA and Britain suggest that one in four women and one in ten men have been raped or sexually assaulted at some time in their lives. Outcomes following rape include physical trauma, *sexually transmitted diseases* and *HIV* infection, pregnancy, psychological sequelae (eg, post traumatic stress disorder, *depression*, sexual dysfunction and *suicide*), and frequent use of health care services in the years immediately following the assault.

Rape may be defined as "nonconsenting sexual relations with another person, obtained through physical force, threat or intimidation",[2] where neither the gender of the victim or assailant nor the type of sexual act are specified but where the potential outcomes remain the same. An increased awareness of rape by health care professionals, with the development of acceptable interventions to lessen physical and psychological morbidity, and mortality, is required.

References

1 Brownmiller S. *Against our will – men, women and rape*. London: Secker and Warburg, 1975.
2 Groth AN, Burgess AW. Rape: a sexual deviation. *Am J Orthopsychiatry* 1977; **47**: 400–6.

GF

Rationality (from Latin to think/calculate) (i) reasonableness, not being irrational; (ii) possessing reason, the quality (difficult to define or measure) alleged to distinguish humans from other animals.

KMB

Rationing Finding and justifying a reason for limiting the allocation of scarce *resources* to some but not all potential beneficiaries.

See also: Cost containment; effectiveness and efficiency; health economics; justice; National Health Service; needs; queuing; parsimony; priorities; purchasing; public policy.

KMB

Realism Since consideration of medical ethics is usually stimulated by a problem case but conducted away from the actual management of the case, or without personal contact with the individuals concerned, there is a danger that theoretical, procedural or abstract issues may dominate the debate, and thus make it academically fascinating but clinically and practically useless. Techniques such as group *role play* may help to keep everyone's feet on the ground.

See also: Practice.

RH

Reality principle According to Freud, natural impulses tend to seek satisfaction or release, consciously or unconsciously (the pleasure principle). But circumstances and society (the reality principle) normally teach us when to delay gratification.

KMB

Reason (from Latin to think) (i) a cause, motive, explanation or proof; (ii) the power to generalise, infer, deduce, compare and draw conclusions; (iii) intellect, as opposed to emotion or sensation; (iv) intuitive knowledge of universal and necessary truth, as opposed to sense-based understanding; (v) scientific knowledge as opposed to faith or superstition.

KMB

Reasonable person standard What does a *patient* need to know, about possible *risks* and benefits, to give valid *consent* to *treatment*? Traditionally, this was determined by a professional standard – by medical *consensus* about what should be told. More recently, especially in the USA, less in the UK, courts have begun to judge *informed consent* by a patient standard – what a "prudent patient", or "reasonable person" in the patient's circumstances, would want to know. But what is "reasonable" may be contested, and in practice the best advice (subject to the *therapeutic privilege*) may be that of Lord Bridge in the Sidaway case: "to answer both truthfully and as fully as the questioner requires".

See also: Risk–benefit analysis.

KMB

Reasoning Human thought working from what it knows towards a conclusion, is often contrasted with animals simply associating ideas or impressions. But while human reasoning at its most sophisticated and systematic (eg, in *logic* or science) is beyond the capacity of other species, much that passes for human reasoning is disconnected or illogical, and denying rudimentary reasoning to (at least) primates and some domestic animals (eg, because they lack speech or self-consciousness) requires considerable and contestable philosophical ingenuity.

Reference
Sorabji R. *Animal minds and human morals*. London: Duckworth, 1993.

See also: Emotion.

KMB

Reassurance Few people come as patients to the health care system without significant anxiety, and one of the tasks of professional care is to allay this as much as is possible or appropriate. This is unlikely to be possible without fulfilling at least some of the patient's expectations ("He didn't even examine me properly") and finding out what it is that the patient is really concerned about (as opposed to what the professional is concerned about) and addressing this in a positive and open way.

RH

Rebuttal (from French to hit/drive back) a counter-argument/proof given in reply to a defending assumption/argument. In law, "innocent until proved guilty", and an adult's *decision-making capacity* are rebuttable assumptions.

KMB

Receptionists are the receivers of clients in health care as in any other organisation, but have a particular *responsibility* because of the vulnerability of the client (ill, anxious), the need for consistency and safety (sorting out the seriously ill from the seriously concerned), the relative scarcity of health professional time, and the unpredictability of *emergencies*. The receptionist may be seen as the dragon at the gate, piggy in the middle, or a vital conduit of information and care between patient and professional. As members of a *team* who may not have formal health care skills but who often have considerable local knowledge they may be the vital "eyes and ears" of a *practice* team and may be able to represent patient views. The same ethical problems exist for them as for others in the team, though cast in different shape. For instance, *confidentiality* in family practice and team care is easier to understand than to honour, and the receptionist may be in possession of secrets about patients which those patients would not wish to share with the other health professionals.

See also: Ancillary staff.

RH

Reciprocity Giving and receiving, and acting for mutual benefit are basic to human interaction. "Do as you would be done by" is a version of the *Golden Rule* and much teaching to children about moral ideas comes through reminding them what they would expect from others. Many models of the professional–patient relationship suggest one or the other side as dominant, and the patient as receiver and professional as giver. But the bow needs the violin as much as the violin needs the bow, and an ethics based on caring or on relationships puts a high value on mutual concern and benefits, which often come to the fore in *long term care*.

Reference
Noddings N. *Caring: a feminine approach to ethics and moral education*. California: University of California Press, 1981.

See also: Care; doctor–patient relationship; empowerment; mutuality; power.

RH

Reductionist thinking attempts to reduce one kind of explanation to another, typically moving from more complex to simpler concepts or components – eg, reducing biological to chemical explanations, or discussing morality in terms of animal behaviour or of *behaviourism*. In medicine, reducing a patient's existential predicament to his biopsychosocial problems and thence to their physicochemical components is inappropriate, since each of these requires attention in its own terms. In medical ethics, decontextualised ethical theorising can also be inappropriately reductionist.

KMB

Reflection is an activity for which there is as yet little time set aside in health care and health care training, but which is a vital aspect of moral analysis and practical medical ethics.

RH

Refusal of treatment Where an adult patient is capable of understanding a *treatment* decision, it will be unlawful to give the care unless he consents. Thus, patients have the right to refuse treatment. They may do this irrationally, even though it may be a question of life and death. The courts have suggested that the degree of understanding required to be competent to refuse treatment may be higher than that needed to give a valid *consent*. The position is different for those under the age of 18. For them, withholding consent will not necessarily prevent treatment going ahead because those with parental *responsibility*, and the courts, may give valid consents.

Reference

Montgomery J. *Health care law.* Oxford: Oxford University Press, 1996: chs 10, 12.

See also: Child, status of.

JMo

Regulation is a means of ensuring that the behaviour of individuals and specific functions are conducted according to a set of explicit rules. Such regulation may be imposed by statute, by a professional or management body, or by a person charged with responsibility for the matter or persons concerned. Regulation provides a formal means of ensuring *accountability* and will define appropriate conduct and procedures. It can be a means of ensuring that ethical principles are observed, but risks losing a valuable discretionary element in individual circumstances that may not have been predicted when the regulations were established. On the other hand it may protect individuals from having to make decisions that go beyond their competence or authority.

The very process of regulation may require considerable resources, especially in monitoring adherence. A balance has to be struck in order to avoid burdensome procedures that distract from the issues concerned, while ensuring that conduct is appropriate. Utilisation of scarce resources in the application of regulatory procedures raises concerns about *priorities*. Over-regulation may also undermine *trust*, and can discourage individuals from taking *responsibility* for their actions. Within the *National Health Service* recently there has been a trend for increasing regulation in the areas of *risk management* and clinical risk management, training of doctors, and in the conduct of medical practice, through clinical and medical *audit*, the use of *guidelines* and contracts for *purchasing*, and the issuing of executive letters by the NHS Management Executive. *Self regulation* is a particular means whereby a professional body regulates its members within defined professional codes of conduct.

AJP

Reincarnation (or metempsychosis, palingenesis, or transmigration of

215

souls). Being reborn, according to the merits or demerits of one's past lives, in higher or lower human or animal form, is an important idea in Eastern religions, and appears in Pythagorean, Platonic, and even one early Christian philosophy (that of Origen), as a stage in the soul's journey to its ultimate destiny.

See also: Afterlife; religion and philosophy, Eastern; self.

KMB

Relationships, ethics based on Most ethical frameworks rely on key overriding concepts such as *duty* or specific *principles* or focus on individual *virtues*. In some branches of medicine, especially community based practice, what happens between people is seen as important as what happens within individuals. An examination of interactions and relationships is both morally important and practically helpful. The *placebo* effect bears witness to the fact that a positive attitude to the prescriber makes the prescription more powerful: a complaint is more likely to come from a person who is not only damaged, but also feels slighted.

Reference
Campbell A, Higgs R. *In that case. Medical ethics in everyday practice*. London: Darton Longman and Todd, 1982.

See also: Doctor–patient relationship.

RH

Relativism (i) the observation that many beliefs about what is true, right or good, are culturally, socially or psychologically relative; (ii) the belief that there are no universal criteria of, but only different perspectives on, such matters. While all such suggested universal criteria are philosophically contestable, (ii) does not necessarily follow from (i) and is itself only one perspective.

KMB

Religion and philosophy, Eastern The major religions of India, China and surrounding countries are Hindu and Buddhist. But China has been both Confucian and Marxist, some countries are mainly Islamic or Christian, and others have local religious traditions, from the Jain in India to Shinto in Japan. While Western religions have one God and Book, Eastern religions may have many gods or none, and different religious traditions may merge or be adhered to simultaneously. Truth is not the unequivocal and demonstrable possibility of Western religious and scientific orthodoxy. The basic ethical rules of most Eastern and Western religions often agree on practical questions (eg, abortion and euthanasia). But Hindu and Buddhist ideas of *karma* and release from the wheel of rebirth emphasise freedom from desire (the wheel of Western capitalism) through mental as well as moral discipline. Eastern and Western attitudes to individuals, *autonomy, truthtelling, death* and animals may differ. But while Eastern and Western religions arose independently, they have many concerns, concepts and practices in common. Western science, technology and political *philosophy* (Ghandi, Mao) have influenced the Eastern religions, while Eastern religious philosophy in the 19th century (Hegel, Schopenhauer) and more popular religion in the 20th century, have gained ground in the West. A Korean may have a Presbyterian work ethic, an American citizen may be a *Zen* or Tao-influenced environmentalist, while ethnic minorities and expatriates sing their Lords' songs in strange lands. Practical resolution of medico-moral questions at home and abroad may require sensitive exploration of unfamiliar religious beliefs and practices.

See also: Buddhism; Christianity; Hinduism; Islam; Marxism; Sikhism.

KMB

Religious statements Medicine is not practised in a vacuum and cannot be isolated from the *moral* values of the community, with which the medical practitioner should be acquainted. Moral values may be expressed not only in legislation but also in the official statements of religious bodies; and medical ethics, while having an *autonomy* of its own, is informed not only by moral philosophy, but also by moral theology.

Public debate on medico-moral questions is influenced by legislation, by the authoritative statements or guidelines of statutory, public and professional bodies, and in other ways, notably Church statements on moral issues. Such statements, issued by different Churches, vary in authority.

Thus, typically, the Church of England produces statements occasioned by or anticipating a particular moment in the development of policy, practice or law. These do not claim universal applicability, nor are they framed as exhaustive moral treatises on the subject under consideration. Anglican moral theology appeals to reason in the interpretation of scripture and tradition, and the need to take adequate account of the results of empirical investigation and of the ethical judgments and practice of those clinically involved. Although these statements are often in the form of reports commissioned by the archbishops or official Church bodies, their conclusions are not regarded as morally binding upon individual Anglicans. However, a statement may gain in authority if supported by resolutions of the General Synod.

Free Church statements appeal to the Bible, the tradition of the Church, contemporary experience and the relevant empirical evidence. If approved by the authoritative assembly of the Church concerned, they express its teaching at that particular time.

But conscientious dissent is respected. The Church of Scotland adopts a similar position, but as a national church takes account of, and speaks for, the views of more than its formal membership.

The Roman Catholic Church claims greater authority for its statements than do other Churches. Such statements argue their case by appealing strongly to scripture, to patristic teaching, to previous authoritative statements, to the Church's tradition and to human reason. They may be addressed to the whole Church, or to "all men of goodwill", and include *papal encyclicals* and statements issued by regional or national hierarchies. The critical reception given by many Roman Catholics to some moral statements in recent years has challenged the expectation that such statements will not be questioned or debated within the Church.

Statements of import for medical practice are also made by many other religious bodies, but it is often difficult to judge what authority they carry without learning more about the particular religion or sect, and about what belonging to it means to the adherent concerned. In most of the other world religions, as in *Christianity*, a variety of interpretations exist; but for some religious groups, such as *Jehovah's Witnesses*, statements are specific and authoritative.

In the major Christian Churches, despite their differences, there is ecumenical agreement that Christian moral reflection must be based upon scripture, the tradition of the Church, the moral experience of individual believers and the results of relevant empirical inquiry – all worked upon by reason – even though different Churches may give different emphasis to each of these resources.

A notable example of *consensus* was the then Archbishop of Canterbury's 1976 lecture to the Royal Society of

Medicine ("On Dying and Dying Well"). This highlighted agreement not only between the Church of England and Roman Catholic Church, but also between the doctrine of *extraordinary and ordinary means*, the English common law doctrine of *necessity* and the medical aphorism of "not striving officiously to keep alive". The fact that such agreement exists should be noted, because this (together with the fact that all Church statements do not have the same authority) is not always fully appreciated by the media.

In Britain, development of the study of medical ethics owes a great deal to the informed participation (especially in extracurricular symposia on the subject held in medical schools during the 1960s and 1970s) not only of many clinicians, but also of moral theologians, most notably G R Dunstan, one of the editors of the 1977 *Dictionary of Medical Ethics*.

Reference
Boyd KM, Callaghan SJB, Shotter EF. *Life before birth: consensus in medical ethics*. London: SPCK, 1986.

See also: Buddhism; Hinduism; Islam; Sikhism.

EFS

Repeat prescriptions are issued in *general practice* as a method of providing long-term medication in regular amounts which are small enough to be safe and prevent waste but large enough to allow the patient to live as normal a life as possible without constantly having to consult a doctor. The prescriptions are issued on an agreed basis without the patient being seen, unlike other forms of prescribing. Although this can be seen as a form of symbolic *contract* between doctor and patient, there is a danger that without a *routine* of periodic checking the prescription may become inappropriate, and possibly dangerous or wasteful.

RH

Reproduction The process of producing offspring. In mammals, including humans, all reproduction is sexual and involves the fusion of two distinct genetically haploid gametes (oocytes and spermatozoa) to generate a genetically unique diploid zygote. Asexual reproduction (parthenogenesis) cannot occur in mammals, because during gametogenesis and/or the earliest stages of fertilisation some genes are modified epigenetically and stably in a pattern that depends upon their parental origin (parental imprinting). These epigenetic modifications affect the subsequent expression profile of the genes, such that any zygote/embryo having only maternally derived copies of the genes (a parthenote) will die because of its abnormal gene dosage. Reproduction in eutherian mammals also involves internal fertilisation and development (viviparity), the development of a chorioallantoic placentation system, and the production and use of milk postnatally. In most mammalia, coition is restricted to the period of maximum female fertility. In higher primates, willingness of the female to copulate is not coupled tightly to fertility and reproduction. This biological uncoupling has been developed further in humans by social regulation. Thus, traditionally fertility and reproduction have been controlled through social, legal and religious codes and customs, with strong taboos and sanctions. Latterly, the regulation of fertility has been controlled increasingly through a wider range of contraceptive and abortive methods or by the use of fertility-enhancing techniques such as *in vitro fertilisation* and other assisted conception technologies. This enhanced ability of individuals to control the dissociation of their sexual and reproductive activities, together with the involvement of third party interventions in the reproductive and sexual acts, has challenged established ethical, social and legal traditions. It has made possible – or more public – atypical partnering and/or parenting patterns (more transient partnering; same sex partnering and *"parenting"; surrogacy*; gamete and embryo *donation*). In some of these cases, the genetic relationships between parents and their offspring may not be straightforward.

Reference
Johnson MH, Everitt BJ. *Essential reproduction* (4th ed). Oxford: Blackwell Science, 1995.

See also: Abortion; contraception; culture; fetus and embryo.

MHJ

Research is the systematic acquisition or pursuit of knowledge. It may be rather arbitrarily divided into pure or basic research and applied research (eg, *clinical research*). The fundamental tools of research are the *scientific method* and the principles of scientific enquiry, while the details vary according to the subject and the available methodology. The question to be addressed must first be carefully defined and a hypothesis formulated in the light of existing knowledge. (What is the idea? Is it interesting? Is it important?) It then needs to be determined whether there are methods available to test the hypothesis in a measurable way. (Is it doable?) If so, experiments are done to validate or falsify the hypothesis by rigorous test, controlling for irrelevant variables, and using statistical analysis where appropriate. (Test it.) The results obtained are then reviewed and discussed in the context of the existing body of knowledge; alternative hypotheses are considered and, where necessary, tested for in a discriminant manner. (Prove it. Is this the only possible explanation?) The results should then be presented for *peer review* and publication, where they may be further examined by others, reproduced or challenged, and serve as a springboard for further enquiry.

(Demonstrate to others what has been done and place it on record.)

It is important to appreciate that, while hypotheses are inevitably derived from the particular perspective of the investigator (and are thus subjective), the objective data have supremacy. There are many examples of beautiful ideas destroyed by ugly facts. Data must be gathered so that they provide a complete and valid test of the hypothesis. It behoves the researcher to be prepared to abandon cherished and plausible notions if they are denied by the evidence. Moreover, the data remain, even if the interpretation is superseded by subsequent findings. Scientific principles and methodology are universally applicable, irrespective of the conceptual framework from which they are derived. Thus, alternative or unconventional views on science can and must be tested according to the rules of evidence and established scientific principles and methodology, despite a commonly held lay view that science supports orthodoxy. Iconoclasm, or the challenging of assumptions, is an essential check to the dominance of fashionable or conventional views, but can only be of value if it applies accepted standards of proof and does not ignore existing knowledge.

Ethical obligations on the researcher include honesty in revealing the methodology so that it can be reproduced or checked by others, distilling without distortion all the results of experiments and reporting them in the context of existing knowledge. Publication of results is an obligation as part of *accountability*. There has been much interest in and concern about scientific *misconduct* recently, notably *plagiarism* and *fraud*. This may result from actual or perceived pressures on the scientist to succeed, as judged by receipt of research grants or by *authorship* of scientific papers.

Personal motivation may be driven by ambition or need to justify or obtain salaried position, as well as by the spirit of enquiry. Various institutional measures, supervision of inexperienced investigators and *peer review* can provide a partial check for scientific misconduct, but are scant protection against the determined fraudster. Ultimately, the test will be the reproducibility of the work by others, though not all work outside centrally important areas of study will be checked in this way.

Work involving *animal experiments* has particular controls to safeguard the interests of animals and to avoid unnecessary or gratuitous suffering and waste. Work involving human subjects such as clinical trials and research and *epidemiological research*, and the use of *volunteers* requires *disclosure* and *consent*; it is regulated by *codes*, such as the Helsinki code, and is overseen by *research ethics committees*. Research is distinct from *audit*, in which the application of knowledge is appraised. There may be interesting and even important areas of scientific enquiry that could only be addressed by methods that necessitate a denial of human or animal rights; such research is considered unethical, emphasising that the pursuit of knowledge has limits and does not override basic rights. Examples that are often quoted include research done during the Nazi period and involuntary research on prisoners.

There is a continuing public and political debate, focused on *resource* distribution, about what is an appropriate balance between goal-orientated applied research, seeking immediate specific gains, and curiosity-driven research. The latter may provide a platform of basic knowledge on which applied research can be based and an opportunity for serendipitous discoveries, many of which prove to be as important in achieving practical outcomes as in increasing understanding.

See also: Experimentation.

AJP

Research ethics committees (RECs) There is now consensus that clinical investigators should not be the sole judges of whether their proposals conform to generally accepted ethical standards, and that they should be subject to independent ethical review. The Royal College of Physicians (RCP) states that the objectives of RECs are "to maintain ethical standards of practice in research, to protect subjects of *research* from harm, to preserve the subjects' rights and to provide reassurance to the public that this is being done". It further states that "all medical research involving human subjects, including the use of fetal material, embryos, and tissue from the recently dead" should come before a REC (with the possible exception of some un-intrusive research), which should take care not to hinder good research.

REC members should "be people of goodwill, with a high regard for the human personality, for truthfulness and for continued advance of science in the interest of society". Membership should be "broad and not exclusively medical", with at least two lay members "persons of responsibility and standing who will not be overawed by medical members", one of whom must be "independent of the institution or health authority served by the committee". Members, normally unpaid, are expected to spend an increasing amount of time studying applications and attending meetings that may last for hours.

Important concerns of RECs include:

- The distinction between research and medical practice.
- Scientific quality of research. "Badly planned, poorly designed

research that causes inconvenience to subjects and may carry risk is unethical". The REC should satisfy itself that this issue has been competently assessed.

- Potential risks and potential benefits; and, where there is a risk, the ready availability of compensation for injury due to participation.
- Consent procedures for research subjects, especially those with difficulties of understanding, eg, children and the mentally ill, who should not be allowed to be therapeutic "orphans".
- Investigators who flout the committee should be reported to the appropriate authority, such as an employer or professional association having disciplinary powers.

In the UK the committee system is authoritative but not statutory. In the USA, the uninformative term Institutional Review Board (IRB) is used for RECs. In some countries there are RECs for studies involving animals.

References

Council for International Organizations of Medical Sciences in collaboration with the World Health Organization (CIOMS/WHO). *International ethical guidelines for biomedical research involving human subjects.* Geneva: CIOMS, 1993.

Department of Health (DOH). *Local research ethics committees* (1st ed). London: DOH, 1991.

Royal College of Physicians (RCP). *Guidelines on the practice of ethics committees in medical research involving human subjects* (3rd ed). London: RCP, 1996.

See also: Animal experiments; audit, clinical; clinical research and trials; codes; risk assessment.

DRL

Resources Any economic activity can be seen as a more or less efficient transformation of inputs into outputs. The outputs in the case of medical and nursing care include some combination of the relief of suffering, the cure or alleviation of illness, and the prevention of disease. The main inputs are shown below in diagrammatic form:

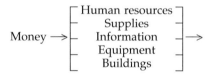

Starting at the bottom of the diagram, buildings provide the setting in which much health care takes place. Along with equipment these are sometimes classed as capital resources. Expenditure on them falls irregularly. Think, eg, of a hospital like the Chelsea and Westminster Hospital in Fulham, where some £150 million was spent on the building before a single individual was treated. Because such expenditure is "lumpy" and does not have to be repeated in that particular location for many years, its cost will often be amortised (or charged out) over a period. Similarly with equipment; though its life is usually shorter than that of buildings, especially as it may be superseded relatively quickly, so its cost will need to be written off over a much shorter period. (In the *National Health Service*, capital expenditure was until quite recently disregarded as soon as it had been incurred and was not charged to operations. No commercial organisation could ignore capital costs in this way and there is now an attempt to include them.) Obviously, neither buildings nor equipment remain immaculate and trouble-free, so they need to be maintained – a form of running as opposed to capital expenditure.

Supplies, such as drugs and dressings or food, differ from equipment in that they are consumables. Even if they are not used up, they sooner or later become valueless.

The most important resources of all in health care, typically accounting for some 75% of running costs, are people. While some may object that classifying people as an economic resource is dehumanising, doing so has the advantage of highlighting their overwhelming impact on performance. Care can be poor no matter how impressive the buildings and equipment. Capital resources exercise a constraint, but good care is what matters. Human resource management (as the personnel function now tends to be called, copying the Americans) is therefore crucial.

Increasingly, information is worth identifying as a resource. At the most basic level, the out-patient consulation depends on having the notes. As information systems become more sophisticated, eg, allowing instant access to large databases, they, like the other key resources, have to be managed.

Money is in one sense the most versatile of all resources for health care because it is generic, convertible into any of the "real" resources, like manpower, supplies, information, equipment, and buildings, provided that all these are actually available.

Not surprisingly, the *management* of resources has ethical dimensions: security of information, eg, or acting with integrity towards staff, while remembering who the whole activity of health care is here to serve.

See also: Cost containment; priorities; public health; public policy.

RJM

Respect (i) To treat another person with consideration (particularly concerning that person's *values* and goals) regardless of age, *gender*, ethnicity, and class would be a general ethical requirement. Lack of it has made the word prominent in the poetry, songs, and public statements of black people in the UK, but there are probably few who feel that they are always treated with the respect that they deserve, particularly when experiencing health

care. This sad lack of *reciprocity* would appear to be resolvable: respect is a renewable resource.

In its more positive sense respect is concerned with providing opportunities for people to demonstrate, activate, or regain their *autonomy*, even when they are, as a result of illness, not easily able to make their own decisions without help. Individuals and groups should be provided with the necessary moral space in which to grapple with difficult choices and achieve their full *potential*, whether as professional or lay people. In its negative sense respect enjoins people to refrain from harming or interfering with certain valuable entities (such as "respect for life"), although such pleas can never be *absolute* by their very nature when they arise in situations of moral *conflict*. These situations have arisen because of contradictory or competing *claims* which themselves have to be heeded and assessed, whichever argument is finally decisive.

(ii) Respect or reverence for persons, the sublime in nature, and the moral law is a key term in *Kantian ethics*.

See also: Golden Rule; self.

RH/ALl

Responsibility There are three key meanings in ethics. (i) A person is responsible when answerable for something or someone else and liable to be called to account, usually related to a particular *role* or position in which he finds himself. This may have been the result of a conscious decision or action, but need not be: for instance, everyone may without warning have a citizen's responsibility to act, say, after witnessing a crime. Equally, others such as health care professionals may be unable to shed this role and its responsibility even if off duty: but being off duty and unprepared would normally provide no defence against a complaint that the task had not been done to a professional standard. (ii) The more common use of deserving blame or credit for an action or situations. ("Are you responsible for running us out of antibiotics this weekend?") (iii) In general ethics, the state of being a free moral agent, and so morally accountable for what one does.

A defensive approach might lead a person or a system to try to shift the responsibility for action or blame elsewhere, but understanding is growing of the shared stake in, and so shared moral responsibility for, a good outcome in health care. Although this attitude of *mutuality* is not without *risk* and may increase the *vulnerability* of both parties in the *doctor–patient relationship*, it is clear there are at least two different sets of *expertise* to bring to that relationship, and so shared responsibility. Just as the law, with ethics, becomes ever sharper about the responsibilities of the professional, so in ethical circles the responsibilities of a patient (or parent) are increasingly of interest.

See also: Accountability; blame; order of preferences; professional responsibility.

RH

Resuscitation The process, over minutes or hours, of restoring or improving physiological function in a person who would otherwise die or suffer permanent disability. Resuscitation may be considered using an ABC system, problems with the Airway, Breathing or Circulation. If the airway is obstructed, no matter how well other body systems are working they will fail for lack of oxygen; if breathing is inadequate, the supply of oxygen to tissues may be so severe as to cause loss of function, which may be irreversible; even if the airway and breathing are satisfactory, there must be a sufficient amount of blood, circulating sufficiently rapidly, to carry it where it is needed.

The process of resuscitation involves rapid identification of the process that is failing and its appropriate treatment. In the case of a cardiac arrest, management is easily taught and undertaken. Sometimes the problem is more subtle, requiring diagnostic skills and a considerable pharmacological and technical armoury.

What are the philosophical concerns about resuscitation? There is a strong feeling towards the sanctity of life, and not attempting to prolong a life which could be prolonged, may be morally indistinguishable from taking life.

When might it be permissible not to attempt resuscitation? Respect for the *autonomy* of the subject means respecting a wish not to be resuscitated. Reasons for such a wish may include intractable pain, known progressive disease or simply a feeling that life is complete. If resuscitation is likely to be futile it is not morally obligatory. *Non-maleficence* demands that patients who are near death and have a very poor quality of life, or a progressive fatal disease, should be spared the indignity of resuscitation attempts. When resuscitation is required however, it is often impossible to ascertain the patient's wishes, or even know much about prognosis.

Justice demands that equals be treated equally so if one person is resuscitated, everyone in a similar state should be, the decision uninfluenced by irrelevant factors. However, distributive justice may demand that the *resources* devoted to resuscitation be deployed elsewhere, where they will be more useful.

See also: Intensive care; transplants.

PG

Reward Modern life is based around the arrangement of wages given for work done. Health care is considered to be "rewarding work" by the general public, that is, in some sense worthwhile and valuable in a way which goes beyond the wage paid. In the past it is possible that caring was considered to be reward enough in itself, enough that is, to allow nurses to receive low pay and informal carers none at all. The mystique surrounding medicine allowed doctors a better deal. With the reduction of long-term employment in health care and academic work, as in other walks of life, there are opportunities for reward from difference sources but also for creative confusion on the part of the unscrupulous. Medical ethics may need to examine this area in order to suggest guidelines.

Rewarding patients or *volunteers in clinical research and trials* can potentially coerce the vulnerable (ill, impoverished) and is generally frowned upon, although expenses incurred should be covered. Sometimes the distinction between expenses and reward is deliberately or unintentionally blurred.

RH/AJP

Rhetoric (from Greek to speak) the ancient art of speaking effectively, particularly in legal or political verbal combat, in order to persuade. Often contrasted with philosophy's search for truth through questioning and *dialectic* (the art of discussion or discourse) – although philosophy also can be rhetorical. Modern rhetoric includes study of the origin and development of language.

KMB

Rhythm method *See* Natural family planning.

Rights A view of social relationships developed in Roman law and mediaeval theology and asserted as human (and other) rights from the 18th century onwards. Moral rights, like (but more expansive and less enforceable than) legal rights, are either negative (eg, not to be tortured) or positive (eg, to health care). Both kinds of rights entail *duties*: but while duties correlative to negative rights are possible for all, duties correlative to positive rights may not be obviously assignable to specific people, or may require unavailable *resources*. Rights are often claimed when relationships go wrong, but also may be invoked to defend human dignity against injustice or inappropriate *paternalism*.

See also: Equity; human rights; justice.

KMB

Risk is an anticipated harm. The perception or fear of danger is what drives people to doctors to ensure their own *wellbeing*. Yet entering the *healthcare system* has specific moral as well as practical hazards. *Illness*, defined as a feeling a person can no longer control or explain, also puts at risk one's ability to make choices, and the physical circumstances (going to bed, having help with bodily functions, etc) enhances the infantilising of the patient and or the paternalism of the professional. However, every person probably has some view of the rank of possible harms (or "risk budget" in Charles Fried's words): the professional's views and the patient's are likely to be different as to what constitutes a significant risk, and these should be articulated and exchanged.

Reference
Fried C. *An anatomy of values*. Cambridge, Mass: Harvard University Press, 1970.

See also: Emergency; harm; primum non nocere; non-maleficence; risk assessment; risk management.

RH

Risk assessment is the formal, or unconscious, process by which people assess the pros and cons of a particular action or intervention. Formal risk assessment is used to determine policy decisions in *public health* and *public policy*. More commonly, an individual will decide to do or not do something based on his view of the level of *risk* attached. Often, this is strongly influenced by his perception of the *probability* of a hazardous outcome, the severity of that outcome, the ability to control risk and the importance of intervening. These perceptions are strongly influenced by prior experience, recent publicity and levels of awareness of implicit risk. Fear of flying, as opposed to driving a car, may be disproportionate to the probability of death. A person may seek a high level of protection against some harms (eg, AIDS, BSE) while being careless about crossing roads. Individuals or advocacy groups may seek policies or procedures on an implicit belief in a risk-free society, particularly in media debate. Attempts to reduce risk for one hazard to a minimum may inadvertently lead to a perversely increased risk (eg, measures to restrict excessively the practice of *infected doctors*, and that breach their confidentiality, leading to concealment).

See also: Sick doctors/healthcare workers.

AJP

Risk–benefit analysis weighs the relative *risks* and benefits of an intervention, assessing the *probability* and degree of each in forming a judgment. Informally, these assessments inform decision-making in health care (such as *clinical judgment*); more formally, risk–benefit analysis is used in regulatory decisions, such as in licensure of *drugs* and *risk management*. It is also used in *resource* management and assessment of cost-effectiveness. While seemingly objective, such analysis necessarily involves moral judgments about the acceptability of a type and

level of risk for a given benefit. These will be affected by context, eg, greater risk may be considered acceptable in attempting to treat an otherwise fatal condition, and lesser risk in trying to prevent disease in a healthy individual or population. The extent to which regulatory bodies can predetermine acceptable risks on behalf of individuals (eg, drugs) or society (eg, vaccines) is affected by the acceptance of a form of *paternalism*, in which *experts* make such judgments.

See also: Regulation; risk assessment; safety.

AJP

Risk management Policies and procedures designed to reduce *risk*, especially in the workplace. Some are derived from legislation or are means of minimising risk of subsequent litigation. They are formally the responsibility of senior managers, delegated as appropriate, and include training, record keeping, and documentation of policies and untoward events. Increasing *regulation* on this in the health service, as elsewhere, poses challenges in maintaining a balance between demonstrable *safety*, efficiency, and cost effectiveness. Clinical risk management is a newer concept, which identifies prodecures that may carry actual or legal hazards and minimises them through formal safeguards and protocols; a cousin of *defensive medicine*?

AJP

Risk register As a result of government guidance, social service departments within the UK are required to maintain a register of children considered to be suffering from, or at *risk* of, significant *harm*, and for whom there is a child protection plan.

Registration follows a *case conference* of all the relevant disciplines.

The guidance makes it clear that children may be registered before their birth.

Debate persists as to the efficacy of the system. Tensions surround the lack of protection afforded parents and the obstacles to child care and family support that an emphasis on child protection generates.

Reference
Department of Health. *Working together under the Children Act 1989*. London: HMSO, 1990.

See also: Child abuse; child, status of.

FEE

Role is a social position involving particular *rights* and *obligations* which should be performed and which in turn in some senses define the role. Any theory to be useful must acknowledge the fluid nature and the blurred boundaries of such a construct, made more problematic by the wider use of the word, closer to its theatrical origins, to indicate the sort of position taken and performance currently given by that person. A nurse or doctor has a clear social position, but then may find himself in turn in different roles (as researcher, teacher, friend, etc), which may cause *conflict* or confusion, particularly if not acknowledged or understood, but which may be further complicated by having of necessity to carry several roles, or change them within one interaction. Clarification of these, and their particular *responsibilities*, at the least prevents misunderstanding, but may also unpack an apparent moral dilemma.

A person may like to meet a professional who is genuine, but both might reflect on the *tradition* and ritual of the roles to which they are committed and which may be sources of comfort as well as conflict. The doctor may have experienced what it's like to be ill or to have to pick up his children from school; the patient is a free citizen who may go elsewhere for help, or decide not to be a "patient" after all. Unreal commitment to a role may be an example of Sartre's bad *faith*: distancing oneself from a role may help to prevent *stress*, but as a persisting strategem may reduce satisfaction.

See also: Persons; role play.

RH

Role modelling is one way in which professional training proceeds, with the person in training following the thoughts and actions of the teacher, like an apprentice. In the best hands it is a powerful educational method, but has the danger that *attitudes* and behaviour which should be subjected to (ethical) analysis or reflection may not receive the attention they require.

RH

Role play is a useful method in education, particularly in small groups, to explore problem cases. It may be done by two or more players taking the part of the main protagonists while the rest of the group watches, or it may take the form of a discussion with each person in the group being assigned a role. Its value in *ethical debate* lies in individuals confronting the realities of the person whose role they are playing and gaining insight into that person's *attitudes, value* set and way of thinking.

RH

Routines are important for orderly life ("*Habit* is the great flywheel of Society" said William James) and may be particularly so to ensure consistent and appropriate medical care in a way and to a standard which society expects. In medical ethics there may be some important routines (such as checking on the values or interests of the person being least attended to) but routines may also be a trap and may prevent appropriate flexibility, mature thinking and a proper "rounded" or three dimensional assessment of a particular problem.

RH

S

Sacrifice/self-sacrifice (Latin for to make sacred) (i) Sacrifice: term for euthanasia of research animals; (ii) Self-sacrifice: risking one's own life or interests for those of others, a supererogatory action whose moral evaluation may depend on its motive and consequences.

See also: Heroes; supererogation.

KMB

Safety It is one of the prime duties of a doctor to ensure the safety and thus the welfare of the patient, and those who do not would be considered to have failed in their *duty of care*. Particularly this is so where a professional may have other duties or different roles in relation to someone who is vulnerable or at *risk* (such as a child at risk of abuse). Psychologically, safety is allied to a feeling of *trust*, and important and sensitive disclosures are unlikely unless the person who wishes to unburden himself feels the environment is appropriate and his confidence or self-esteem is not likely to be abused.

Safety has many medical connotations denoting a need to protect patients and/or staff from *risk* of *harm*, including biosafety, *radiation safety*, *blood and blood products*, safety of drugs, infertility treatments, genetic manipulation, foods, environmental safety, and personal safety.

Biosafety *procedures* are used to protect from inadvertent or excessive exposure to radiation and to minimise spread of infection between patients and/or staff (*infection control*). Measures, including *screening*, are used for blood and blood products to avoid transmitting *hepatitis* viruses and *HIV*. *Drug* safety is assessed in preclinical *experimentation* and in *clinical trials*. Regulation of drug licensure to the *pharmaceutical industry* by

(inter-)national bodies requires toxicity testing in *animal experiments* and demonstration of safety in human trials before a licence is granted. Tests to minimise risk of *fetal* malformation were made more stringent after the thalidomide experience. Novel *infertility* treatments are regulated to avoid risk of fetal damage or other adverse outcomes for the infant. The safety of *genetic* manipulation has been of great concern and is thus also heavily regulated. Food safety and environmental hazards are a focus of public concern in the light of *epidemiological research* or potential hazards, such as BSE. Following increasing numbers of attacks on health care professionals, measures have been instituted to ensure the personal safety of staff. Similarly, hospitals, traditionally regarded as places of safety, need increasing security measures to protect against, eg, the abduction of babies.

In all these cases, given that complete safety can rarely be assured, it is necessary to determine an acceptable level of relative protection from risk; an acceptable level may depend on circumstances – eg, the risk of radiation induced disease set against the cure of *cancer* or of using hazardous drugs in treatment of life threatening disease. Similarly, security measures need to be balanced against the freedom of movement of patients and visitors in hospitals. Economic considerations may influence the extent to which infection control measures are practicable without jeopardising patient flows and the utilisation of limited *resources*.

RH/AJP

Sale of organs Shortages in the availability of donor organs for *transplantation* affect the affluent as well as the poor. Some agencies have addressed the shortfall of transplant kidneys by recruiting suitable living donors, offering payment in return for a transplantable organ. Typically, the donors are among the world's poorest citizens, compared to whom the intended recipients are among the wealthiest. Frequently the parties' respective countries of origin reflect the same disparity of wealth.

Commentators have generally condemned the practice, though for varying reasons. Politicians simply denounced the practice's supposed intuitive abhorrence, whereas other critics[1,2] deplored an unfettered manifestation of the *market*. With few exceptions,[3] most agree that the practice constitutes a categorically indefensible *exploitation* of the donors' *vulnerability*, for whom the cash rewards involved are effectively irresistible. Claims that the poor should not be denied an opportunity freely to *consent* to improve their material circumstances have been generally regarded as unconvincing, and as succumbing to the objection that "free choice" is effectively meaningless in such extreme poverty.

References

1 Brecher B. The kidney trade: or, the customer is always wrong. *J Med Ethics* 1990: **16**, **3**: 120–23.
2 Evans M. Kidneys for sale: the real evil. *Inst Med Ethics Bull.* 1989; Mar: 13–15.
3 Richards JR. From him that hath not. In: Kjellstrand CM, Dossetor JB, eds. *Ethical problems in dialysis and transplantation.* Dordrecht: Kluwer, 1992: 53–60.

ME

Sanctioning Although a sanction is usually used as a penalty or *reward* for a particular behaviour, in *general practice* sanctioning is sometimes used to describe the process where someone ratifies the *patient* as being really ill, or "gives permission" in a broad sense for a particular form of *(illness) behaviour*.

RH

Sanctity of Life This essentially religious concept has its basis in the notion that life is a gift from God. An additional factor within Christianity is the belief that humans are created in the image of God. In non-religious circles the term is used to indicate the utmost respect with which human life should be treated.

BHo

Scepticism (Greek for thoughtful, reflective) (i) attitude that sees the truth on both sides of a philosophical question and refuses to come down on either (in Greek philosophy, Pyrrhonism); (ii) doubt regarding religious or other claims made by authority.

KMB

Scientific method is the term applied to the means of scientific inquiry used in *research*. It is the systematic testing of an hypothesis by the acquisition of data that may support or refute that hypothesis. The two principal approaches to the methodology of science are *induction* and falsifiability, the latter formulated and developed by Karl Popper. In some ways these are descriptors of the process of scientific inquiry rather than its determinants. The two are complementary and are in many ways used in conjunction rather than in opposition. The inductive approach takes the existing body of knowledge and attempts to derive from it general empirical rules and principles. Popper's view is that a hypothesis is put forward and then an experiment is performed to attempt to falsify it. If it cannot be falsified it can provisionally be accepted as corroborated or proven, pending further or different tests. In practice, much basic and clinical research is predicated on this approach – eg, the "null" hypothesis used in statistical analysis. An important extension of this view is that a hypothesis that cannot be falsified is not acceptable since it can never be subjected to a test of its veracity, regardless of its plausibility, interest or value as an idea. This concept is at the heart of some of the debate between science and anti-science.

AJP

Scope A term used to distinguish those to whom or which a moral obligation is owed from those to whom or which it is not owed. Thus a stone cannot fall within the scope of an obligation not to kill because it cannot be killed. An embryo cannot fall within the scope of an obligation to respect *autonomy* because it is not autonomous. Determining the proper scope of application of *moral* obligations is of obvious moral importance.

RG

Screening "The presumptive identification of unrecognised disease or defect by the application of tests, examinations or other procedures which can be applied rapidly to sort out apparently well persons who probably have a disease from those who probably do not. A screening test is not intended to be diagnostic. Persons with positive or suspicious findings must be referred to their physicians for diagnosis and necessary treatment."[1]

There are two main screening strategies: mass screening – of large unselected populations in clinics organised specifically for the purpose, eg, cervical *cancer*; and opportunistic screening or case finding – where the patient has initiated the contact, eg, with a general practitioner, and the health professional takes the opportunity to search for other diseases or *risk* factors, eg, measuring blood pressure or asking if they smoke.

Screening is usually carried out on apparently healthy people from the general population. Thus it differs from traditional medicine in that it seeks to detect disease before symptoms appear and before an individual decides to seek medical advice. Screening therefore raises considerable ethical issues and responsibilities, and requires justification. A screening programme should meet the following criteria: is the condition an important health problem? Is there a safe, reliable test available? Is the test acceptable to the population? Is there effective treatment available that is acceptable to patients? Does earlier treatment improve the prognosis? Are facilities for diagnosis, treatment and follow-up available? Is there a recognisable pre-symptomatic or early symptomatic stage in the natural history of the condition at which screening tests can be applied, and is the natural history of the disease adequately understood? Is there an agreed policy on who should be treated? Can the target population be reached? Is the screening programme part of a continuing process? Is the overall cost reasonable, eg, cost effective?

Deciding whether a screening procedure or programme meets all these criteria can be problematic. Eg, a test may incur some *pain* or have side-effects but these may be seen as justifiable given the risk of the disease. Also, screening tests vary in their reliability. In choosing an appropriate test the costs of maximising sensitivity, ie, obtaining positive results in those who have the condition (minimising false negatives) must be weighed against specificity, ie, obtaining positive results only in those who have the condition (minimising false positives). Other dilemmas can arise over efficacy and appropriateness of treatment, and wider societal implications related to insurance, employment or health costs, eg, in screening for conditions where financial *resources* are not available for *treatment* or may result in resources being redirected from other health care.

229

References
1 Commission on Chronic Illness. *Chronic illness in the United States*. Vol 1, *Prevention of chronic illness*. Cambridge, Mass: Harvard University Press, 1957.
Holland WW, Stewart S. *Screening in health care*. London: Nuffield Provincial Hospitals Trust, 1990.

See also: AIDS; autonomy; carriers; genetic disorders; public health.

AA

Secrecy implies deliberate concealment and is both linked and contrasted with *confidentiality*, where a secret is openly shared with a professional.

See also: Privacy; professionalism.

RH

Self Personal identity remains a conundrum of great interest. Who is this "I" who speaks, and writes? Am I the same "I" as I was as a child and will this "I" survive? How can I be sure that other people really exist, or if this is accepted, how can I really know who they are, or what they feel or think? Can I really know these things about myself?

Common sense thinkers in health care may find this type of questioning not to their taste, but the moral issues of personal *identity* continue to raise problems in clinical care. Some concern the more abstruse areas of split *personality* (like Jekyll and Hyde) or split brains (as following commissurectomy in the treatment of intractable *epilepsy*), but many more commonly occur in an apparent alteration of personality following a stroke or major illness, or when elderly people are sometimes described as "becoming even more like themselves" as they get older. But everyday discourse now assumes that there are also different levels of *consciousness* within normal "healthy" thinking which suggest more than one sort of everyday self. For instance, we accept the idea of a repressed thought or feeling, of flashes of insight coming from somewhere we don't quite understand, of memories both created by stories retold and rediscovered through smells.

Even the consciously accessible self may change: sociological theory suggests that one's conception of oneself is constructed by social experience (seeing oneself reflected in others' reactions).

Personal identity assumes great importance in medical ethics when it appears to be changed through treatment (eg, by *Prozac*) and when it forms (through *values* and goals) the basis for important decisions, such as when a competent individual makes a choice which is socially unacceptable and not easily understandable by others (such as repeated attempts at suicide).

Competence and respecting *autonomy* as concepts imply both that we can make real contact with the person who is making the choice and that that person is able to make contact with his own "self", yet in clinical practice it is not uncommon to find choosers who have made judgments about themselves that are clearly even at a superficial level quite wide of the mark (such as somatisers). Phenomenological psychiatry joins other branches of physical medicine in not finding it easy to accept the idea of a psychological or motivational subconscious "cause" of serious illness, yet it is not difficult to construct psychosis as a "refuge" or even a "solution" for distress, or to make good sense of some symptoms as arising from a form of blocked communication between a person's body and his conscious mind. All of these aspects we might wish to include in the full "self".

One useful philosophical distinction has been made between the living body (as objectively studied), the lived body (as subjectively experienced) and the lived self (as an entity experiencing, reflecting on, choosing, etc). However, the history of recent

Western thought, plagued by the Cartesian division between mind and body, is wary of further unhelpful watertight compartments. While the difficulties inherent in thinking about thinking or reflecting on oneself led previous generations to construct a belief in God, modern secular society struggles with a concept of mind and consciousness that ultimately may remain elusive. Self reference may be too much for us: we may simply not be able to grasp fully who or what "we" are.

The practical conclusion for ordinary choosers remains that individual purposes and *perspectives*, in so far as they can be ascertained and assuming that they are attainable, remain the cornerstone of good decision-making in health care, but that we are probably still a very long way from realising this ideal of self-expression in everyday practice.

References

Glover JI. *The philosophy and psychology of personal identity*. Harmondsworth: Penguin, 1988.

Higgs R. Shaping our ends: the ethics of respect in a well led health service. *Br J Gen Pract*, 1997 (in press).

See also: Persons and personhood; respect; self creation.

RH

Self awareness concerns the extent to which a person is in touch with his own needs, and aims (particularly emotional). The outcome of some conditions is dependent upon self awareness: clear ethical decision-making is hard without it. It is difficult to help a person without insight, whether patient or professional, to make progress.

RH

Self consciousness as it is used in everyday speech describes a form of shyness but in medical ethics it indicates one of the key characteristics of a human *person*, that he is aware of his own existence as a separate entity and as something over which he has some control and for which he has *responsibility*. Babies appear to go through a process of developing it; the assumption that (higher) animals also have it may be problematical for medical ethics but seems an increasingly tenable position.

RH

Self creation is a concept which suggests that we are in some sense the products of our own aims and activities, under the influence of both conscious and unconscious drives and motivation. Its importance in medical ethics is to help all involved in a difficult decision to understand what the important aims and values of an individual might be, so that the decision made will be coherent with the "*self* which is being lived".

RH

Self defence Actions using such force as is reasonable in the circumstances, as the individual believes them to be, in defence of himself,[1] his rights[2] or his property.[3] Ethically, justification of use of force is by a subjective test, which in law is judged on the strength of the evidence.

References

1 *Beckford* v *R* 1987 3 All England Law Reports 425.

2 In English law, the draft penal code leaves open for common law to develop a defence of necessity, whereas in the USA, the general principle is codified in statute.

3 Criminal Damage Act 1971.

AH

Self determination Understood as choosing, deciding and acting for oneself, "self determination" is an alternative term to *autonomy*. *Moral* agents are self determining and in most if not all moral theories it is a *prima facie* moral obligation to respect the self determination of other moral agents in so far as such respect is compatible

with equal respect for the self determination of all potentially affected.

RG

Self harm *See* Self mutilation.

Self-induced illness is usually used
to describe a condition which is
brought on by conscious and deliberate action on behalf of the *patient*, as
distinct from hysteria, which would
clinically be considered to stem from
motivation beyond the patient's control and into which he has little or no
insight. Self-induced illness may vary
enormously. At one end of the spectrum there is deliberate self harm
(such as wrist-cutting) where the injury and the cause are not concealed,
and forms of illness (such as factitious
fever) where a patient at one level
knows what he is doing but is attempting to conceal it and so denies
he is doing what he is doing. At the
other end there are illnesses related
to lifestyle, such as *alcoholism*, or conditions related to overwork. Questions about *responsibility* and *autonomy*
of will are key, although people vary
as to where the first group sit on the
"mad/bad/sad" scale. However, the
concept begins to fall to pieces when
it comes to illnesses related to lifestyle,
as it becomes apparent in the biopsychosocial model of *disease* and illness that most conditions have
multiple causation and that we probably have more influence over our
state of health than we think we have.

See also: Münchausen syndrome; parasui-
cides; self mutilation; smoking.

RH

Self interest Concern with what is
important to oneself. Self interest may
be to the exclusion, or at the expense,
of others' interests (selfishness). But
rational ("cool") self love, equitable
concern for others' interests, and even
religious self denial can be claimed as

manifestations of self interest, depending on how the self and its
shorter or longer term interests are
regarded.

KMB

Self mutilation To mutilate is to de-
prive of a limb or essential part of the
body, to maim, or to damage. "Self"
refers to the individual. Thus self mutilation is the infliction of wounds or
the separation of bodily assets by the
individual. These wounds can range
from the cutting of limbs and faces to
the severing of limbs and the removal
of eyes and testes.

Self mutilation can be considered
to have two separate forms: damage
that is inflicted by the individual; and
damage that is carried out by a third
party with the cooperation of the individual. This note relates only to the
former.

When considering self-inflicted
damage it is essential to be aware of
factors such as the *culture* and social
organisation to which the individual
belongs. To view all self-inflicted
wounds as irrational behaviour or
part of the pathology of a *mental illness*
can be misleading. Self-harming behaviour may be a feature of the "rites
of passage" of social groups and apparent self-mutilating behaviour, eg,
self flagellation, may be carried out
during religious activities.

It is generally assumed that self
mutilation is a characteristic normally
associated with women. D'Orban
quotes research by Gunn (1991) that
32 per cent of women and 17 per
cent of men had self-harming histories
prior to admission to prison.[1] Two
studies, however, reported by Tantam
et al, indicated that more men self
mutilated than women.[2]

Tantam *et al* point out that "repeated self wounding is one of the
symptoms of borderline *personality*
disorder in the DSM-III-R (American
Psychiatric Association, 1987) or of

other 'flamboyant' personality disorders" (page 197). Self mutilation, however, is not confined to those with a personality disorder. Gunn states that self mutilation can also occur as part of the delusional process of those suffering from a severe psychotic illness.[3]

References
1 D'Orban PT. Female offenders. In: Gunn J, Taylor PJ, eds. Forensic psychiatry: clinical, legal and ethical issues. Oxford: Butterworth-Heinemann, 1993.
2 Tantam D, Whittaker J. Self wounding and personality disorder. In: Tyrer P, Stein G (eds) Personality disorder reviewed. London: Gaskell, 1993.
3 Grounds A, Gunn J, Mullen P, Taylor PJ. Secure institutions: their characteristics and problems. In: Gunn J, Taylor PJ, eds. Forensic psychiatry: clinical, legal and ethical issues. Oxford: Butterworth-Heinemann, 1993.

See also: Mutilation.

MB

Self regulation This term may be applied either to an individual or to a profession collectively. In both cases, the keynote is discipline and the ethical imperative is good conduct based upon the ideals of virtue and character applied to the demands of professional practice. The claim to be a "professional" requires personal *accountability* to an educated conscience and submission to the authority of a regulatory professional body, such as the *General Medical Council* in the UK, which includes a leavening of "lay" members, is in turn answerable to the people it exists to serve through statute law, and issues ethical advice to the profession.

Reference
Good medical practice. London: General Medical Council, 1994.

See also: Authority; character; colleagues/collegiality; conscience; discipline; law; professionalism; statutory bodies; virtues.

SM

Semen donation Sperm from anonymous donors has been used for many years in the treatment of *infertility* with a significant male factor. The selection and counselling of donors is quite rigorous and controlled by the *Human Fertilisation and Embryology Authority* (HFEA). Sperm donors have no rights or responsibilities in law with respect to children born using their semen. A maximum of ten children may be conceived using sperm from any individual donor. Concern has been expressed regarding the possibility of consanguinity in future relationships of children born using donated sperm. The HFEA keeps a register of the details of children born as a result of donated sperm. However, they are not allowed to release identifying information regarding the donor.

ALo

Sex change Sex reassignment surgery in a biological man or woman, with an absolute conviction of belonging to the other sex. Preparation is paramount and antagonistically rigorous, excluding all without ineradicable conviction; there is a trial of cross gender living and hormone treatments. Half will proceed to undergo surgical re-assignment. For men, this means removal of testes and penis and creation of an artificial vagina; for women, mastectomy, hysterectomy, oophorectomy and fashioning of a penis. Those with pre-existing psychiatric problems do less well. Suicide has been reported in up to two per cent of postoperative patients. Legally they remain as their biological sex and are often marginalised in an intolerant society.

Reference
Isaacs A. Sex and sexuality. London: Cassell, 1995.
Kaplan HI, Sadock BJ. Synopsis of psychiatry (5th ed). Baltimore: Williams and Wilkins.

VC

Sex, determination of In strict biological terms, sex involves any process whereby genetic material from two individuals is mixed to produce a genetically novel individual. In mammals, however, sex is reserved exclusively for the reproductive process in which two individuals of opposite sexes (female and male) produce from two different gonadal tissues (ovaries and testes) two different haploid gametes (ova and spermatozoa). These are then brought into proximity at coition, fertilisation ensues, and a diploid genetically unique zygote results. This process of reproduction is sexual, and the two individuals are described as being of different (opposite) sexes. The term sex is thus used to describe these individuals.

The basis of sex determination in mammals is genetic, the activity of a small piece of the Y chromosome (called SRY and situated towards the end of the short arm in humans) being responsible for the activation of a male developmental pathway. The primary step in this pathway, which involves many other genes on the autosomes and X chromosome, is the creation of a testis. The developing testis then produces two hormones (androgen and Mullerian Inhibitory Hormone: MIH) which in turn act upon the embryonic rudiments of the internal and external genitalia to promote the development of the male reproductive tract. Thus, genetic sex leads to gonadal sex and thus to phenotypic (including genital) sex. In the absence of the SRY activity, a female developmental programme appears to activate by default.

At birth, it is phenotypic sex (external genitalia) that is used to diagnose a baby as male or female. However, genitalia may be ambiguous or may be discordant with either or both chromosomal and gonadal sex. Thus, some XY individuals lack a functional SRY region and some XX individuals express a translocated SRY region. In other individuals, testis or ovary development may occur inappropriately or elements of both gonadal tissues may form in one individual: such a situation is described as primary (gonadal) hermaphroditism. In other individuals, the sex of the chromosomes and gonads is concordant, but the genitalia are either inappropriate or intermediate in structure: such a situation is described as secondary (somatic or genital) hermaphroditism. These hermaphroditic or *intersex* conditions can be problematic in a society which is highly gendered, and in European and derived cultures such individuals are usually considered as candidates for medical and/or psychiatric intervention. In other societies, intersex or hermaphroditic individuals may be accommodated socially within a third gender.

Both the brain and the behaviour of non-primates are also "sexually determined" as male by the testicular endocrine secretions. It is unlikely that this is also the case in humans, in whom there is a considerable emancipation of *gender* and sexuality from determinative genetic and endocrine processes. However, although cultural learning plays a major role in the development of gender and probably in the development of sexuality, some genetic and endocrine influence cannot be excluded.

References
Johnson MH, Everitt BJ. *Essential reproduction* (4th ed). Oxford: Blackwell Science, 1995.

MHJ

Sex education probably provokes more controversy than any other element of the school curriculum. What, how much, and when are interminably debated, with strongly held views, derived from culture, personal experience, and moral positions, being expressed in the media and the political arena. In the meantime, since many parents are uncomfortable in taking a lead role in raising and addressing the issues, schools attempt to prepare children for sexual experiences. This is usually conducted in a biological context, in which it may be felt that a level of objectivity and seriousness can be achieved. However, the moral tensions and the personal skills needed to cope with the emotional aspects and with sexual experiences in adolescence may not be adequately covered; homosexuality, masturbation, and other diverse sexual practices may receive scant or no attention. Any attempt to focus on such issues may arouse parental or social opprobium, and teachers may feel ill-equipped to deal with such topics. Adults tend to underestimate the need for sound information, preparation and guidance, and overestimate the age at which this should be given. The vacuum will be filled by information and attitudes of dubious quality from other children and other indirect sources. It may be hard to make a consistent linkage between sex and moral codes, especially in a multicultural society, while social images and *peer pressure* may provide conflicting messages. Sex education and *health education* are strongly intertwined regarding prevention of unwanted pregnancies and of *sexually transmitted diseases*. Indeed, the emergence of *AIDS* has reinforced the need for effective sex education, and has catalysed the development of substantially improved programmes, although these are patchily implemented and are hemmed in by statute. The topic of sex education raises important questions regarding the acceptability of the *paternalistic* approach usually adopted, which allows little *autonomy* for the developing child and adolescent and which, while well-intentioned, may not necessarily be *beneficent*.

See also: Homosexual.

AJP

Sex therapy A collective term for the eclectic techniques used to deal with sexual response, sexual desire and relationship problems, by an equally eclectic group of professionals. In Victorian times it involved barbaric practices designed to reduce sexual desire, which was perceived as dangerous. Modern day therapy may be conducted with individuals, couples and groups. The standard format, established by Masters and Johnson, involves male-female co-therapists treating a male-female couple. The use of sexual surrogates for clients without a regular or cooperative sex partner remains controversial. As the societal norms change in relation to sex, so the techniques designed to address perceived sexual problems reflect these changes.

Reference
Kilmann PR, Mills KH. *All about sex therapy.* New York: Plenum Press, 1983.
VC

Sexual practices Sexual acts independent of sexual orientation and as diverse as those involved in them. The main categories are vaginal, oral, anal, and masturbatory sex, but individuals or groups may practise other varieties; acceptance of sexual practices may vary according to societal, *gender*, or orientation norms. To quote Dr Alex Comfort in *Medical World News* (November 1974): "There is no norm in sex. Norm is the name of a guy who lives in Brooklyn."

With the advent of *HIV* and *AIDS*, detailed knowledge of sexual acts has become essential. It has enabled the production of a hierarchy of high to low risk sexual practices with respect to infection transmission.

Reference
Isaacs A. *Sex and sexuality.* London: Cassell, 1995.
VC

Sexually transmitted diseases (STD)
The range of conditions that are associated with sexual contact is broad

and ever increasing. Worldwide, sexually transmitted infections are one of the greatest causes of morbidity and, with the advent of the human immunodeficiency virus (*HIV*), of mortality. Although the traditional venereal diseases of syphilis, gonorrhoea, and chancroid have shown a decline in incidence in the developed world since the Second World War, there has been a marked increase in other conditions, especially chlamydia, herpes simplex, and human papilloma virus. Globally, the incidence of STDs continues to rise. The discovery of HIV, the causative agent of the acquired immune deficiency syndrome (*AIDS*), marked a new phase in sexually transmitted disease pathology, treatment, and prevention.

The tension between the needs of the individual patient and the public health needs of society is particularly marked in this field. Partners of patients with STDs may themselves be infected and infectious. Some conditions may be carried asymptomatically. If left untreated, long term consequences can be serious for the patient and the infection may be spread to others. Issues of *partner notification* and *contact tracing* can be highly sensitive. Legal issues such as under age sex, illegal sexual practice, *drug misuse*, and commercial sex work must be acknowledged and appropriately handled. Such matters may prevent patients from seeking treatment or advice. A legacy of social and moral perceptions about the nature of STDs has served to stigmatise both the conditions themselves and the individuals who have acquired them. Such attitudes may hinder efforts to prevent and cure.

STD clinics in the UK exist to provide a service that is confidential, non judgmental, and safe for patients who wish to seek advice and treatment. Staff work under specific legal controls outlined in the Venereal Diseases Act 1978 to ensure a completely confidential service. Increasingly such clinics are widening their remit to one of sexual health and provide services such as *contraception* and colposcopy together with treatment and *health education*.

See also: Carriers; confidentiality; prostitution; stigma.

JAn

Shadow is a concept useful in two ways in medical ethics.

(i) Jung used the word to describe the less acceptable or darker sides of the *self*, particularly concerned with personal motivation, some of which may not be accessible to conscious control. Do we ever therefore have completely good motives? Is something good done for a bad reason still something good?

(ii) In balancing moral principles, one principle may become predominant in a particular context, but the others nevertheless remain in consideration, and may need to be given different prominence as the situation changes. For instance, a person in a psychiatric crisis may be temporarily taken into hospital against his will to prevent major harm to himself or others: but respect for his *autonomy* continues to be just as important, although temporarily in "shadow". In follow up, specific adjustment may need to be made both in the professional–patient *relationship* and in the moral balance sheet.

RH

Sick doctors/healthcare workers Many doctors dread the thought of treating a *colleague* whose illness is such as to pose a real threat to the safety of that individual's patients.

Ethical challenges arise from the interaction of competing interests. Society's interests are not served by practising doctors whose judgment or skills are impaired to the extent that they threaten the *welfare* of others. From that perspective the public good and public safety are paramount – a presumption which underlies the "Fitness to practise" procedures of the *General Medical Council* (GMC).[1] Such procedures have the force of law.[2]

However, it cannot be in the interests of society to pursue the paramount aim of optimum public good and safety without regard to the interests of the sick doctor who may face loss of job and *stigma*, and who may also be having difficulty in facing up to the need to seek treatment because of the fear of disease itself.

Any system of regulation that fails to recognise the doctor's interests risks driving such individuals away from seeking help and a possible conspiracy of silence until some major event occurs. By that stage the situation may not be remediable and patients may have suffered. A balance has to be struck and that balance is reflected in the GMC's guidance to the profession.

There is in our view no doubt that a doctor who becomes aware that a colleague may be sick, has an overriding duty to report that concern to the relevant "authorities", which may include an employer and also the General Medical Council. Similarly an individual doctor who realises that he is impaired and possibly unfit to practise has a professional obligation to seek help. The establishment of schemes such as the "sick doctor scheme", and the GMC procedures, are recognition by society of a need to enable doctors to seek help, in confidence and in a manner that will not automatically result in loss of position or employment, all of which may have devastating consequences both for that individual and any dependents.

The National Counselling Service for Sick Doctors was set up in 1985. Staffed by volunteers from the medical profession, it is a confidential, independent counselling service

supported by the medical profession. It aims to provide advice and help at an early stage to doctors who appear to lack insight into the nature and potential seriousness of their illness. The counselling service is considered to be a humane and helpful scheme that benefits not only the doctors who are ill, but also the patients they may be treating.

The doctor who treats the sick colleague may experience an ethical dilemma, particularly if that colleague insists on continuing to practise. First, the consequences of inaction may risk, or result in, actual harm to patients. Second, preventing that individual from working may have a devastating impact on the prospects of recovery, if the hope of return to practice is removed. Third, matters of patient *confidentiality* can arise from the consultation.

These factors have been deliberately placed in the above order. While the normal ethical principles governing patient confidentiality apply they cannot justify inaction on the part of a doctor treating a sick doctor if patients are at risk. Similarly, the concern not to harm one's patient by removing hope has to be overridden by the principle of a duty to society as a whole. An additional difficulty for the treating doctor is that he may not always be in a position to make a judgment on the *risks*. In our view the treating physician should not attempt to carry the burden alone but should seek guidance from the National Counselling Service for Sick Doctors and the General Medical Council. However, the overriding presumption should always be in favour of the protection of the public.

A system of professional *self regulation* underpinned by a professional code of ethics can be effective only if the public are confident that the system protects their interests, and doctors are confident that the individuals

237

affected will be treated in a humane and responsible manner, with the aim of rehabilitation wherever that is possible. In permitting the profession to self-regulate, in the interests of the public, society accepts a moral and ethical obligation to enable the profession to operate systems that achieve that end.

References
1 The General Medical Council. *Professional conduct and discipline: fitness to practise.* 1993: 39–42.
2 The Medical Act 1983 and Health Committee (Procedures) Rules 1987 SI 1987 No 2174 (HMSO).

See also: AIDS; blood and blood transfusion; boundaries; burnout; difficult patients; infected doctors.

KC/RHa

Sikhism was founded by Guru Nanak (1469–1539) in the Punjab, India. In 1992 it had approximately 18 million followers worldwide.

The Sikhs (disciples) believe in one God and in reincarnation. Sikhism strongly opposes caste divisions, smoking tobacco, and taking non-medicinal drugs. The holy book is Guru Granth Sahib.

Devout Sikhs, called Khalsa (pure), wear as symbols of baptism, the five Ks: Kesh (long hair); Kangha (comb); Kirpan (sword); Kacha (short trousers), and Kara (steel bracelet). Sikh men take the last name "Singh" (Lion) and women "Kaur" (Princess). The men wear turbans to protect themselves from environmental hazards.

Non-Sikh doctors should be tactful when asking about *smoking* and should not run for cover if a Sikh patient – man or woman – is found wearing a sword.

Reference
Qureshi B. *Transcultural medicine.* London: Kluwer Academic Publishers, 1994.

See also: Transcultural medicine.

BQ

Silence A lack of spoken or written *communication* is considered by the thoughtful to be usually of some significance: we may be annoyed by a letter that goes unanswered but be aware that a question that evokes silence may be particularly pertinent, painful or complex, and so the questioner who breaks the silence will possibly destroy an evolving line of thought or impose his own answer. Equally in ethics a view unexpressed, whether by a patient, in group discussion by a quiet participant, or in general by a social group whose "voice" has yet to be found or heard (such as a *minority* group not attended to by the majority) may be particularly important for a full ethical response. In all these situations it could be considered a shared *responsibility* to enable the silent to speak, but in reality it often falls to the interlocutor with ethical insight to bring this to pass, and so should be a particular duty for work in medical ethics.

RH

Sin A religious concept, related to but distinct from *fault, pollution,* and crime; popularised and impoverished by its traditional identification with specific outwardly recognisable (especially sexual) sins. Sin chiefly consists in not resisting the tendency to turn away from *God, truth,* and *freedom,* to inertia, self-deception, and compulsive self-justification.

KMB

Situation ethics (USA, mid 20th century) a reaction against dogmatic or theoretical ethical systems, that claims that what is right or wrong in one situation may not be so in another, and that the moral features of each situation have to be judged on their respective merits, in the light of their possible consequences, and guided by love.

See also: Context.

KMB

Skills are part of the education triad of knowledge, skills and *attitudes*. Skills in detecting and analysing an ethical issue, in handling arguments and clarifying concepts join with *communication* and *management* skills as a vital part of good professional work. That such individual skills may be clearly taught and explicitly tested is not in doubt: whether the best ways have been found to integrate specific and acquired abilities into broad professional conduct is not so obvious. There are skills involved in being a *patient*, and education, experience and class may make a difference here too.

RH

Slippery slope This describes a form of argument where one action, in itself possibly permissible, might nevertheless lead to other similar actions being taken which would be undesirable, there being no clear way of preventing the slide from one to the other or, even if there are clear *boundaries*, it is likely, *human nature* being what it is, that people will cross them without noticing or caring. "One thing leads to another". It is also called a wedge argument, and is particularly employed by those resisting a *change*, because the existing prohibition or boundary is seen as clear. (The clinical example is voluntary *euthanasia*, where the fear is that it may lead to involuntary acts, or even wholesale destruction of unwanted people.) For those wishing to examine such arguments, it is worthwhile to see whether there really is a slippery slope, and how slippery in reality it is, and whether clear points of arrest in the slide exist. There will usually be found to be an equally slippery slope in the opposite direction (for instance, in the above situation, that rejecting a request

from a terminally ill person in pain to be allowed or helped to die may lead to people becoming hardened to suffering in others) and often the bottom of the slope is described in heightened or inappropriate language.

See also: Double effect; intention and motive; treatment.

RH

Smoking Inhaling tobacco fumes is now seen on good evidence as a habit likely to exacerbate or even initiate a number of medical conditions, such as ischaemic heart disease, arterial disease, chronic bronchitis, and lung *cancer*. Mothers who smoke *risk* having smaller (and possible more immediately vulnerable) babies. These medical risk factors have influenced some areas of public opinion to see smoking as antisocial, since it is smelly and it is hard for another person in the proximity of a smoker not also to inhale (passive smoking). Bans on smoking in public places such as theatres, hospitals, and on public transport are now commonplace. Tobacco is an addictive substance and smoking is a style of life at which it is easy to point a finger, so at the extreme smokers currently risk being stigmatised as doing (and so also in some senses as being) *evil*. A multitude of ethical problems have declared themselves. In clinical work, where the outcome is worse for smokers and treatment is borne by the public purse, these individuals may find themselves being given a lower priority for treatment or are being refused admission to a *treatment* programme. Smokers prohibited from smoking in hospital may refuse to attend for necessary treatment or care. In *public health* there are questions about who should carry the cost of treating smoking related diseases, how much should be diverted from treatment to preventive programmes, and to what extent promotion of smoking, especially to the young, should be tolerated. Is smoking reduction a form of treatment to be paid for by the NHS? Huge profits are to be made from tobacco sales. In the USA litigation against tobacco companies has been initiated and had limited success. Whether it is appropriate to use some of these funds from profits or litigation for healthcare research or other academic pursuits raises key questions. The threat to Third World people could be seen as only just beginning. Evidence from the West is that governments may tacitly or even openly encourage smoking when there are times of national crisis or stress such as war, and particularly in individuals serving in vulnerable positions. In the UK governments have recently consistently raised revenue by imposing heavy tax on tobacco and smokers could argue that they are paying (or even overpaying) their way in health care in this regard. But patterns of smoking are changing: it is no longer in any sense a predominantly male habit and younger generations in Western countries have not been put off smoking. There seems no logical reason for smokers to be seen in a particularly negative light where other lifestyles (eg, overworking, overeating, or underexercising) pose equally significant risks of some conditions, except that less work has been done on the effects that anxious, greedy, or fat people have on others. More thinking needs to be done on *limits* and *boundaries* of *responsibility* for health, who should pay for what in health care, and the distinction between treatment and *punishment* or revenge in lifestyle or dependency related conditions.

See also: Bias; blame; dependency; health education; peer pressure; stigma.

RH

Social aspects of medicine Medicine as a profession and as a set of activities cannot be understood independently of its social context. There have been two main sociological approaches: one that accepts the definitions used by medicine and the other that stands outside these definitions. The first is sometimes referred to as sociology in medicine and includes the social patterning of health and illness within populations, the social meanings attached to particular diseases, social reactions, and the differential use of health care by different social groups. At a micro level, this approach is concerned with *illness behaviour* and lay health beliefs. Ethical issues include inequalities in the burden of disease and access to health care associated with *poverty* and social deprivation.

The second approach is often referred to as the sociology of medicine and looks at medicine from the outside. Theories about the relationship of medicine to society include the functionalist, in which medicine contributes to the harmonious running of society by defining the social roles of *patient* and doctor. Various conflict based theories stress the oppressive role of medicine as an agent of social control, *Marxist* writers in particular arguing that medicine serves dominant capitalist interests. Others like Illich accuse medicine of iatrogenesis at the clinical, social, and cultural levels. A third set of theories claims that the epistemological basis of medicine is historically and culturally specific, and that the diagnoses and treatments of all medical systems are a product of dominant theories at the time. Sociologists working within this approach have examined medicine as a profession, what medicine does, how it organises itself, and how it relates to other professions and to society at large. They have analysed topics such as systems of health care, health policy, and hospital organisation. At a micro level, this approach has been concerned with the specific ways in which doctors dominate and control their patients, and with related issues such as consumerism and the empowering of clients. Ethical issues include the harmful effects of medicine.

See also: Behavioural sciences; consumerism; culture; doctor–patient relationship; empowerment; epidemiological research; health, illness and diseases, concepts of; human rights; iatrogenic disease; illness behaviour; politics; power; public health; public policy.

NBr

Social construct Social constructs are perspectives or theories that are shared within social groups. Different social groups may have different constructs, but good *communication* relies on shared understanding of constructs. To the extent that *patients* and doctors do not share the same social constructs, having been socialised differently, communication is often impaired.

See also: Emergency; concept of; illness.

NBr

Social contract A hypothetical agreement, among equal individuals or with rulers, to respect certain principles, rules, *rights*, *duties*, because this is for the common good, any alternative being less desirable. While individuals rarely if ever predate societies, the idea of a social contract can help to investigate what they (and modern society) might reasonably agree to; and it has been used for this purpose, with varying conclusions, by many philosophers (notably Hobbes and Rawls).

KMB

Socialism Political philosophy advocating social control of wealth for the common good – formerly, through state ownership and universal welfare provision funded from taxation, more

recently through government regulation, insurance, and state welfare provision where this is most efficient and/or necessary for social cohesion and morale (eg, a national health service).

KMB

Social work There is no totally satisfactory definition of social work. In essence it is an institutionalised form of the Judaeo-Christian ethic of caring for the stranger. Indeed, within the UK many of the roots of social work arrangements for child care, with families, and offenders originated within specific Christian organisations. The underpinning belief is the value of every individual. The other principal historical thread of social work is the system of Poor Laws dating back to the 16th century with their cyclically changing emphasis on control and care. Social work within the developed world has been largely based, in this century, on social administration, psychoanalytical influences, community work, and advocacy.

Society's perspectives of those in need, whether through poverty or as a result of vulnerability, have always swung between those of nuisance and compassion. Social workers are invariably motivated by the latter.

Areas of tension surround the manner in which social work is perceived. This reflects society's frustration at such matters as not being able to guarantee that people will not kill children, to control the feckless or to discriminate between the deserving and the undeserving. Fuelling these issues is the relatively open and undefensive manner in which social work is practised.

There are questions about the degree to which social work is a profession. Steps to rectify that situation are hampered from both within and outwith social work.

There are also problems about the content and length of training. A great deal of time is spent in practice placements while there is insufficient time to acquire the intellectual rigour to deal with the complex cultural, moral and psychological issues.

Social work is delivered through statutory, private and voluntary organisations. Private services are more common in North America than other parts of the developed world. This is changing.

Reference
British Association of Social Workers. *A code of ethics for social work*. Birmingham: BASW, 1986 (under review).

See also: Adoption and fostering; case conference; child abuse; child, status of; group work; multidisciplinary teams; risk register.

FEE

Society, views in medical ethics
Many ethical dilemmas regarding personal or *public health* are resolved by clinicians with their *patients*. It has been suggested that society should be more involved and that doctors should not have such a powerful role in decisions that properly belong to society. In practice, it is hard to determine what society's view is.

Some debates on headline issues such as abortion and euthanasia are regularly discussed in the media and by politicians; such debates may be provoked by particular cases or by lobbying from *pressure groups*. While these debates may lead to changes in *public policy*, it is moot as to whether such debates genuinely represent the views of society, since they are often conducted in a reactive and often polarised manner, remote from the clinical coalface and from the personal dilemmas. Views that are unpopular with the media or the perceived majority view, or that are too complex for presentation in the media, may be inadequately rehearsed. Policies may be forged to please a particular view or lobby and the public may not have the opportunity to consider and express its views.

In some situations the issue may be a matter of *law*, and the exercise of the judicial process may present a resolution of an ethical issue; yet this is heavily dependent upon the adequacy of statute to clarify complex ethical matters. Such cases may draw attention to the limitations of the law and lead to modifications of statute by parliament.

Many personal ethical issues may have to be resolved rapidly and privately to protect *confidentiality* in the clinical setting; there is little time or opportunity, nor formal process, by which to consult others. Thus, clinicians are often left to resolve these matters with patients and *colleagues* according to their conscience. While this may be seen as reinforcing the *power* that clinicians exert, there is no practical alternative; this places a heavy duty upon clinicians to exercise judgment not only on their own behalf but also as surrogates for society's views.

See also: Accountability; facts vs values; moral judgment; politics; religious statements.

AJP

Solipsism (from Latin for alone) in popular usage, the view (or acting as if) I alone exist; hence egocentricity or selfishness. In philosophy, the theory that it is impossible for someone to know how the world seems from the point of view of another person or member of another species.

KMB

Somatisation is a word used to describe the process whereby an emotion is expressed or experienced by a person as a physical symptom (soma, Greek for body), and therefore the symptom is falsely considered to originate in a physical illness. The somatiser may be considered to have little or no insight into this false attribution or *displacement*. He may not be reassured by negative findings, and may go from doctor to doctor to try to gain relief or to find a physical diagnosis or explanation. The result may be a "thick case file", and leads to much unhappiness in patients and professionals, but whereas some (such as Balint) have recommended trying to help a person perceive the origins of his symptoms, if he lacks insight the only satisfactory way may be to try to limit the medical interventions to those that are as simple or least harmful as possible.

See also: Balint Movement; mental illness.

RH

Sophistry (from Greek for wise, clever) originally applied by Plato to Socrates' opponents, philosophers who charged fees for teaching the arts of successful argument. Subsequently applied to any clever but fallacious argument used with the intention to deceive and persuade, eg, through ambiguity or obfuscation.

KMB

Specialism refers to the division of clinical practice into discrete specialties, where clinicians have particular training and expertise, against the background of general skills. Many clinical specialties are organ-based, such as cardiology and neurology, but others are system-based (immunology), technique-based (anaesthetics, cytology), disease-based (infectious diseases) or treatment-based (*transplants*). Patients may be referred to specialists by *general practitioners*, by general physicians or surgeons, or by other specialists, either for a consultation or for those specialists to take on responsibility for patient care. Increasingly, as *medicine* becomes more complex and as knowledge expands, specialism is necessary to ensure that patients with

disorders in multiple organs or systems obtain optimal advice and care. However, generalists are still needed in hospital to retain an overview for some patients. Yet the general physician and surgeon are less common, being replaced by specialists who do general work to a limited degree. It is moot whether general physicians/ surgeons themselves have such particular skills (breadth) to be considered a separate specialty.

See also: Hospital medicine; National Health Service; medicine.

AJP

Speciesism late 20th century term (analogous to racism and sexism) for views that give priority to the interests and wishes of human over other species on the assumption that humans are superior and that other species may be used for human and not their own ends.

See also: Animal experiments; ecology and medicine; persons and personhood; self consciousness.

KMB

Spina bifida *See* Neural tube defects.

Spiritual healing Two predominant forms exist in western Europe. One involves the "laying on of hands", or direct bodily contact, and the second, or "absent healing", is accompanied by prayer and meditation. In the UK, the Confederation of Healing Organisations monitors and supervises the practice of healing in medical settings. It issues strict guidelines and abides by a code of ethics (eg, not to promise cure) drawn up in conjunction with the British Medical Association. Over one hundred well documented studies, some strictly controlled, suggest that spiritual healing is more than a *placebo* response. Some studies, especially those undertaken with plants, animals, and cellular material,

243

suggest that an exchange of substance occurs between object and subject.

References

Aldridge, D. Spirituality, healing and medicine. *Br J Gen Pract*, 1991; **41**: 425–7.

Benor D. Survey of spiritual healing. *Complementary Med Res*, 1990; **4**: 9–33.

PP

Spirituality When people are unwell and need to be cared for they may have a range of physical, emotional, psychological and social needs. When these various needs have been recognised, and attended to, they may be aware of a further area of need relating to the spiritual dimension of a person and which may be described in various terms including soul, spirit, inner being, the real me or my beliefs.

Spiritual relates to the way in which a person makes sense of life experiences (the search for meaning[1]) and does not always mean the same thing as religious which has more to do with the outward expression of a person's spiritual experience or belief system.[2] If people are to feel cared for as persons then, for many, it can be important that this aspect of care is properly respected and responded to. The health service nationally and most *National Health Service trusts* have appointed chaplains to their hospitals to provide for, and co-ordinate, this aspect of care. This is in keeping with the Department of Health *Patient's Charter* Standard relating to the importance of "Privacy, dignity, religious and cultural" aspects of care.[3]

The key principles, ethically, would seem to be *autonomy* and *respect* for the individual and his belief system especially when different from one's own. Sensitivity and perception of spiritual need are important, together with a recognition that the individual may have a different personal value system arising out of his spiritual understanding. Thus what may be ethically/legally permissible in a particular society, *culture* or profession may not be acceptable to certain adherents of a particular religious, or non-religious, spiritual belief system.

Areas of controversy would include *abortion*, *donation* of organs, *consent* to *treatment* or non-treatment. In all of these circumstances a person's belief system may affect what he considers to be in his best interests from a spiritual perspective.

References

1 Frankl VE. *Man's search for meaning*. London: Hodder and Stoughton, 1987.

2 King M, Speck P, Thomas A. The Royal Free interview for religious and spiritual beliefs: development and standardisation. *Psychol Med* 1995; **25 pt 6**: 1125–34.

3 Department of Health. *The Patient's Charter.* London: HMSO, 1991; 51–1003.

See also: Buddhism; Christianity; Islam; persons and personhood; religion and philosophy, Eastern; religious statements.

PS

Splitting is a term variously used to refer to (i) headaches, (ii) marital separation, and (iii) more or less radical discontinuities in the *personality* of individuals who may have no psychiatrically diagnosable condition. Ordinary people asked to do extraordinary things may resolve this internally by such a process.

The phenomenon of "acting out of character", formerly attributed to "the devil having got into me", but nowadays often excused as "not being myself", or flatly denied, with the relevant behaviour being attributed to (or projected on to) others, raises psychological and philosophical questions about the nature of the *self*, and also moral questions about responsibility. "Know thyself" is one of the oldest maxims in ethics. But as Goethe remarked, "If I knew myself, I'd run away".

See also: Displacement.

KMB

Sport, drugs in Since the earliest days of sporting competition many substances have been taken by participants in the belief that they would enhance performances. As more powerful medicines became available after the Second World War, so more sportsmen experimented with more drugs. Sports authorities responded by banning drugs – because their use is unfair and a danger to health. The ban gave the false message to sportsmen that the banned drugs must be able to enhance performance. At the same time, the incentive to take drugs – the chance of making a lot of money – was rapidly increased.

Reliable scientific evidence of performance enhancement was until recently available only for one drug – oxprenolol, a beta-blocker – in one group of sportsmen – middle-grade pistol shooters (top-level marksmen's performance deteriorates). In 1996, however, a properly conducted clinical trial confirmed for the first time that supraphysiological doses of testosterone increase muscle size and strength. Yet education materials do not mention the lack of evidence of performance enhancement for the remaining 98% of banned drugs, concentrating instead on their possible lethal side-effects. Very few sportsmen are seen to drop dead from drug taking, however, so the misdirected educational message does not work.

Is it unethical to take drugs in sport? Yes, but only in the sense that the rules of sport are broken. Drug use does not necessarily deprive opponents unfairly of any reward. For amateurs, there are few rewards: taking part in a healthy and socially beneficial activity is surely more important than winning and a drug taker, if mentally normal, would derive little satisfaction. Professional sport is closer to the circus: the spectacle is all, since it brings in the (television) money. If properly informed sportsmen take drugs to improve their performance, so be it. Problems may arise if sportsmen take drugs for actual medical conditions that are also drugs considered to affect performance.

The ethical issues in drug use in sport arise from there being no clear information that any benefits from most banned drugs are just placebo effects: chalk pills taken by sportsmen who believed in their value would be just as effective. It is arguable that the rules are not applied even-handedly and – being designed, and applied, to maintain an artificial image of sports that brings great profit to their elites – are more unfair than sportsmen who break them.

RN

Status, moral How persons or things are seen to stand against one another morally has practical consequences. Eg, whether (and to what degree) a hospital patient is regarded as a moral *patient* or *moral agent*, or a *fetus* as a *person*, or an animal as the subject of a life will influence how they are treated in terms of their own and others' *rights* and *responsibilities*.

KMB

Statutory bodies regulate the training, registration, and disciplining of professional groups. The *General Medical Council* (GMC) is the archetype, established in 1858 to enable people requiring medical care to distinguish qualified doctors from imposters and "quacks". By operating a public register of appropriately qualified members, the GMC made the delimitation of a group of approved medical practitioners a matter of public record. Subsequently established bodies fulfil this function for other therapies.

Through standard-setting in education and ethical conduct and removing from registration practitioners who breach those standards, statutory bodies protect the public and safeguard the corporate reputation of their profession. Any therapy in which the diagnostic process is integral to the application of the therapy and whose practice involves invasive or potentially harmful techniques should be subject to statutory regulation. Some complementary therapies have not yet achieved such statutory recognition.

Although primarily seen as a means of public protection, the establishment of a statutory body and professional register benefit practitioners by defining a discrete area of knowledge, clarifying the status of those on the register and protecting their livelihood from the encroachment of unqualified practitioners. Statutory bodies confer respectability through legal recognition and provide *patients* with means of redress. Other disciplines can refer patients with confidence and without fear of incurring legal liability to statutorily regulated professionals. Attainment of statutory recognition is seen as vital to the wide acceptance of any therapy.

Doctors, dentists, opticians, pharmacists, nurses, midwives and health visitors, osteopaths, and chiropractors are statutorily regulated. Training standards in chiropody, dietetics, medical laboratory sciences, occupational therapy, orthoptics, physiotherapy, and radiography are set by professional boards, which also publish registers of qualified practitioners. The Council for Professions Supplementary to Medicine (CPSM) is the coordinating statutory body for these groups.

See also: Complementary medicine; medical education; nursing; professionalism; self-regulation; unqualified practitioners.

ASo

Sterilisation is the process of rendering a person unable to produce gametes (eggs or sperm) available for *reproduction*. Operations are usual in either sex, but chemical agents have been used, and sterility may follow therapeutic irradiation.

Despite population pressures, *coercion* or involuntary sterilisation are not usually considered ethically acceptable.

JAM

Sterility is the inability to conceive. This condition may be acquired by deliberate intention in individuals whose family is complete by dividing the vas deferens in the case of the man (vasectomy) or the fallopian tubes in the case of a female. Involuntary sterility may lead to the condition of *infertility*.

ALo

Stigma In Goffman's terms, stigma refers both to an attribute that is deeply discrediting and to the social reaction to this attribute.[1] This social reaction then spoils the individual's normal *identity*. Stigmatised attributes tend to evoke feelings of fear and repulsion in others, and to be associated with a range of other, negatively evaluated, attributes. Eg, people who are blind may be regarded as loners or have sadness and depression attributed to them. Clearly these latter attributes may be spurious. A stigmatising attribute may be discreditable, when it is not immediately visible and therefore only potentially stigmatising, or discredited, when it is visible or otherwise known about.

If stigmatised individuals accept the dominant social values they may feel a sense of shame and may respond in one of three ways: by attempting to pass as normal, by minimising the significance of the stigmatising attribute, or by withdrawing from social activities with "normal" people. However, not all stigmatised individuals accept the dominant judgement of their condition. In these cases, they may respond in one of two ways: with retreatism or with political activism. In the former, the individual has a negative self-image but does not aspire to normal activities. The latter response tends to be collective and aims to reject the dominant judgment by changing the way in which the stigmatised condition is perceived and labelled. Recent changes in terminology have resulted from this kind of political activism (eg, replacing the word "crippled" with "disabled").

The identification of a stigmatising illness often depends on a medical diagnosis, and it has been argued that the medical profession does not merely identify, but in some cases actually creates, stigmatised conditions. This argument has been advanced most often in relation to *mental illness*.

Reference

1 Goffman E. *Stigma: notes on the management of spoiled identity.* Englewood Cliffs, NJ: Prentice-Hall Inc, 1963.

See also: Advocacy/activism.

NBr

Stress The notion of stress as a negative, psychological force has given rise to numerous definitions which vary in their emphasis of the relative importance of external stressful events, (stressors) and individuals' cognitive appraisals and responses. An integrative model which relates the intensity of stress experienced to the negative discrepancy between external demands and the response capabilities of the individual, where a failure to meet the demands is perceived as important, has been found useful in relating stress to disease and illness.

Potential stressors range from cataclysmic events and major life traumas through to chronic strains and daily hassles. In *health care systems* identified stressors include the *roles, relationships, communication* systems, structure, and culture of the organisation. Other frequent stressors are breaking or receiving *bad news*, working with difficult patients or staff and managing loss and *grief*.

Perceived personal control is a major factor in determining response to stressors. When individuals perceive that they can take effective action against stressors they are less likely to experience stress than when they can not. This has implications for paternalistic models of health care which reduce the lack of control experienced by patients. Authoritarian organisations that leave carers with little personal control over their physical, psychological, or social environment are likely to add to stress particularly where roles, power or status in the organisation are ambiguous, illogical or unclear.

The stress reaction is characterised by fear, anxiety, and *anger* and is accompanied by physiological changes which may increase the risk of illnesses such as cancer and cardiovascular disease, and reduce survival times. Stress impairs cognitive activity, reducing daily efficiency by lowering concentration and attention levels or by altering motivation or mood.

Mediators such as high levels of social support, adoption of internal coping strategies, and high self-efficacy can moderate and buffer the impact of stressors. The use of *denial* or external coping aids such as alcohol or drugs is more likely to increase the stress experienced and is associated with increased *suicide, risk*, and *burn out*.

Maintaining a high *quality of life* with little stress requires a balance to be reached between the available resources and stressors which provide a stimulating environment, heighten arousal, and prevent boredom. Since many stressors in health care are intrinsic to the work (eg, sick patients) and constitute part of its attraction, it may be counterproductive to decrease these. Rather, there is a need to identify and remove avoidance stressors such as the intensity and chronicity of staff work patterns, and to increase available resources by developing individuals' internal coping skills and increasing patient *autonomy*.

Sources of stress are interactive, so even when stress related to health care is of primary concern, it must be viewed in the context of wider social stressors. The latter may contribute to the variations seen in the degree of stress experienced by those in comparable health care settings. Psychological *support* for individuals in distress may help where stress prevention has failed.

See also: Paternalism.

BHe

Strike, the right to It is generally considered in free societies that workers have the right to withdraw their labour as a last resort in resolving disputes with employers on wages or terms and conditions of service. Many health care workers have traditionally waived this right because of their vocational approach and in order to avoid causing harm to their patients. In the more combative industrial relations setting now found in some countries, some groups (eg, nurses in the UK) have now reserved their right, as they feel that their goodwill has been exploited.

See also: Nursing.

AJP

Students need to be aware of the ethical responsibility of being a doctor. Formal ethics teaching as part of the core medical curriculum is in its infancy and its importance is a matter of debate.

The primary aim of the undergraduate medical course is: "to gain an understanding of health and disease, and the prevention and management of the latter in the context of the whole individual in his or her place in the family and society."[1]

This requires a clear, objective appreciation of the ethical dimensions of every clinical encounter. Such awareness is not an innate ability, but a discipline that needs to be taught. Without the concepts and language of ethics, the most reflective student will find it difficult to make sense of the compromises that are constantly being made between different ethical principles (*autonomy, paternalism, beneficence, non-maleficence, justice*).

Traditionally, students have learned the "correct" attitude to patients by adopting the example set by the seniors. However, this perpetuates the system where doctors have little value for, or a poor formal understanding of, the ethical issues in their daily work. This deficiency has led to a call for a proper education in medical ethics. There is no consensus on who is qualified to teach, nor how this subject should be taught. Methods range from lectures on ethical topics (mental *competence, euthanasia, abortion, contraception*) by academic ethicists, to seminars where the ethical dimensions of real or proposed case histories are discussed, to workshops where students listen to patients, their relatives, and other members of staff and discuss their experiences of health and disease.

The potential for *conflict* arises as ethically aware students start to question the actions of their ethically naïve seniors. This might be resolved if both students and teachers listen and learn from each other.

See also: Clinical teaching; doctor–patient relationship; medical education; nurse education; role modelling; teaching of medical ethics; uncertainty.

References

1 General Medical Council. *Undergraduate medical education. The need for change.* London: GMC, 1991.

Claxton AP. Introduction to ethics – 1. Tools of the trade. *Student BMJ* **2**: 410–11.

Claxton AP. Introduction to ethics – 2. Personal autonomy. *Student BMJ* **2**: 455–6.

Claxton AP. Introduction to ethics – 3. Do no harm. *Student BMJ* **3**: 12–13.

AC

Subjective in popular usage, a partial, self-centred view. But, arguably, all knowledge is ultimately from a subject's point of view and objectivity relies on inter-subjective consensus.

KMB

Subjectivism the view that *moral judgments* are simply matters of opinion or taste. There are sophisticated (if debatable) philosophical defences of this. The claim "it's a very personal opinion", sometimes made in popular debate (eg, about abortion), is less defensible since it blocks further examination of the quality of the moral arguments.

KMB

Substituted judgment The attempt to determine what a patient who lacks *decision-making capacity* would have decided, had he possessed it. Best made by those who know the patient best who can also lay aside their own interests and judge impartially. It may be difficult to satisfy these criteria, or for others to know how well they are being satisfied in a particular case. Substituted judgment substitutes for the patient's, not clinical, judgment.

KMB

Suffering In relation to medical ethics, suffering presents itself most obviously as disease, which may be as much a mental construct as a physical symptom. As such, it is always experienced in particular cultural and social contexts, so that, while there is a general agreement that medical intervention should alleviate pain so far as possible (including the assistance of pain-alleviated *death*), suffering is pain occurring to individuals with their own beliefs and feelings about its nature and purpose. Thus suffering might be regarded as a trial (in the *Christian* case, often to be offered and borne on behalf of others), as a test (eg, in *Islam*), as a necessary working out of previous behaviours (eg, *karma* in Asian religions), as redemptive (eg, in *Judaism*), as transient and illusory (eg, in *Buddhism*). "Suffering" is not an abstract concept, but a personally evaluated experience; medical intervention, therefore, should be sensitive to the individual construction of experience, which may affect both diagnosis and treatment.

So far as alleviation is concerned, there is an equally widespread agreement that intense suffering is not an *emergency* that would justify meeting a patient's plea to put an end to it, ie, to be killed. Whereas, eg, in the case of a driver trapped in a burning car, his plea might be heeded by someone who knows that the situation is hopeless. The concept of emergency is truly exceptional.

Less easy to handle in medical circumstances are *priority* decisions in relation to suffering, eg, the allocation of finite *resources*: to what extent do the degrees and/or the numerical incidence of some kind of suffering determine where resources are to be allocated? Does arthritis have priority over heart transplants? Such questions require a prior agreement on what kind of ethical constraints are to be employed in the discussion. A major concern of medical ethics in relation to suffering is to ensure that these prior ethical debates and agreements are in fact engaged in and undertaken.

References

Bowker J. *Problems of suffering in religions of the world* (4th ed). Cambridge: Cambridge University Press, 1995.

Bowker J. *The meanings of death*. Cambridge: Cambridge University Press, 1993.

See also: Euthanasia.

JBo

Sufficient/necessary conditions A necessary condition for something is one without which it cannot be; a sufficient condition is one which, if present, ensures it will be. Eg, manual dexterity is a necessary but not sufficient condition to be a neurosurgeon – other necessary conditions are required which, together with manual dexterity, may be jointly sufficient.

KMB

Suicide is death by one's own hand. Suicidal acts have been documented throughout time and are still a source of intrigue and burden. Suicide, attempted or completed, is a complex phenomenon. No single theory can account for the behaviours. Look-back studies often identify a range of factors which form the bases of management and intervention protocols. It is unclear whether suicidal behaviours form a continuum from ideation, attempts through to acts, or whether these are discrete entities. Theories range from psychological to sociological, legal and ethical. Psychodynamic theory explains suicide as internalised anger, pain, panic or punishment. Durkheim's early work identified three kinds of suicide, namely altruistic which occurs in people who are very sensitive to social group norms, egoistic suicide which emerges when, on the other hand, the individual withdraws from the social group, and anomic suicide, which occurs as a result of sudden change such as job loss, bankruptcy.

Suicidal epidemiology is often limited, given that there is a reluctance to report suicide, record it or document it.

Suicide is often shrouded in myths that impede intervention and are not grounded in fact. These include assertions that people who talk about suicide do not attempt suicide. On the contrary, studies reveal almost three-quarters of those who attempt suicide mention it. Suiciders are not necessarily depressed and talking about suicide does not necessarily trigger the behaviour. Men outnumber women in a ratio of about 3:1 for suicide, yet this is inverted for suicide attempts. The latter half of this century has seen a dramatic increase in suicide among the young.

Factors which are associated with increased suicidality include physical illness (such as *cancer*, *AIDS*, and neurological disorders); previous history of suicidal behaviours (with the highest risk occurring in the first few months after the initial attempt); family history, and previous psychiatric history. All these are exacerbated by factors such as unemployment, low social support, and *depression*. The means of suicide vary from culture to culture and between the sexes. Men often choose more violent means and this may in part account for the higher rate of completion among males.

Management and policy in relation to suicide needs to be broad and sensitive to individual issues. The mental health burden of all elements of suicidal behaviour (from ideation, disturbing thoughts through acts, completions and bereavement) carry a specific load. Survivors are themselves at heightened risk of suicide and support after a suicide is vital.

There are often presumptions that suicide is a negative behaviour to be avoided at all costs. These are challenged in the comprehensive literature on end-of-life decision-making, covering, as it does, *advance directives*, personal control (*autonomy*), and *euthanasia*. Suicide is a complex and emotion-ridden phenomenon.

References
Bohme K, Wedler H, eds. *Suicidal behaviour: the state of the art*. Regensburg: Roderer Verlag, 1993.

Hawton K. Assessment of suicide risk. *Br J Psychiatry* 1987; **150**: 145–53.

See also: Mental illness; parasuicide.

LS

Supererogation (from Latin for beyond what requires to be paid) going above and beyond the call of duty; doing what others might admire you for doing but would not blame you for not doing. What counts as supererogatory depends on one's moral yardstick: eg, some unpaid overtime may be supererogatory from a *contractual* but not from a covenantal perspective.

See also: Covenant.

KMB

Supervision Professional training in health care should aim to produce a competent professional, able to act in isolation, and to monitor his own performance. While this gives impetus to strong *internalisation of standards*, it denies the reality that few of us, if any, are entirely able to reflect satisfactorily on our own work (even if we have the time set aside to do so), and that standards, if in question, need to be demonstrably checked. With the changing of traditional relationships between seniors and juniors in health care, there appears to be a need for a model of supervision separate from the *management* line, whereby individuals could reflect on their own work in a non-judgmental atmosphere with a peer. This may take different forms, and be part of mentoring, professional *group work* and *support* systems.

See also: Reflection; routines; traditions.

RH

Support, staff Staff support aims to maintain the physical and mental health of carers by increasing their capacity to cope with work *stress* and thus prevent *burnout*. Identification of potential stressors and the strategies required to cope with these allows support to be targeted directly at increasing personal coping skills. The provision, in individual or group settings, of educational programmes and communication-skills training can be beneficial. Staff support groups which offer peer support for those suffering crises or chronic difficulties can be a useful adjunct but cannot replace direct skills enhancement. In isolation no support can substitute for necessary changes being made to the demands and constraints of *health care systems* that promote high stress levels.

See also: Communication; group work; management; wellbeing.

BHe

Surgery uses judgment, manual skills, instruments and implants or *transplants* to repair injuries and remove dead, dangerous or disabling tissues. Newer procedures aim either to improve function by modifying or replacing anatomical structures or to change body-image by altering physical appearance.

Operations benefit individual rather than *public health*, cost more per intervention than most medical treatments and depend upon *teamwork* and facilities for *anaesthesia*, asepsis, *intensive care* and *blood transfusion*. Surgery is becoming safer, less invasive, more precise and specialised, but also more complex and costly. Increasingly surgery is perceived to be a low-priority, luxury component of health care in developing countries but a *"human right"* in industrialised countries.

Surgeons inflict deliberate wounds in order to improve the duration and quality of patients' lives: the principle "first, do no *harm*" is therefore of prime importance, particularly for immunocompromised patients.

The major ethical problems of surgery centre around relationships between risk to life or organ and potential benefit; financial costs and benefits to individuals and society; *informed consent*; fitness of the surgeon to practise; *audit* and *accountability*; *triage* of mass casualties; inequalities of access to, or imbalances between need for and supply of, surgical services (low-technology emergency surgery, high-technology cardiovascular or transplant surgery, super-specialties); training and recognition of surgeons for work in differing circumstances;[1] training for new techniques (minimally invasive surgery, microsurgery) and the role of surgery as a "shop-window" to validate and commend preventive primary health care in developing countries.

Personal qualities in a surgeon (aggression and ability to take calculated risks versus caution, confidence in *clinical judgment* versus humility) as well as training, experience and physical and mental stamina may influence his results.

In most industrial societies surgery is organ or system-based. In addition, developing countries need "specialists in common conditions" who can deal safely with the surgical problems disclosed by a local community diagnosis. Conventionally trained surgeons argue a case for training these "community surgeons" in locations where appropriate pathology and methods can be seen and where costs are controlled (health budgets of less than five US dollars per person per year are common).

Everywhere, however, choices are needed between *"good"* and *"best"* techniques, and between what is possible and what is wise. The principle "first, do no harm" requires choices (made deliberately, not by default) which minimise *risks* to individual *wellbeing*, and make ethical use of limited *resources* (eg, Perkin's traction for open fractures of the femoral shaft).

Reference

Watters DK, Bayley AC. Training surgeons to meet the surgical needs of Africa. *BMJ* 1987; **295**: 761–3.

See also: Primum non nocere.

ACB

Surrogacy in the context of fertility describes the use of a third party to assist a couple in conceiving and bearing a child when the commissioning woman is either lacking a uterus or is unable to use her own uterus for medical reasons. The surrogate may conceive using the commissioning male's sperm by intrauterine insemination in which case the resulting child will be genetically related to the surrogate mother. Alternatively, *in vitro fertilisation* (IVF) or "host surrogacy" involves the use of the egg and sperm from the commissioning female and male respectively. IVF occurs and the resulting embryo is implanted in the surrogate's uterus. In this situation the child bears no genetic relation to the surrogate mother. However, in law the commissioning couple will need formally to adopt the resulting child. Clearly there are a large number of ethical and moral dilemmas facing both the commissioning couple and the surrogate. A number of surrogates feel an overwhelming sense of attachment and connection with the child and there have been a number of cases in which the surrogate has felt unable to allow the commissioning couple to adopt the resulting child. Provided extensive and very careful and skilled counselling is undertaken by all parties involved and appropriate legal and practical arrangements are considered the technique can be most successful.

See also: Adoption and fostering; infertility; paternity.

ALo

Surrogate markers are indirect measures of the efficacy of a treatment that are used in clinical practice and especially in *clinical trials* to predict or anticipate a desired clinical outcome. Examples include the reduction of blood pressure to prevent stroke in hypertensives, or preventing arrhythmias in patients at risk of sudden cardiac death; changes in *laboratory tests* include reducing cholesterol to prevent arterial disease, and monitoring CD4 cell count in assessing the natural history or efficacy of antiviral therapy in *AIDS*. Their use requires that the marker has a proven relationship with the disease and that treatments that affect the marker will also affect clinical outcome; several examples have cast doubt on the wisdom of assuming this.

AJP

Surveillance is the systematic monitoring of the incidence or prevalence of disease, infection, or factors that contribute to disease. It is complementary to *epidemiological research* and uses some of the same tools. It may involve passive monitoring, analysis of data collected for statutory purposes (eg, *notifiable diseases, sexually transmitted diseases*), or actively seeking data from clinicians or clinical pathologists. Surveillance can enable more effective planning of preventive initiatives and provision of treatment *resources*, especially if trends are changing, eg, due to spread of infection or the impact of control measures. Data from individuals are generally aggregated or provided without personal identifiers and therefore avoid problems of *confidentiality*.

Anonomysed *screening* of markers in *blood* samples taken for another purpose has been used to follow trends in infectious disease but caused some controversy when used for HIV/*AIDS*. The system used ensures that the results cannot be traced back to an individual (since they have not

have given explicit *consent*). The concern was that individuals found to have HIV infection could not be informed. However, if this form of surveillance is combined with freely available named testing for those who wish it, knowledge about the level of infection in defined groups in defined areas derived from such studies can inform personal choices and is thus able to give a balance of advantage to *public health* and the individual.

See also: Münchausen syndrome by proxy.

AJP

Symbolism is the expression of the actual and something too that underlies the actual. It is common in all forms of human *communication*, and is in particular part of the power of the visual arts and poetry, but also of dreams, jokes, and everyday conversation. What is being expressed as well may be psychologically repressed and therefore not consciously accessible to the communicator, or may be part of an accepted (but equally often unquestioned) system of signs which has accreted historically but is understood personally. For instance, a doctor's white coat symbolises cleanliness and so freedom from infection, but would now also represent a particular clinical or objective approach or even (via the media's "the men in white coats") a controlling *paternalism*, and so those who wish to create an atmosphere of *intimacy* or relaxation in a consultation might signal this by not wearing one. These forms of communication are not only enriching but necessary for a full clinical and moral assessment. This is part of a recent *tradition* in studying *doctor–patient* interactions which should not be lost.

RH

Systems theory approaches the organisation of phenomena by looking at the connections or relationships between different parts of the system,

253

rather than just the properties of the parts themselves. It is thus a form of *holism*, but gains its importance in health care particularly because of the pervasive influence of *reductionist thinking* in *medicine*. Thus, a *person's* symptom might be seen as a reflection of that person's set-up (social or environmental), and professional responses might be understood likewise (eg, chaotic behaviour creating a chaotic reaction). Seeing the *family* as a "system" might enable a general practitioner to understand the unusual importance of a symptom or condition to members of that family group. For instance, a helpful question here might be: "what would your mother or father have thought about that?". In ethical work this might give insights into the *values* of an individual where a line of thought or action otherwise appeared problematical.

RH

T

Teaching of medical ethics Until 30 years ago ethics was taught in British medical schools on an ad hoc and occasional basis only. In the 1960s and 1970s extra-curricular medical groups, run principally by medical *students*, were set up in most medical schools. In 1980 the *General Medical Council* (GMC) stipulated that ethics should be taught to all medical students. The Pond Report, published by the Institute of Medical Ethics in 1987, made specific recommendations on how such teaching might be carried out.[1] The GMC's 1993 recommendations for undergraduate *medical education* place ethics as part of the core medical curriculum.[2]

In Britain ethics teaching is, generally, more firmly established in nursing than medical school curricula, and such teaching has been an integral part of most medical schools in North America for over ten years. There are currently about half a dozen Master of Arts courses in Britain in health care ethics (often combined with *law*).

Four goals of teaching are frequently identified: changing students' *attitudes*, principally towards taking ethical issues seriously; increasing awareness of the ethical components of clinical practice; improving ability to analyse ethical dilemmas; and enabling the professional to act in a way consonant with the results of such analysis.

There is much variation in the methods of teaching, and disagreement about the best approaches. Some of the key issues are: the extent to which theory should be taught before analysis of actual cases; the extent to which health care workers need explicit knowledge of ethical theories (such as *consequentialism* or *Kantian ethics*); the most appropriate methods of analysis (eg, a principles approach versus the approach of *casuistry*); and whether or not ethics should be taught in association with other subjects, such as law or *communication* skills.

References
1 Boyd KM. *Report of a working party on the teaching of medical ethics.* London: Institute of Medical Ethics, 1987.
2 General Medical Council. *Tomorrow's doctors.* London: General Medical Council, 1993.

See also: Ethical debates; medical education; nurse education; perspective; relationship; teamwork; virtue.

TH

Teamwork is increasingly required in the delivery of clinical care both within and between different sectors, eg, *primary care* and *hospital medicine*, health and social services and statutory and voluntary bodies. Medical teams, or firms, are groupings of clinicians in one or more *specialties* for patient care and training of junior doctors. Teamwork is most overtly embodied in formal *multidisciplinary teams*, but informally and implicitly is needed for optimal care of all patients. Effective teamwork requires a common information-base and shared values, as well as respect for professional roles. *Procedures* and *guidelines* can help to secure harmonious and effective work within teams. Patient *empowerment* is perhaps the ultimate expression of teamwork in response to health problems.

AJP

Technology in medicine comprises the tools that extend the doctor's skills. Diagnostic technologies include radiological imaging, endoscopy to visualise interior cavities of the body, and the electronic monitoring of physiological functions in various organs. Data from these technologies and from bedside observations can be processed by *computers* to produce statistical probabilities for diagnosis and prognosis, making the computer an additional medical technology. Therapeutic technologies include ventilators, kidney *dialysis* machines and artificial joints, various surgical devices, and *radiotherapy*.

Almost all technologies involve some *risk*. The balance between these burdens and the expected benefits is determined by technology assessment. Even effective technologies are of benefit to only a limited range of patients, and concerns about the human and financial burdens of technology usually apply to inappropriate use when benefits are small.

BJ

Teleology (Greek for logic of ends) metaphysical theories about ends, goals, purposes, and purposiveness. In ethics, teleological arguments are concerned with consequences and outcomes.

See also: Consequentialism; utilitarianism.

KMB

Terminal care The terminal phase of any chronic life-threatening condition is characterised by a profound and progressive weakness with no improvement or active curative intervention. The aim of terminal care then is to control or minimise distressing symptoms, maintain the patient's *dignity* and comfort until the end, and support him emotionally and spiritually. Practical emotional and pastoral support are also offered to the family before and after *bereavement*.

See also: Death; hospice movement; palliative care; spirituality; suffering.

VM

Terrorism Violent action designed to provoke public panic and force political change. Breaching medical *confidentiality* by disclosing information relevant to preventing terrorism may be morally justified in order to save the lives of potential victims, and not disclosing such information to the authorities can be a criminal offence.

KMB

Theology – theism/deism is the philosophical, mystical, or practical study of the content of religious and particularly theistic belief. (Theism is belief in a divine creatory who – but not according to the more rationalistic deism – is involved in human history.) It includes study of the scriptures (biblical theology), of doctrine (dogmatic theology), and of metaphysical arguments (philosophical theology). Moral or practical theology and Christian ethics include the study both of medical ethics and of the pastoral care of the sick and dying. Despite recent use of "theological" to mean "hair-splitting", theology's frequently *narrative* approach may make it more accessible to a wider audience than philosophy's often more conceptual approach.

See also: Religious statements.

KMB

Therapeutic privilege An exception (which a doctor must be prepared to justify) to the normal rule of providing as much relevant information as a patient requires or requests. Information likely to psychologically damage or needlessly distress a patient (particularly a mentally impaired patient) may be withheld or minimised. Applies when seeking *consent* to treatment, but not to research.

See also: Deception; lying.

KMB

Tolerance has a number of important meanings in medical practice. An individual may become used to *pain*, and neurological mechanisms may reduce his actual perception of it. Likewise, in using a drug, a person may feel less of the good effect as time goes by and may need to increase the dose to gain the same good effect, thereby risking an increase in unwanted side effects, or an overdose if starting again after a break on the dose level at which he stopped. All these share with the ethical concept the idea of putting up with something (or someone) which may be alien or in some senses unwanted as an acceptable burden for the sake of a greater good. Tolerance could be seen as one of the *virtues* of a mature individual or group, and is an absolute requirement in a multicultural society or in a situation where *minorities* hold differing views about right conduct. Intrinsic to *professionalism* is the ability to deal with, help and (to whatever degree possible) understand individuals whose views, actions or needs are different from the professional's own, while delivering a consistent service. Most individuals find that there are some people, or groups of people, they find it difficult to cope with. For professionals these have been labelled in the medical literature as *"heartsink patients"*, although the time is overdue for a parallel literature on "heartsink doctors".

One of the insights of the *Balint* movement was the suggestion that such intolerance indicates something important about the professional as well as about the patient: and further, that which it indicates about the professional may be more important. Everyone should examine their antipathies. The greater challenge for ethical thinking is to what extent one should tolerate people or approaches which are viewed not only as wrong but as themselves intolerant or encouraging intolerance, such as those expressing or advocating racial hatred. Even racists need doctors: but "if you're not part of the solution you're part of the problem".

See also: Culture; difficult patients; discrimination; ethnicity; gender; prejudice.

RH

Torture and medicine The World Medical Association's (WMA) *Declaration* of Tokyo defines torture as "The deliberate, systematic or wanton infliction of physical and mental suffering by one or more persons acting alone or on the orders of any authority, to force another person to yield information, to make a confession, or for any other reason".[1] A British Medical Association Working Party in 1986, for fear of compromising acceptable medical treatment, added the words "... which is an outrage on personal dignity".[2] In a recent report from Amnesty International torture was reported to have occurred in about 65 countries.[3] The extent to which doctors are involved is difficult to assess but the evidence of two authoritative publications suggests it is not insignificant.[3,4]

The spectrum of medical involvement in torture may include: examining detainees beforehand to ensure "fitness to be tortured"; monitoring them during torture to advise torturers when to continue or when to desist or treating them after torture knowing or suspecting they will be tortured again when they have been "patched up". The last of these raises a particularly difficult ethical issue if the doctor wishes to act in the best interest of the victim. Doctors have been known to devise techniques of torture, physical or mental, and even to take part in it themselves. Incorporated within the WMA's definition would be *complicity* in authorised physical punishment such as whipping, amputations or *capital punishment*. Complicity would also include failure to protest about or report known or suspected instances of torture; doctors are frequently reported to have ignored signs of torture when examining victims.

Why do doctors get involved in torture? Some are coerced by direct or indirect means, eg, threats to themselves or their families; some believe the end justifies the means, for instance, when "important" information may be extracted; others become involved for complex psychosocial, cultural or political reasons. Leaving aside *coercion*, which may be pardonable, the almost universal view is that doctors should never be involved. The Tokyo Declaration starts off: "The doctor shall not countenance, condone or participate in the practice or torture", but this may be the counsel of perfection. In some despotic countries a protesting or non-compliant doctor could easily become the victim of retribution. It takes *courage* to speak out. Those who do need the strongest possible support from official medical organisations, which should vigorously assert their opposition to the use of torture, encourage doctors to inform when they suspect it is taking place, support them when they protest, and protect them against possible recrimination, appealing if necessary

to international bodies such as the WMA to apply their authority.

References
1 World Medical Association. *Declaration of Tokyo*, 1975.
2 Working Party of the British Medical Association. *The torture report*, 1986.
3 Amnesty International French Medical Commission and Valérie Marange. *Doctors and torture. Collaboration or resistance*. London: Bellew Publishing, 1991.
4 British Medical Association Working Party on Torture. *Medicine betrayed. The participation of doctors in human rights abuses*. London: Zed Books in association with the BMA, 1992.
Downie RS, Hare RM. Symposium on the ethics of medical involvement in torture. *J Med Ethics* 1993; **19**: 135–41.
Various publications of Amnesty International, London.

See also: Punishment; quietism; war.

RHf

Trade off may be important in practical ethics as a way of reaching *compromise* where *conflict* or disagreement prevents a necessary decision being taken. Something may need to be given up or let go of in order to achieve something else which appears to be, in *context*, more important. Where decisions have to be taken because of time or resource constraints, perfectionism may be fatally inhibiting: but equally there is a *slippery slope* inherent in compromise which must be recognised, and *boundaries* set. Even moderation can be taken to excess.

RH

Tradition Custom and practice which are handed down from one generation form the framework within which the new generation develops its work. Rapid *changes* in the fabric or purposes of society may challenge tradition (whether through evolution or revolution), but for professional groups and patients in health care the assumptions and expectations created by the tradition of Western medicine define good practice and enable

257

choices to be made within an assumed *contract* or *covenant* without explicit or time-consuming re-negotiation. For instance, the tradition of *confidentiality* enables people to present difficult or painful secrets with *trust* that the secret will be kept. Research evidence suggests that lay people may have a higher regard or perhaps a better appreciation of the need for and value of these traditional features than the professions themselves, and may therefore need a greater say in preserving them.

RH

Traditional medicine is an umbrella term currently loosely used to cover various forms of medicine and health maintenance practised by indigenous healers in developing countries as well as by those in developed societies who follow in the footsteps of unqualified lay practitioners in pre-industrial rural communities. Present day herbalists, for example, are descended from those who used remedies based on the healing properties of natural products of the fields and woods. Other healers consider that most illnesses can be cured by drinking or immersion in mineral waters. Others believe that musculoskeletal misalignment is at the root of most types of physical or mental distress. Spiritual healers believe not only that bodily ills are influenced by states of mind, but that the soul or essence of the individual requires support. In some cases this still takes the form that was common in the middle ages of exorcising the devil. These have perhaps more in common with the traditional medicine practices of so-called witch doctors in many parts of the world where Western-type medicine has only made a partial penetration.

The practices of others, such as acupuncturists, originated in the early civilisations of Asia, rather than those of Western Europe. Other practices, such as reflexology and aromatherapy, have evolved from earlier systems of thought or practice, mainly of far eastern origin. Today these practices are often called *"complementary medicine"* but the distinction between them and "traditional" is not clear. What all the traditional and complementary medicines have in common is that their practitioners challenge to some degree the major underlying scientific theories of disease causation and appropriate *intervention* held by practitioners of scientific or Western-type medicine. Some believe their knowledge to be "complementary" to orthodox Western medicine; others are antagonistic or "alternative".

Popular consumer demand for traditional healing or alternative medicine appears to have increased rather than diminished in recent decades in industrialised countries, as well as maintaining its hold in developing countries, even though orthodox Western-type medicine is undoubtedly the dominant form of practice in most parts of the world today. A perpetuation or revival in demand is particularly apparent where the latter either appears ineffective (eg, in the treatment of chronic disabling conditions) or to ignore a role in *palliative care* (eg, in dealing with terminal illness or bereavement).

Traditional healers in Western societies, if they belong to a formal association of healers with similar views, usually subscribe to the same kind of ethical code of conduct as does the medical profession proper. Many, however, do not go through any form of recognised training or belong to a *professional* body. Consequently, their patients do not have the same degree of legal protection against exploitation or abuse as they would have in their relationship with a medical practitioner registered by the *General Medical Council* in the UK or equivalent body in other national jurisdictions.

Given that many people today wish to secure the services of both orthodox and traditional healers in their treatment, a variety of ethical dilemmas can arise. These include issues arising from the sharing of information given by patients in confidence, the responsibility for the patient's wellbeing in situations where recommended procedures may conflict, and payments made to one another in connection with referrals or recommendations.

Reference

Stacey M. *The sociology of health and healing.* London: Unwin Hyman, 1988: 152–76.

See also: Acupuncture; chiropractic; chronic disease; developing world; empowerment; exorcism; healing; palliative care; spiritual healing; treatment; unqualified practitioners.

MJ

Tragic choices are those that, whatever is chosen, result in great suffering or death for some persons or other living creatures. The term was originally used as the title of G Calabresi and P Bobbit's classic study (1978) of society's allocation of scarce health care and other resources.[1]

Reference

1 Calabresi G, Bobbit P. *Tragic choices.* New York: WW Norton, 1978.

KMB

Training, vocational Tension exists between education, as a broadening of knowledge and ways of thinking, and specific training for areas of professional work, where proven *skill* and an agreed consistent response may be high priorities. This tension is seen in undergraduate *medical education* and basic *nurse education*, and again in vocational training for *general practice* in the UK. The general public wants and deserves professionals who are not only competent but also good communicators, kind, responsive and reflective, and who can be demonstrated by their standard of

work to be so. The emphasis should probably be on phases in a life-long training programme, in which ethical thinking would play a part both as content of a course and in the external validation of such a programme. "Vocational" implies a calling: at the very least a professional should be prepared to reflect on the relationship of his life to his work.

RH

Tranquillisers The term tranquillisers is generally used to refer to a drug such as a benzodiazepine, like diazepam (Valium) or lorazepam (Ativan) used to treat anxiety in whatever context it arises. The term major tranquilliser is sometimes used for drugs otherwise known as antipsychotics, used in the treatment of major *mental illness* such as schizophrenia and mania. Both types of tranquilliser have unwanted effects. The benzodiazepine group can cause over-sedation, with impairment of psychological performance. Long-term use carries a risk of *dependence*. The major tranquillisers have a long list of side-effects, of which the most serious are disorders of muscle activity. Before commencing either type of medication the patient must be as fully informed as possible of the benefits and the risks attendant on what he is being prescribed.

See also: Informal consent; psychopharmacology.

ML

Transcendence (from Latin for to climb or pass over) refers to what is "above" the world or beyond human understanding (contrasted with, but not necessarily exclusive of, what is "immanent" or present in the world and to human reason); psychologically, "self-transcendence" means overcoming self-centred views or one's own *limitations*.

KMB

259

Transcendental meditation A mental technique whereby the internal repetition of a sound (mantra) takes the individual's attention from the outer surface of the mind, the level of turning thoughts, into the deep tranquil centre. This tranquil centre is said to be part of the transcendental structure of the universe. After spending time at this level of mind the meditator returns refreshed and re-energised. This technique has an application in the treatment and support of people undergoing stressful situations.

PF

Transcultural medicine is concerned with both the substance and the *communication* aspects of medical encounters between a doctor or health worker of one ethnic group and a patient of another. It embraces the physical, psychological and social aspects of care as well as the scientific aspects of *culture*, religion and *ethnicity* without getting involved in the politics of segregation or integration.

Transcultural medicine means dealing with patients from different cultures, religions and ethnic backgrounds. Therefore attention to the detail of transcultural issues is essential for the practice of modern medical ethics.

Broadly speaking, in every country there are: populations from three distinct cultures – western, eastern and westernised eastern; six major religions – *Hinduism, Buddhism, Sikhism, Judaism, Christianity* and *Islam*; four persuasions – liberalism, secularism, agnosticism and atheism, and four ethnicities – Caucasian (Europeans, Middle Easterners), Asiatic (Indians, Pakistanis, Bangladeshis, Sri-Lankans), Negroid (Africans, Caribbeans) and Mongoloid (Chinese).

During history-taking cultural differences in language, gestures and diet should be considered. Eg: (i) the German language has no word for "chest pain". The substitute words are "breast pain" or "heart pain"; (ii) eye contact is essential in western culture but it is considered rude in eastern culture; (iii) English food has low fibre but Indian diet has high fibre. The former may lead to constipation but the latter to the "hurry with curry" syndrome.

Health workers should be aware that a gelatine capsule may not be acceptable to devout Jews, Muslims, Hindus, Sikhs and vegetarians because gelatine is made from the bones and skins of animals, including pigs and cows. In Islamic countries and India, capsules made from rice paper are used.

Ethnic epidemiology is significant not only in the diagnosis and management of disease but also for the distribution of resources and medical training. Eg: (a) pernicious anaemia is the most common cause of vitamin B_{12} deficiency in the British white population but it is rare in Africa and Asia; (b) sickle cell disease is common among Africans and Caribbeans; (c) beta thalassaemia and G6PD deficiency occur particularly in Mediterranean people; (d) Tay–Sachs disease and Niemann–Pick disease are both common in infants of Ashlcanazi Jewish origin.

Reference
Qureshi B. *Transcultural medicine*. London: Kluwer Academic Publishers, 1994.

BQ

Transparency is a style of behaviour of individuals or groups, especially in *management*, where the way in which things are decided and done is quite overt and open to observation, and hence to challenge. It can also be applied to medical decision-making. It is a means of demonstrating and achieving *accountability* for one's actions and decisions, and can also assist in teaching and training.

AJP

Transplants Organ transplants are used to treat those suffering terminal disease of kidney, heart, lung, and liver. Diabetic patients may be cured of their dependence on insulin by a successful pancreatic graft.

Success has come through understanding the biological mechanisms of graft rejection, and the development of effective immunosuppressants: these drugs protect the transplant from rejection yet do not dangerously suppress antibacterial immunity in the host. Three-quarters of such grafts now survive for more than three years. Fit recipients are spared a lingering death, and their *quality of life* with a transplant is usually normal. State allowances are reduced, and the majority return to work and pay tax; transplants are expensive but cost-effective when compared with the cost of chronic life maintenance (eg, continuous hospital care, or haemodialysis).

In the West most organs are obtained from heart-beating, brain dead *cadavers* admitted to *intensive care* units with stroke, head injury or brain tumour.[1] Organs remain alive (despite *death* of the brain) if artificial ventilation and oxygenation of the blood is continued, and the circulation supported. If the clinical criteria for the diagnosis of *brain stem death* are satisfied, removal of organs from the corpse may proceed while the heart is beating. Near-universal adoption of brain stem death (as opposed to cessation of heart beat as an indicator of death) has allowed the removal of physiologically near-perfect organs. Hearts, lungs and livers have to function satisfactorily immediately after transplantation (though delayed renal function can be supported by *dialysis*); transplantation of these organs would not have developed without heart-beating donation being possible.

Cadaver organs are in short supply: in the West, waiting lists grow inexorably; in developing countries the lack of dialysis and transplant facilities causes a high mortality from renal failure. European initiatives to improve the supply include changing the *law* on organ removal to a "contracting out" form (Belgium, Austria), and professionalising the transplant coordinator-run intensive-care support programme (Spain).[2]

In India, a market in kidneys developed in the mid-1980s. Relatively poor donors sold kidneys to fee-paying recipients; surgeons and their "donor agents" made large profits.[3] The ethical debate on the permissibility of organ sales ranged from the *absolutist* (medical) view that commodification of the human body is always ethically wrong, to the contextualist, libertarian approach which sees selling an organ as an autonomous right and a useful act, benefiting the impoverished donor and his family. The absolutist view was favoured by most governments who legislated against organ sales before 1990. The Indian government followed suit in 1994 when the Upper House legislated against all forms of paying for organs, at the same time legalising cadaveric organ donation.

In the People's Republic of China, the State allows and encourages the use of executed criminals as organ donors.[4] Evidently the practice has increased since the end of the Cultural Revolution. Although there has been a recent outcry against the practice, it is not clear how the medical profession in China may be persuaded to re-establish an ethical code of practice, free of government interference, and which acknowledges *human rights* as a foundation of medical ethics.

Many ethical problems, caused by the shortage of organs, will be solved when a method is found to transplant animal organs (*xenografts*) safely and successfully to man.

References
1 Conference of Medical Royal Colleges and their Faculties in the United Kingdom, 1976.

261

Diagnosis of brain death. *BMJ* 1976; **2**: 1187–8.

2 New W, Solomon M, Dingwall R, McHale J, eds. *A question of give and take: improving the supply of donor organs for transplantation*. London: King's Fund Institute, Research Report 18, 1994.

3 Daar A, Sells R A. Living non-related donor renal transplantation – a reappraisal. *Transplantation Rev* 1990; **4**: 128–40.

4 Organ procurement and judicial execution in China. *Human rights watch Asia*, 1994, Aug.

See also: Sale of organs.

RAS

Transvestism A distinct entity, not to be confused with drag or transsexual cross dressing. The wearing of opposite sex garments, often associated with sexual arousal, most commonly described in heterosexual men. Beginning in childhood or adolescence, adult cross dressing is pursued in privacy, but may involve a partner or social gatherings.

Reference

Kolodny RC, Masters WH, Johnson VE, *Textbook of sexual medicine*. Boston: Little, Brown, 1979.

VC

Treatment is an intervention offered by clinicians in the control or cure of disease or its consequences. Usually a *patient* presents with symptoms, the clinician makes a diagnosis and sets out treatment options. Patients are increasingly *empowered* to decide whether to accept treatment or to choose an option. At any stage they can elect to stop or change treatment or to seek other advice. The clinician's duty is to ensure that the patient understands the nature of his disease and its prognosis, and the impact and risks of intervention (*disclosure*). These will affect treatment *compliance*. Ethical tensions may arise if the treatment that he wishes is contrary to the clinician's advice, if the patient has a psychiatric disorder impairing his *decision-making capacity*, if the treatment is unavailable or exceeds available *resources*, or if the patient (or a *child's* parent) refuses life-saving treatment (eg, *Jehovah's Witnesses* and *blood transfusion*). Treatment given to people who are currently well to prevent future disease also raises different issues than the treatment of disease that has already expressed itself, such as in the treatment of symptomless hypertension or the use of *prophylaxis*; *immunisations* raise similar issues but with the additional *public health* rationale.

Most treatment decisions that create ethical dilemmas are where the patient is incompetent or unable to convey their wishes. Clinicians may need to decide whether it is appropriate to start or to stop a treatment if they consider it futile or too hazardous. While they may be able to use the patient's previously stated intentions, especially if formulated in an *advance directive*, or to consult *next of kin* or significant others, they may ultimately have to make a decision on the patient's behalf. It has been argued that there is a difference between witholding treatment (eg, not starting antibiotics for pneumonia, or not ventilating a patient in respiratory failure) and withdrawing treatment (eg, discontinuing life-sustaining therapy, turning off a ventilator, witholding food or *hydration*); a particular case is the issue of do not resuscitate or *DNR orders*. However, others consider the difference between acts of commission or of omission to be arbitrary, each constituting an active denial of treatment. The question relates to what is obligatory and what is optional, and what are *extraordinary means* in terms of *risk–benefit analysis*. The issue abuts with *euthanasia*, the foregoing being considered "passive euthanasia" by some. The active causing of a patient's death is distinguished technically from treatment decisions that inevitably lead to or hasten his death (such as giving opiates in pain control in doses that risk respiratory arrest); the distinction is one of intent, though this may not be articulated explicity. While there are clear *guidelines* for patients with *brain stem death* and *persistent vegetative state*, there are many more instances where the clinician must be guided by their *clinical judgment* and assessment of *quality of life*. These are areas where the conscientious clinician acting to relieve suffering may be at risk of breaching the law or contravening religious dictates, and may be considered to be "playing God".

See also: Active/passive distinction; appropriate technology; burdensomeness; competence; double effect; fertility; futility; intention and motive; proxy.

AJP

Triage has become a widely used term to describe processes involved in assessing priority in relation to the need for health care and the availability of scarce health care *resources*. Triage was originally used within military and disaster contexts to direct health care according to whether the individual was likely to survive with minimal or extensive medical intervention. Today, triage is also practised in many "open access" settings, often by nurses, to assess when and where patients should receive care. This includes accident and emergency departments, telephone advice/triage services and emergency ambulance services. There are many different systems in operation, each with their own protocols and training methods; few have been formally evaluated. Triage decision-making should be judged in terms of *equity, justice* and *accountability*, as well as clinical effectiveness and patient satisfaction.

References

Jones C, Hall G. The moral problems involved in the concept of patient triage in the A&E department. In: Sbaih L, ed. *Issues in accident and emergency nursing*. London: Chapman and Hall, 1994: 150–64.

Winslow GR. *Triage and justice*. Berkeley: University of California Press, 1982.

See also: Catastrophe; emergency; war.

JRD

Trials *See* Clinical research and trials.

Trust is basic to health care by the very nature of the relationships required between professional and *patient*, between professionals themselves, and between the service and the general public. Legally this is often typified as a *"fiduciary" relationship*, and underpins the professional "secret" of *confidentiality* and enables *consent*. The analogies are with close personal *relationships*, and are in some contrast to the relationships set up in commerce. This makes concepts like *"contract"*, *"market* forces" and *"consumerism"* difficult to integrate into health care.

Traditionally, the professional is trusted to put the patient's *interest* first (which may mean in some cases above the professional's own interest) and holds some things (such as confidential information) "in trust". *Conflicts* in this area are key issues in medical ethics, and more interest is now being paid to this by philosophers. Trust probably always involves an element of *risk*, and judgments about appropriateness: in this sense, as in others, professionals in health care need to be trustworthy. The use of the word recently in Britain to describe independent health care provider units may not have been intentionally ironic, but inappropriate *management* styles and budget restrictions have reduced trust between some professional groups and between units and the general public to a new low level.

See also: Professionalism.

RH

Trusts The UK *National Health Service* has introduced NHS Trusts as the organisational units for statutory providers of health care. They are allowed a degree of independence, as opposed to the earlier centrally run system, eg, in determining strategic direction, and local pay, terms, and conditions. In practice, their independence is constrained by the purchasers, who determine the contract income and set out a service specification, by national policies or directives, and by professional regulation. When introduced, the establishment of NHS Trusts was feared to be a first step towards privatisation; in the event, they have turned out to be a further internal reorganisation. However, the "*market*" concept has introduced competition in place of cooperation and joint working and has fostered new *management* styles in some Trusts, loosely derived from commerce, requiring attention to *business ethics* appropriate for the health sector.

See also: Purchasing.

AJP

Trustworthiness underlines the assumption that workers in health care, of necessity being given access to intimate and detailed knowledge of an ill person's physical and psychological state, must be particularly able to discharge that trust, and must be seen to do so (through professional regulation if necessary). This should include the capacity to handle appropriately and sensitively the moral dilemmas caused by having to play more than one *role* (eg, as clinician and researcher), deal with groups working under very different rules (eg, managers, the press), take *responsibilities* in new sets of relationships (eg, with families and clinical teams), and show appropriate *commitment* to their work.

RH

Truth Philosophers dispute whether truth is what fits the facts (correspondence theory), what hangs together (coherence theory), or what works (pragmatic theory), or some combination of these. *Logic* uses the word in various technical senses (eg, t-condition, t-value). For religion, truth may be found in a state of being, a way of acting, or a relationship. In medical ethics, telling a patient the truth about his prognosis calls for an ability to translate its scientific into its existential meanings.

KMB

Truthtelling *Honesty* underpins scientific activity and the moral life in general, and yet doctors have traditionally been given some latitude in not being open to *patients*. It is still commonplace worldwide for physicians and relatives to suggest that knowledge of a serious or lethal diagnosis should be withheld from a patient, on the basis that honesty would harm by destroying hope. The importance of respecting a patient's *autonomy* has challenged this approach in Western medicine recently: if someone does not know what is wrong, how can he make an appropriate choice about the treatments on offer to him, including whether to accept *treatment* at all? The law of *consent* in Britain and the USA requires that the person be informed, and to treat without consent risks the charge of *assault*. There are possible *harms* of both telling and not telling: whereas such harms may be able to be worked through on a personal level and can be influenced by a good professional–patient relationship, the corrosive effect of loss of *trust* between health professionals and the general public is considered by some to be a more serious issue and less easily remedied. The traditional professional-led approach to decisions is changing: choice in health care is more commonly now seen as a *partnership*, with the professional offering technical expertise tailored to a particular individual, but the final choice being made by the informed individual user of the service. As such, there is a place for the patient also to choose how much he wants to know.

Recent focus has been on the *skills* needed to be open about different diagnoses, and the way in which a professional's own concerns or anxieties may obstruct good *communication*, and need handling in their own right. Although the management of conditions such as *AIDS* has demonstrated good standards of *openness* in care in adults, questions remain about how best to approach dying children, the *elderly* (who may be used to a different approach) or those with restricted understanding. The scarcity and expense of professional time poses continuing threats to good communication, but fuels research into other ways of informing users. Full *respect* for individual *choice* will also have to face the challenge of an individual who chooses not to be fully open with the professional, or who chooses not to hear or not to be told in the first place.

Reference

Higgs R. On telling patients the truth. In: Lockwood M. (ed) *Moral dilemmas in modern medicine.* Oxford: Oxford University Press, 1985.

See also: Breaking bad news; child; disclosure; doctor–patient relationship; empowerment; lying; mutual participation model; mutuality; paternalism; therapeutic privilege.

RH

U

Unborn child *See* Fetus and embryo.

Uncertainty is a state where there is no evidence to inform a specific decision, eg, regarding *treatment*, and is a key precondition for the conduct of *clinical trials*, where it is uncertain whether a new treatment is better than the existing standard. The uncertainty must be shared by patients and clinicians to avoid denying patients the

best current treatment and to avoid *bias* in patient selection. It permits *randomisation* between treatment options or between treatment and *placebo*, if no treatment currently has been proven. There is strong pressure in medical practice to be sure about diagnosis and *treatment* and to reassure. However, understanding that we do not know whether one treatment is superior to another until proper clinical trials have been conducted is central to scientific medicine; and being aware how little there is which we can be objectively certain about in clinical practice (and how difficult it remains to bring the general certainties to bear on a particular situation) is the marker of a mature health professional. Some approaches make a virtue of the *ambiguities* and uncertainties of clinical interaction; for instance, through deepening or broadening the assessment by not closing down too soon on a single diagnosis. People tolerate uncertainty to different degrees, both as patients and professionals. Educational and sociological literature suggests that medical *students* go through a phase of "black and white" thinking; learning to tolerate uncertainty is a key feature of vocational training.

See also: Equipoise; training, vocational.

RH/AJP

Unconscious, the According to Freud and others, mental activity related to past experience, fears, wishes, of which the waking *self* is not, or may not want to be, aware. Its contents may be brought into consciousness (or the subject may be persuaded that this is the case) by psychological therapies, including study of dreams or slips of the tongue.

KMB

Unconsciousness implies that a patient is unaware of his surroundings and is unable to react to them in a psychologically meaningful way. A sleeping person is unconscious but rousable; *coma* is unrousable sleep-like unconsciousness. A person in coma has his eyes closed, speaks no recognisable words and obeys no commands. Many patients in coma have reflex pupil reactions and eye and limb movements. Only in the deepest level of coma are there no responses, and it is misleading to describe all patients in coma as unresponsive. Different levels of coma, and of other types of altered consciousness, are defined by the Glasgow Coma Scale, from a score of three for deepest coma to 15 for fully alert. The brain mechanisms for wakefulness and awareness can be separately damaged, resulting in patients who are awake but not aware–unconscious but in a *persistent vegetative state* (PVS).

BJ

Understanding has several implications including knowledge, integration of that knowledge, comprehension of the meaning of what is known and, crucially for medical ethics, a sympathetic (albeit sometimes tacit) perception of what a person's aims or *values* may be in a given situation. Confronted with a chooser making choices that do not appear the best but are strongly held, a clinician may be helped by "taking a values history" or gaining some grasp of the underlying *meaning* of these choices. The French have: "Tout comprendre est tout pardonner". Respecting the autonomous but unusual choice of a competent individual may require the type of understanding that "gives the benefit of the doubt".

See also: Autonomy; competence; empathy.

RH

Uniqueness That an individual *person* has no like and is in a moral sense irreplaceable is central to good medical practice. Whatever the future of genetic engineering or *cloning* it is currently inconceivable that two people could see the world exactly alike. *Illness* may be perceived as a threat to uniqueness (by reducing an individual's control over personal decisions): becoming a case may undermine it still further (because that individual is now part of a group with the same characteristics).

See also: Cases; context; particularity.

RH

Universalising In ethics (especially *Kantian*) asking what would happen if everyone else acted in a way, or followed a rule for action, which one is thinking of adopting. If their doing so would lead to self-defeating or otherwise untenable consequences (eg, if everyone told lies, any advantage in lying would be lost and social life would be impossible) the act or rule may be morally unjustifiable.

KMB

Unqualified practitioners pose a problem to any organised system where standards are maintained by proven professional competence, backed up by a professional code and the sanctions of a supervisory body that can penalise or remove the qualification to practise. However, every patient knows that there are good doctors and bad doctors (and that these are extremes), and it is possible to meet non-doctors, or practitioners without qualifications, who are natural healers or who seem more in touch with the needs of sufferers. The range of alternative practitioners has increased and, with some well-publicised exceptions, has posed no greater threat to public health and welfare than the mistakes of professional health care. Moral or legal problems remain, however, about referral by one type of practitioner to another, and who takes *responsibility* for a bad outcome; about who should receive financial support where public funding is involved; and about the evaluation of *outcome* and the standards used, and who sets these. It may be that the stage is set for a rerun of the 19th century obsession with this debate.

See also: Association, rule against; complementary medicine; traditional medicine.

RH

Utilitarianism Consequentialist theory, based on maximising utility, or the greatest happiness of the greatest number. Developed by British philosophers Bentham (in a more quantitative form) and Mill (in a more qualitative). Rule utilitarianism (weighing the consequences of acting according to a general moral rule) may be less unsatisfactory than Act utilitarianism (weighing the consequences of my doing a particular act), but translating either into practice is far more difficult than the utilitarian *rhetoric* of *politics* often admits.

See also: Consequentialism.

KMB

Utility (i) What is of use or useful. But evaluation of what is useful depends on knowing what it is useful for, to whom, and how much it matters to them. Moreover, someone or something not useful to me may be greatly valued by me, eg, an elderly cat, or an amateur painting by a deceased friend. (ii) A public utility is something not just useful but necessary to the community, equitable provision of which Government has a moral duty to ensure.

KMB

V

Vaccines *See* Immunisation.

Validity refers to the logical form of a deductive argument, rather than to the truth or falsity of its contents – its premises and conclusion. If an argument has a valid form and all its premises are true, its conclusion must be true. But it may still be valid when either a true or a false conclusion is deduced from false premises.

See also: Logic.

KMB

Value means the worth of something. It is routinely used in medicine to indicate the level of a particular chemical in a laboratory test, but has regained its more general meaning in the assessment of different forms of clinical intervention (evaluation), often linked closely to cost and thus to effectiveness; and in relation to moral values, linked to thinking in *virtue*-based ethics. Individuals or groups may give different ordering or priorities to particular moral values, which may lead rational individuals to make radically different choices in similar circumstances. There may be differences between the ordering of the values of professional groups and those of the broader society or *culture* of which that group is a part, and individuals within that group may make differing choices depending on the *role* that they are playing or the responsibilities that they see themselves to have. The importance of making these *conflicts* explicit is that a group in which different individuals are explicitly "taking care" of different values may be very effective. For instance, there may be conflict between a practitioner giving precedence to patient choice and the practice manager focusing on health promotion or the possible remuneration obtained from each activity, and if this is not understood resulting conflict may make the group dysfunctional.

Values have recently entered *politics*, inappropriately hijacked by right wing thinking (where "family values" are supposed to show the triumph of

267

family integrity over individual choice). It is probably more true to posit an individual set of values that may be strongly influenced by the history and culture of that particular family. Thus "taking a values history" in a clinical situation posing difficult moral choices may enable a clinician to understand the particular viewpoint of the patient or other players. Clinical *systems theory* may suggest that questions such as "what would your mother or father have wanted you to do?" may tap into a seam of choice of which the individual may only be half aware.

Scientists consider that their work is value free, and social scientists under the influence of Weber may aim to provide descriptions that do not express the values of the author. However, there is increasing doubt as to whether this can be achieved in the mainstream or social sciences.

See also: Perspective; responsibility.

Reference
Pratt J. *Practitioners and practice: a conflict of values?* Oxford: Radcliffe Medical Press, 1995.
RH

Vasectomy is a relatively minor operation aiming to cause permanent sterility in men. Many are carried out under local anaesthesia. There is no known adverse effect on health or sexual activity.

Fully *informed consent* is essential and it is preferable to involve a partner in the preparatory discussion though whether people have the right to preserve their partners' ability to reproduce would be controversial.

See also: Contraception; sterilisation.
JAM

Veil of ignorance In Rawls' theory of justice, rational individuals in a hypothetical state, "under a veil of ignorance" concealing their own identity, interests and powers, are asked to

choose what sort of social institutions they would consent to by imagining which such arrangements would be most advantageous to them if they were to find themselves in the worst position. Rawls concludes that they would accept arrangements not unlike those of liberal Western democracies with welfare provision, despite the social inequalities of such democracies.

Reference
Rawls J. *A theory of justice*. Oxford: Oxford University Press, 1972.
KMB

Veracity is another word for truthfulness.

See also: Truth; truthtelling.
RH

Viability is a concept used especially in relation to the ability of very premature infants to survive: it is the point at which a *fetus* can become an infant. As techniques improve for sustaining the life of very low birth-weight infants, the limit of viability decreases. It does not mean fully independent living, but a significant chance of survival without permanent damage or disability. It raises issues of *risk–benefit analysis* and of *resource* allocation, as the hazard of death or disability may be high and life-sustaining treatments may be extremely costly. It is also relevant to decisions about late *abortion* and the gestational age after which an infant is regarded as stillborn.

See also: Prematurity.
AJP

Videos Teaching by example and learning by watching are important parts of health care training. Increasing concern for patients' *privacy* and the "natural scarcity of the best" suggests that learning from videotaped examples will increasingly become a key mode in teaching health care professions. In addition, it is important for each individual learner to be able to review his own performance, particularly in terms of *communication* skills. The video or audio-taping of interviews, and their discussion with a mentor or teacher, is now standard procedure in a number of areas. The moral issues arise because this is a further potential threat to patient *confidentiality*, through sharing with another, and through the preservation of an interview on tape for who knows how long. Fears that some patients might not disclose fully, and others "act up", in the presence of a camera demonstrates that these are not negligible concerns. Good practice suggests therefore that a patient should have the procedure explained, should be able to refuse without detriment to his care, should sign a *consent* form, should know with whom the information on the video may be shared, and should be able to ask – and be assured – that the video will be erased afterwards. The review of videos of patient and doctor by a third party as part of a diagnostic or treatment schedule is in its infancy, but shows promise. Operations on videos, sold without patient consent because identification was thought impossible, caused a political storm in the UK in 1996.

RH

Violence enters the moral arena of medicine in several ways. Some *disease* processes in medicine make patients confused and frightened and therefore violent, because they perceive attempts to help them as threats against them. Some medical treatments in the past and the present could reasonably be seen as unnecessarily violent, and a form of legally sanctioned medical *assault:* some treatments for *mental illness* could be seen in this way, and rightly cause disquiet. (The onus of proof of clear benefit and absence of more humane alternatives rests firmly with the medical participants.) Violent behaviour may be a symptom of paranoid psychosis (the delusion is that someone is "plotting" or "out to get me" in a systematic way), or of lack of control in *psychopathy*. The moral status of "treatment" in the first instance (which may actually just be social control, at considerable cost to the patient) and of *"illness"* in the second (where the debate is whether a psychopath is mad or bad) may need to be explored. Danger may sanction certain forms of intervention to protect both the patient and society, but the professional has also himself and his other patients to consider. Some would argue that violent behaviour, in the absence of cause, disease, or illness, puts a person outside health care, others that a violent patient is still a patient with real needs. Practical foresight seems important both in making sure that health service premises are safe and that personnel have access to help and ways of raising the alarm. The so-called "law of overwhelming force" suggests that most potentially violent patients are subdued by an overwhelming number of calm and unaggressive individuals. Managers and employers have particular responsibilities in regard to facilities and staffing levels.

RH

Virtue can be thought of as moral excellence. As a technical term in *philosophy*, virtue ethics indicates thinking which starts with considerations of particular qualities or *character* traits (such as *honesty, kindness, courage*, etc) rather than concepts like *utility* or *duty*. It would ask "what is a good doctor?" rather than "what does a good doctor do?", and as such could help discussion of health care ethics from an internalised, value-based perspective rather than that of obeying external rules and directives.

269

Different *virtues*, or ranking of them, have appealed to different thinkers and cultures, so this mode of thinking may not provide easy solutions but rather an increased complexity. There may be differences within a group at any one time: for instance, the qualities of a charge nurse in a psychogeriatric ward might well differ from those of a casualty sister. There is a link with professional *practice* (as a form of organised social activity) and individual *roles*, and virtue ethics may shed light on areas where good professional conduct may appear to conflict with other areas, such as *law*. MacIntyre, an influential modern exponent, also pointed to the importance of narrative and *tradition* in this approach.[1] Most philosophers have taken an interest in virtue but the most important probably remains Aristotle, who saw close connections between human flourishing (*eudaemonia*) and acting virtuously. The problems remain for the modern philosopher, as to what form this flourishing should take, who would define it, and how to make judgments about the link between character and action. With modern insights into the messier aspects of motivation, there must always remain questions when "good chaps" go into action.

Reference
1 MacIntyre A. *After virtue*. London: Duckworth, 1982.

RH

Vivisection The use of living animals in invasive scientific procedures. The term, which literally means "cutting alive", was in use before the advent of *anaesthesia* and still carries connotations of the cruelty that early surgical experiments on conscious animals must have involved. As such, the word is used mainly by those opposed to *animal experiments* ("anti-vivisectionists").

JAS

Voluntary (from Latin *volo* to will) – of one's own free will, not coerced or unduly influenced by others; and hence an important element of *informed consent*. In Platonic and Kantian thinking, no one can do wrong voluntarily, ie, not to will the good is to misunderstand what the good really is.

KMB

Voluntary work is most commonly characterised as work undertaken for the purpose of mutual benefit to the volunteer and the beneficiary of the voluntary work. The benefit to the volunteer will be non-financial although it is good practice among voluntary organisations to reimburse out-of-pocket expenses. The volunteer may gain in other ways from undertaking the work, such as deriving experience that will be useful in applying for paid positions. Ethical difficulties concerned with volunteering most frequently arise when a paid worker is replaced by a volunteer, or when there is a perception of this having happened.

Reference
Savishinsky JS. Intimacy, domesticity and pet therapy with the elderly: expectation and experience among nursing home volunteers. *Soc Sci Med* 1992; **34**, 12: 1325–34.

NBe

Volunteers are people who participate of their own free will in, eg, clinical trials or *donation* of *blood* or sperm; living donors for *transplantation* are normally close relatives. With informed *consent*, volunteers may be considered to be acting at their own risk. Normal volunteers are used for early safety tests of new *drugs* or as donors, while *patients* may volunteer to help investigate new therapies or to provide samples for *clinical research and trials*. While *altruism* or enlightened self-interest may lead people to volunteer, there is a risk of implicit or explicit coercion, notably in organ donation or in some clinical trials. Financial incentives would similarly deny true voluntarism, although in some settings reimbursement of expenses may extend to covering indirect costs or recognition of inconvenience. The use of medical students for research studies has been felt to require particular care for risk of excessive voluntarism in respect of frequency or degree of hazard.

See also: Reward; sale of organs.

AJP

Vulnerability Many modern health professionals see themselves as being strong and useful just because they are in some senses impervious to the conditions suffered by their patients. In this view the "good doctor is never sick" and "patients are a different sort of people". This may encourage medical *heroism* (such as when a doctor or nurse decides to work with patients suffering from an infectious disease for which there is no cure, or to work under fire in *war*) but is challenged both by the statistics of ill health in health professionals, by statistics of professional *burnout* and breakdown, and by common sense. The reverse view has recently been propounded, that a healer's power resides in his vulnerability, since whatever his wound, this wound both reminds him of his humanity and makes him more approachable for those in need. In terms of motivation to practise medicine or to nurse, there is some evidence that unresolved personal issues may play their part.

Reference
Guggenbuhl-Craig A. *Power in the helping profession*. Dallas: Spring, 1990.

RH

W

Want vs need A disabled person would rather spend his mobility allowance on a violin. Should his subjective preferences have priority over what is thought necessary for him as a human being? *Justice* may be said to require that he be permitted to advance his *wellbeing* as he sees fit.

See also: Interest; need; paternalism; rights; welfare.

RCr

War involves the deliberate inflicting of death and injury on others through the pursuit of "politics by other means" (von Clausewitz) and could be seen to present a fundamental contradiction to the ethical practice of medicine. It is now probably the greatest worldwide threat to *public health*. Yet, clinicians are necessarily involved in war, to assess (hence *triage*) and treat the injured, whether on the field of battle or behind the lines, and to manage the considerable psychological trauma. It has been suggested that the presence of the MO (Medical Officer), even though he had limited scope to treat casualties, was important to the troops as "Morale Officer"[1]. Needs also arise from the process of translocating military personnel in large numbers to remote and sometimes hazardous terrain for prolonged periods, such as risk of infection, including *sexually transmitted diseases* (for centuries the scourge of military personnel). Recently military personnel have been seen to be vectors of *HIV* in some African conflicts.

More complex needs have arisen as the machinery of war has become more diverse, through different forms of remote missiles to nuclear, biological and chemical warfare. Much has been learnt from the study of physical and psychological trauma in war and this has informed civilian clinical practice, marginally offsetting the contradiction of medical principles inherent in war. In recent years, organisations of physicians opposed to war, and specifically *nuclear war*, have developed with the objective of reducing the risk of war and of preventing the use of weapons of mass destruction. These organisations apply the principles of preventive medicine to the political arena.

Reference
1 John Pinching. Personal communication.

AJP

Warning Just as an assessment of *risk* is key to many decisions, so it is incumbent on a professional to point out potential dangers to patients and colleagues. In dealings with patients, a professional would normally be expected to be explicit about potential unwanted effects of any medical *treatment* for *consent* to such treatment to be valid, since it is the professional's duty to provide the information on which such consent is based. Although the currency of such exchanges may alter with time and place, (depending on, for instance, expectations of professionals and general knowledge in the community at large), and will be influenced by law (for instance, what has to be stated about a particular pharmaceutical product), nevertheless the onus is on the professional to warn rather than on the patient to ask (contrast *"caveat emptor"* – "let the buyer beware" in ordinary shopping). Since the extent of such warnings may be immense, and time necessarily limited, it makes sense for the professional to concentrate on potentially dangerous or serious side-effects, on the particular concerns of that individual patient, and on possible effects on sexual partners, children or the next generation. The professional should also clarify what the patient should expect from the treatment, what symptoms indicate serious, unwanted effects, and what to do when they occur. The range of normal human behaviour is also a legitimate concern ("Can I drink?" "Should I drive?"). The extension of professional practice to *health promotion* and thus to covering the risks of the patient's behaviour in general, and the need to change it, is a developing field.

There are twin risks of this focus on warnings: such as that the positive effects of treatment may be diminished and that patients may not wish to see professionals who always appear to focus on the negative. However, the risk for the professional is that if such warnings are not given, and noted to have been given, *blame* may be attached with possible serious legal consequences.

In other relationships, such as that between employer and employee, the employer would usually be expected to give proper warnings about deficiencies before suspending or ending employment. Statements should be explicit, clear, in a form that makes sense to both parties, and written down.

Reference
Rottenberg KH, North RL. The duty to warn "dilemma" and women with AIDS. In: Beauchamp TL, Walters L, eds. *Contemporary issues in bioethics*. Belmont, California: Wadsworth, 1994.

See also: Risk assessment.

RH

Water *See* Hydration.

Wealth Wealth consists in possessions with economic value. Should it be permissible to use individual wealth to purchase health care? Or should such care be available to all, free at the point of delivery? A mixed system would permit the private purchasing of non-essential care, such as *cosmetic surgery*, only.

See also: Health care systems; justice; need; poverty; private medicine; wants vs need.

RCr

Wedge *See* Slippery slope.

Welfare A state of being well or doing well could be said to be a general and high aim of human life, seen in the history of Western thought in different guises – from the Greek philosophers' "human *flourishing*" to Christian "salvation" and the Enlightenment's "liberty". The central theme today is an enjoyment of health and prosperity, and thus it is applied particularly to that work that enables people to overcome the threats of *poverty* or ill health. In broad terms the link between these threats means that the welfare of all is a central concept for *public health policy*; in detail the practice of health care makes no sense without it, as any action that does not aim towards patients' welfare (even if constrained by other principles or concerns) would be open to question.

The word has gained a particular political edge since the assertion of the state's role (via social insurance or a *national health service*) in combating the disadvantages suffered by the poor, oppressed, or unhealthy among its citizens. A "welfare state" thus enacts comprehensive legislation to provide (directly or indirectly) state funding for services that aim to improve the quality of its citizens' lives, and a number of examples were set up following the end of the second world war, notably in Great Britain and Europe. However, the mounting costs of such operations and the apparently cumbersome and inflexible nature of some of the necessary systems have recently led the political right, in particular Thatcherism in Great Britain, to reverse this process. Criticisms of welfare-based public policies ("welfarism") include practical issues of expenditure and taxation, definitions of eligibility, and policing national boundaries to exclude the citizens of countries with less comprehensive systems from claiming benefit, as well as broader moral questions as to whether a welfare approach reduces the individual's self-determination or drive

and is an unacceptable form of state *paternalism*. Others claim that evidence of the ill effects of a break up in the welfare state – beggars on the streets, a return to poverty related diseases such as tuberculosis, and the development of a disadvantaged under-class in sections of the richer nations – are there for all who will to see. Most modern democracies are seeing a struggle to find the best dividing line between the public and the private in responsibility for health and social care.

Caught in the political crossfire, it may be more helpful for users and professionals in a health service to return to an examination of the human *needs* to which such services respond, and a re-evaluation of whether what is being provided is responding to the real *need* at the right time in the best way, whatever the differences between individuals. Without an understanding of what makes human beings flourish and "a commitment to the consistency of whatever vision of the good ... we accept"[1] it is likely we shall remain confused and at the mercy of political fashion. The welfare of the professionals and the service itself will also need attention.

Reference

1 Doyal L, Gough I. *A theory of human need.* London: Macmillan, 1991.

See also: Gatekeeping; community care; public policy.

RH

Welfare (individual) A person's welfare is what his *flourishing* or *wellbeing* consists in. Welfare has been argued to be: (i) certain mental states, such as pleasure; (ii) the fulfilment of certain preferences; (iii) certain objective goods, such as health or personal relationships. It is a notion at the heart of many medical ethical problems, and which view is adopted makes a large difference. For example, keeping a comatose person alive on a respirator may be said not to harm him on view (i), but to do so either by overriding a past preference (view (ii)) or by inflicting indignity on him (view (iii)).

Reference
Griffin J. *Well-being*. Oxford: Clarendon Press, 1986.

See also: Aims (personal); cost–benefit analysis; human rights; interest; justice; need; poverty; QALYs; self interest; utility.

RCr

Welfare rights *See* Rights; gatekeeping.

Wellbeing A portmanteau word often used to complement more restricted uses of "health". Roughly equivalent to *"flourishing"* or *"eudaemonia"*.

KMB

Well person clinics Although prevention of illness and disease has always been part of good clinical practice, the extension of such processes to a formal and major part of health service practice, with clinics specially designed for people who are still well, remains in some sense controversial. On the one hand, there may be conditions that can only be prevented, not cured, and the physical deterioration of normal aging may be prevented. Individuals may not know that they are at risk without professional examination and advice. On the other hand, attenders at such clinics are disproportionately the well-off or well-informed (who are at less risk of ill health in general); and it is unclear how much of a limited health budget should be devoted to this work, or who should pay for it. Anxieties raised by such processes may not be adequately allayed if the findings are negative, and this may be yet a further example of medical imperialism and undermining the individual's *responsibility* for and confidence in his own health. If the jury on this issue is still out, there is plenty of evidence that it is being influenced, or even packed, by interested parties.

Reference
Skrabanek P. *The death of humane medicine and the rise of coercive healthism*. London: Social Affairs Unit, 1994.

See also: Health education.

RH

Whistleblowing is the term applied where a member of staff, such as a health care worker or scientist, draws the attention of external agencies or the media to a problem in their institution, such as poor clinical standards, unavailability of care and unethical or unprofessional practices, including *fraud* and *plagiarism*. It is an extreme measure that should only be taken after pursuing normal channels of *regulation* and *accountability*, managerially or professionally, without effect. Codes of conduct and of organisational *confidentiality* should ensure that those with legitimate concerns can raise them without personal disadvantage through proper *procedures* with *due process*, but that they may seek external investigation or attention if these have been exhausted. In the medical profession there is an obligation on doctors to report certain issues to the *General Medical Council*. Measures to protect the whistleblower against explicit or implicit *discrimination*, or against legal challenge, are often regarded as inadequate, and several have lost their jobs and found it difficult to gain re-employment.

AJP

Will (i) Legal or quasi-legal document; (*advance directive*). (ii) A wish or desire imbued with the power or intention to carry it through.

KMB

Wisdom (i) A type of literature, eg, the Hebrew books of Proverbs, Ecclesiastes, Job. (ii) The quality of rightly using knowledge, reason and understanding, either for effective action (*practical reasoning*) or in a religious context, where wisdom (sometimes personified as Sophia) is the way to ultimate harmony. For Socrates, awareness of one's own ignorance is the beginning of wisdom. Wisdom, unlike knowledge, can rarely if ever be communicated directly.

KMB

Women's rights In medical ethics women's rights means the rights of women health care workers and patients to be treated in a non-sexist, non-stereotyped way. For instance, assumptions (often unconscious) that women are inherently emotional, nervous, unstable, or hysterical militate against their being treated as full autonomous human beings. But being equal and different poses extra questions. Do women have extra rights because of this difference, for instance as correlative to their extra duties as being the only bearers of the next generation of society? Should they have the same opportunities, judged in the same (possibly male) way, or are new ways of expression and assessment required: if so, how will these be (or should they be) integrated with current approaches? A particular concern has arisen that *clinical research and trials* have systematically excluded women, despite their relevance to disease in women and into treatments that will be used by women after licensure. One reason given was that drug trials should not include potentially pregnant women to avoid the risk of teratogenicity (and possible ensuing litigation). Studies are now generally designed to include women on the undertaking that contraception is used or pregnancy avoided.

See also: Feminism; gender; silence; yin yang.

Reference
Mills J. *Womanwords*. London: Virago, 1989: 123–7.

ALI/RH/AJP

Work ethic The tendency to make a virtue out of the necessity of working is often traced back to early modern capitalists whose ascetic devotion to economic success (popularly seen as a sign of divine favour) was an unintended consequence of their Calvinist concern over whether they were predestined to salvation. Today, a work ethic is more immediately fostered by concern over job security. Its dangers are those of mistaking the *means* for the end, and possibly wants for *needs*.

See also: Burnout; ends and means; want vs need.

KMB

Wounded healer *See* Vulnerability.

Wrongful life The duty of professionals in medical practice to save life, or to enable *potential* lives to become actual lives, has been challenged recently by some patients who find themselves, following medical intervention, thereby placed in a position of particular or intense *suffering*. They consider these to be lives that are not properly lives or are not worth living, and thus to have been wrongfully preserved or created. Examples might be someone who asked not to be resuscitated, but was; or a fetus with severe physical defects who was born as a handicapped child, when termination of pregnancy was requested by the mother but not performed. Wrongful life is a legal rather than ethical concept and gains its strength from the need to apportion *blame* in order to make someone responsible for the added burden of the costs of medical treatment or personal care. It is thus more commonly invoked where private rather than public health care systems are in operation.

RH

X

Xenografts are animal organs transplanted into humans. Xenotransplantation goes wider and includes the *transplantation* of animal cells into humans, eg, the use of pig fetal islet cells in diabetics and pig fetal neural tissue in Parkinson's patients.

The ethical issues raised by xenotransplantation include: At what stage in the exploration of its scientific feasibility will it be proper to proceed to trials on humans? Should animals be used for this purpose? How should the risk of transmitting new viruses to humans be handled? How should patient consent be organised in view of the risks and of the need for lifetime monitoring?

References

Department of Health Advisory Group on Ethics and Xenotransplantation. *Animal tissue into humans*. London: HMSO, 1996.

Institute of Medicine. *Xenotransplantation: science, ethics and public policy*. Washington: 1996.

Nuffield Council on Bioethics. *Animal-to-human transplants: the ethics of xenotransplantation*. London, 1996.

DS

Y

Yin yang In classical Chinese philosophy express opposites through contrast and difference. Originally the shaded and sunlit side of a hill, the former evoked the dark, negative, and feminine, the latter, the light, positive, and male. They express the interaction and interdependence of diverse features and things through a fluid, complementary, and creative relationship between unique particulars: these are facets of life that find place with difficulty in the "either-or" static polarities of some Western philosophy.

RH

Z

Zen A form of *Buddhism*, found mostly in Japan, but influenced by Chinese Taoism. Through meditation and contemplating paradoxes, practitioners may achieve gradual or immediate enlightenment. A popularised version, introduced to North America in the late 19th century, has found favour with many who were dissatisfied with doctrinal religions.

KMB

Short bibliography

Books

Beauchamp TL, Childress JF. *Principles of biomedical ethics* (4th ed). Oxford: OUP, 1994.

British Medical Association. *Medical ethics today.* London: BMA, 1993.

Campbell A, Higgs R. *In that case. Medical ethics in everyday practice.* London: Daston, Longman and Todd, 1982.

Downie RS, Calman KC. *Healthy respect: ethics in health care.* London: Faber, 1987.

English DC. *Bioethics: a clinical guide for medical students.* New York: WW Norton, 1994.

Gillon R. *Philosophical medical ethics.* Chichester: Wiley, 1985.

Gillon R, Lloyd A. *Principles of health care ethics.* Chichester: Wiley, 1994.

Hope T. *The Oxford practice skills manual: ethics, law and communication – skills in health care education.* Oxford: OUP, 1996.

Mason JK, McCall Smith RA. *Law and medical ethics* (4th ed). London: Butterworths, 1994.

Thomasma DC, Kushner T. *Birth to death; science and bioethics.* Cambridge: CUP, 1996.

Thompson IE, Melia KM, Boyd KM. *Nursing ethics* (3rd ed). Edinburgh: Churchill Livingstone, 1994.

Journals

Bioethics. Oxford: Blackwell.

Bulletin of Medical Ethics. London: Royal Society of Medicine.

Cambridge Quarterly of Health Care Ethics. Cambridge: Cambridge University Press.

Hastings Center Report. Briarcliff Manor, New York: Hastings Center.

Journal of Medical Ethics. London: BMJ Publishing Group.

Index